HEALTH AND HUMAN DEVELOPMENT

JOAV MERRICK - SERIES EDITOR –

NATIONAL INSTITUTE OF CHILD HEALTH AND HUMAN DEVELOPMENT,
MINISTRY OF SOCIAL AFFAIRS, JERUSALEM, ISRAEL

FOOD, NUTRITION AND EATING BEHAVIOR

Pain Management Yearbook 2011
Joav Merrick (Editor)
2013. ISBN: 978-1-62808-970-7

Pain Management Yearbook 2012
Joav Merrick (Editor)
2013. ISBN: 978-1-62808-973-8

Public Health Concern:
Smoking, Alcohol and Substance Use
Joav Merrick
and Ariel Tenenbaum (Editors)
2013. ISBN: 978-1-62948-424-2

HEALTH AND HUMAN DEVELOPMENT

FOOD, NUTRITION AND EATING BEHAVIOR

JOAV MERRICK, M.D.

AND

SIGAL ISRAELI

EDITORS

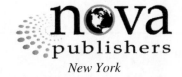

nova
publishers
New York

NOTICE TO THE READER

Library of Congress Cataloging-in-Publication Data

ISBN: 978-1-62948-233-0

Library of Congress Control Number: 2013949350

Published by Nova Science Publishers, Inc. †New York

CONTENTS

INTRODUCTION

IT IS NOT NUTRITION UNTIL YOU HAVE EATEN IT

Joav Merrick, MD, MMedSc, DMSc[1,2,3,4,5]*
and Sigal Israeli, degrees[1,2,3]

[1]National Institute of Child Health and Human Development, Jerusalem, [2]Office of the Medical Director, Health Services, Division for Intellectual and Developmental Disabilities, [3]Ministry of Social Affairs and Social Services, Jerusalem, [4]Division of Pediatrics, Hadassah Hebrew University Medical Center, Mt Scopus Campus, Jerusalem, Israel and [5]Kentucky Children's Hospital, University of Kentucky College of Medicine, Lexington, Kentucky, US

Eating habits are influenced by social, cultural, religious, economic, environmental and individual factors. On the whole, people eat to stay alive and get their nutrition, but they also eat to show belonging to family or other social groups. Eating habits are linked to acceptable patterns of behavior, which differs across countries, cultures and ethnic or religious groups.

The food you eat affects your health and also risk for certain diseases. To eat healthier food, people may need to change some habits and also their environment. But in the Western world habits are hard to change and in many countries there is a reputation for reckless eating. People fill their cups with fatty, sugary, high-calorie foods instead of more nutritious fruits and vegetables that the experts tell us to eat. The result is an increase in obesity, heart disease and higher mortality.

Our eating habits also change over time and across generations. What we liked as kids are not the same we like as adults and what we eat is not what the generation before us ate. In this book you will find examples of the younger generation, who are snacking not always healthy food. Chocolate bars and biscuits between or instead of regular meals can leads to obesity and health problems. As a person grow up and become more aware of the health hazards they also become more concerned with nutrition and health issues, especially if they experience health problems that eventually will make them change their eating habits.

---

* Correspondence: Professor Joav Merrick, MD, MMedSci, DMSc, Medical Director, Health Services, Division for Intellectual and Developmental Disabilities, Ministry of Social Affairs and Social Services, POBox 1260, IL-91012 Jerusalem, Israel. E-mail: jmerrick@zahav.net.il.

Economic factors such as the availability of food and its cost also affect food choices. Government policy or laws also influence or regulate food price and availability and the media also have a big impact on our eating habits. The media can work both ways: ads on certain foods such as biscuits and chocolate may boost sales and change eating habits for our youth in an unhealthy way, while cooking tips on television, videos and easy-to-follow recipes may improve and change eating habits in a more healthy way.

The International Food Information Council Foundation in Washington DC, United States has ten tips for healthy eating (http://www.foodinsight.org/about-ific-and-food-safety.aspx):

- Eat a variety of nutrient-rich foods. You need more than 40 different nutrients for good health and no single food supplies them all. Your daily food selection should include bread and other whole-grain products; fruits; vegetables; dairy products; and meat, poultry, fish and other protein foods. How much you should eat depends on your calorie needs. Use the Food Guide Pyramid and the Nutrition Facts panel on food labels as handy references.

- Enjoy plenty of whole grains, fruits and vegetables. Surveys show most people do not eat enough of these foods. Do you eat 6-11 servings from the bread, rice, cereal and pasta group, three of which should be whole grains? Do you eat 2-4 servings of fruit and 3-5 servings of vegetables? If you do not enjoy some of these at first, give them another chance. Look through cookbooks for tasty ways to prepare unfamiliar foods.

- Maintain a healthy weight. The weight that is right for you depends on many factors including your sex, height, age and heredity. Excess body fat increases your chances for high blood pressure, heart disease, stroke, diabetes, some types of cancer and other illnesses. But being too thin can increase your risk for osteoporosis, menstrual irregularities and other health problems. If you are constantly losing and regaining weight, a registered dietitian can help you develop sensible eating habits for successful weight management. Regular exercise is also important to maintaining a healthy weight.

- Eat moderate portions. If you keep portion sizes reasonable, it is easier to eat the foods you want and stay healthy. Did you know the recommended serving of cooked meat is three ounces, similar in size to a deck of playing cards? A medium piece of fruit is one serving and a cup of pasta equals two servings. A pint of ice cream contains four servings. Refer to the Food Guide Pyramid for information on recommended serving sizes.

- Eat regular meals. Skipping meals can lead to out-of-control hunger, often resulting in overeating. When you are very hungry, it is also tempting to forget about good nutrition. Snacking between meals can help curb hunger, but do not eat so much that your snack becomes an entire meal.

- Reduce, do not eliminate certain foods. Most people eat for pleasure as well as nutrition. If your favorite foods are high in fat, salt or sugar, the key is moderating how much of these foods you eat and how often you eat them. Identify major sources of these ingredients in your diet and make changes, if necessary. Adults who eat high-fat meats or whole-milk dairy products at every meal are probably eating too much fat. Use the Nutrition Facts panel on the food label to help balance your choices.

- Choosing skim or low-fat dairy products and lean cuts of meat such as flank steak and beef round can reduce fat intake significantly. If you love fried chicken, however, you do not have to give it up. Just eat it less often. When dining out, share it with a friend, ask for a take-home bag or a smaller portion.

- Balance your food choices over time. Not every food has to be "perfect." When eating a food high in fat, salt or sugar, select other foods that are low in these ingredients. If you miss out on any food group one day, make up for it the next. Your food choices over several days should fit together into a healthy pattern.

- Know your diet pitfalls. To improve your eating habits, you first have to know what is wrong with them. Write down everything you eat for three days. Then check your list according to the rest of these tips. Do you add a lot of butter, creamy sauces or salad dressings? Rather than eliminating these foods, just cut back your portions. Are you getting enough fruits and vegetables? If not, you may be missing out on vital nutrients.

- Make changes gradually. Just as there are no "superfoods" or easy answers to a healthy diet, do not expect to totally revamp your eating habits overnight. Changing too much, too fast can get in the way of success. Begin to remedy excesses or deficiencies with modest changes that can add up to positive, lifelong eating habits. For instance, if you do not like the taste of skim milk, try low-fat. Eventually you may find you like skim, too.

- Remember, foods are not good or bad. Select foods based on your total eating patterns, not whether any individual food is "good" or "bad." Do not feel guilty if you love foods such as apple pie, potato chips, candy bars or ice cream. Eat them in moderation, and choose other foods to provide the balance and variety that are vital to good health.

Healthy eating is not about strict nutrition rules, but finding a way to get the right nutrition in your food and meals, stay away from unhealthy habits and keep yourself as healthy as possible.

SECTION 1: BREASTFEEDING

In: Food, Nutrition and Eating Behavior
Editors: Joav Merrick and Sigal Israeli

ISBN: 978-1-62948-233-0
© 2014 Nova Science Publishers, Inc.

Chapter 1

MEMORABLE STORIES ABOUT MOTHERS' EXPERIENCES WITH BREASTFEEDING

Cecilia S Obeng, PhD and Adrienne Shivers*
Applied Health Science Department, Indiana University, Bloomington, Indiana, US

ABSTRACT

This chapter explores mothers' experiences with breastfeeding and the impact of breastfeeding on the health of their infants conducted using grounded theory approach. The research was conducted in the state of Indiana in the United States. Data were collected by the authors and a research assistant. A total of 26 mothers were included in this study. Findings Five themes emerged from the data: 1) Breastfeeding education should be part of initial doctor's visits; 2) mothers and their infants falling asleep together while nursing; 3) mothers and doctors should be able to watch the children grow free of health problems; 4) breast pumps and other incentives should be provided to encourage mothers to breastfeed and 5) there is a general lack of information on breastfeeding to which mothers are exposed. The majority of the mothers in this study reported a positive response to breastfeeding their babies. Participants, especially African-Americans, reported that breastfeeding was not encouraged as an option at the time when they had their babies. We found that giving incentives to breastfeed, providing breastfeeding education, and encouragement from health professionals all are crucial toward increasing the likelihood that mothers will breastfeed their children.

INTRODUCTION

The number of infants who die before their first birthday worldwide is astronomical. In the developed world, the United States was ranked 30th in infant mortality in 2005 (1). The United States also ranked much higher than most European countries in infant mortality rates

---

* Correspondence: Associate professor Cecilia Obeng, PhD, Department of Applied Health Science Indiana University, 1025 E 7th Street, HPER 116, Room 296-I, Bloomington, IN 47405 United States. E-mail: cobeng@indiana.edu.

for infants born at 37 or more weeks of gestation. In 2005, it was discovered that one in eight births in the United States was preterm (1).

The preliminary infant mortality rate for 2010 in the United States was 6.06 infant deaths per 1000 live births. In Indiana, where this breastfeeding research was conducted, although statistics indicate that the number of infant deaths declined between 1996 and 2006, the state's infant mortality rate is unnecessarily high. The average infant death in Indiana is 7.87 deaths in 1000 births; the above-stated figure most certainly puts Indiana's mortality rate higher than the national average.

According to United States Center for Disease Control and Prevention (CDC) (2), the four leading causes of infant death in the United States are congenital malformation, disorders related to short gestation, low birth weight, and sudden infant death syndrome (SIDS). Concerning the health of infants and young children, the America Academy of Pediatrics' policy statement document on Breastfeeding and the Use of Human Milk and the World Health Organization document, Infant and Young Child Feeding, note that a mother's milk is best for all infants. Babies of low birth weight are at risk for mortality, and feeding a child with the mother's milk is the best strategy to ensure their survival and wellbeing (3,4). A mother's milk, can adapt to the nutritional needs of babies. Incidence of SIDS, also, is lower in babies who are breastfed (4, 5).

Regarding breastfeeding in the United States, the CDC's (2) Breastfeeding Report Cardindicates the achievement of the 75% target set by Healthy People 2010 for mothers to initiate breastfeeding upon giving birth. Targets as set by Health People 2010 for breastfeeding at six months and twelve months, and for exclusive breastfeeding (i.e., no water, human milk only) at three months and six months, however, were not met by mothers in the United States (2). In addition, the Breastfeeding Report Card stated that although there has been great improvement in babies being born at Baby-Friendly facilities in the United States, the 4% rate attained is considered to be extremely low (2). According to Bartick and Reinhold (5), "if 90% of US families could comply with medical recommendations to breastfeed exclusively for 6 months, the United States would save $13 billion per year and prevent an excess 911 deaths" (3).

Convincing a majority of mothers to practice exclusive breastfeeding will be challenging for healthcare professionals. The World Health Organization document, Infant and Young Child Feeding, indicates that infant feeding is often neglected in the basic training of healthcare professionals such as doctors, nurses, and allied health professionals. Lack of knowledge about breastfeeding among healthcare professionals may lead to a situation where mothers are either not given advice at all or are given advice that may not ensure the child's optimal health. In order to reduce the infant mortality rate, it would be beneficial to improve breastfeeding education, especially among healthcare professionals. Research indicates that breastfeeding helps to prevent many childhood diseases, including obesity (5). The capacity for breast milk to help curb childhood obesity will more likely, then, help to prevent other health-related problems such as asthma, fatty liver disease, and sleep apnea in children (6,7).

The purpose of this paper, therefore, is to: (a) highlight possible attributes that make breastfeeding possible for mothers and the problems that mothers encounter; and (b) provide recommendations that will encourage breastfeeding among mothers.

OUR STUDY

The study took place in Indianapolis (Indiana State's capital) and surrounding towns in 2011, after approval from an Institutional Review Board of Indiana University. Participants were recruited through snowballing and purposeful sampling. To qualify to participate in the study, a participant ought to have had at least one child. There were 40 questionnaires distributed to mothers, and 26 took part in the study, with a response rate of 65%. Some potential participants for this study were contacted through e-mail and, where possible, were met in person. Others also participated through snowballing research approach.

Study design and analysis

The instrument used in this study contained six questions and consisted of both closed- and open-ended questions. The closed-ended questions dealt with demographic information of the participants. The open-ended questions were used as the primary questions of this study. The questions were developed by the lead author after several years of having taught children's health courses in which breastfeeding was a major component. The instrument for this study was pilot tested with 15 participants. This was done in order to make sure the wording and the content of the information were appropriate for mothers who were breastfeeding. None of the mothers who took part in the pilot study participated in the main study. This was done in order to prevent participants from having the advantage of previous knowledge about the questions. The demographic information asked participants their ethnicity/race and the number of children they had. The primary questions asked participants whether they breastfeed their child/children and their best and worst experiences while breastfeeding their child/children. All of the questions used in the pilot study were used in the main study, with the addition of another question that asked what mothers would need to make breastfeeding possible. Participation was voluntary.

To verify whether the information collected from the participants was what they actually said or wrote, the researchers went back to the participants after one week for verification.

This study also employed the grounded theory approach (8). Because the study used grounded theory approach, the data was closely examined and placed into various categories (e.g., participants were categorized by demographic details, and the responses were categorized into specific analytical categories or themes). Comparisons were made to determine differences and similarities in participants' responses.

FINDINGS

There were 12 African-Americans, 11 Caucasians, 2 Hispanics, and 1 Native American in the study. Five themes emerged from the data, and there were three responses that did not fit in any of the five themes. The five themes were: (a) the need for breast pumps and other incentives to encourage mothers to breastfeed; (b) the need for breastfeeding education to be part of the initial doctor's visit; (c) mother and infant falling asleep together while nursing; (d) the desire to watch children grow free of health problems; and (e) the need for more information on breastfeeding. Table 1 below illustrates a thematic summary of the participants' responses about breastfeeding

Table 1. Thematic summary of the participants' responses about breastfeeding

Theme	Group Summary	Individual Quotes
Breast pumps and other incentives to encourage mothers to breastfeed	Participants in this group believed that families being given incentives would encourage breastfeeding.	*"I have no breast pump and I think if I can afford one it will help me a lot to breast feed my child."*
Breastfeeding education should be part of the initial doctor's visit	Participants in this group believed that they were not given advice from the start when they visited their healthcare professional.	*"If I was advice right from day one I would have breastfed my baby up to two years or beyond. I nursed my baby for only one month"*
Mother and infant falling asleep together while nursing	The mothers in this group reported positive experience with breastfeeding when they awoke to see they had fallen asleep with their infants during the nursing period. Three of the mothers said they wished their families had taken a picture of them.	*"Both of us will fall asleep together in the rocking chair."*
Desire to watch children grow free of health problems	Participants reported that they barely reported any health problems when they nursed their children	*"Although she was born almost 11 pounds by nursing my baby her weight stabilized and she grow up perfect in weight and in height"*
Lack of information on breastfeeding	More than one-third of the African-American participants reported that they did not receive the needed information that would have encouraged them to breastfeed.	*"I was not informed enough about breastfeeding otherwise I would have definitely breastfed my child for months. I did two weeks of breastfeeding"*

Responses that did not fit into the five themes include: "When she was almost one year she will like to stand up and nurse"; "He will put his hand on my chest while nursing"; and "When he was older he would nurse on one breast and put his hand on the other breast."

DISCUSSION

This study adopted a strength-based approach that encouraged expectant mothers to nurse their children to enhance their children's health. For instance, six mothers reported that insurance companies covering the purchase of a breast pump would go a long way toward encouraging mothers who return to work after their baby is born to breastfeed. Some mothers suggested that the breast pumps would not only help mothers who work outside the home but also mothers with such problems as small nipples; they noted that mothers with large nipples will also find breast pumps useful. Engorgement mothers, they noted, would also benefit from the breast pump. In addition, participants indicated that including breastfeeding information in prenatal education and teaching mothers the differences between human milk and milk substitutes for infants would go a long way toward helping mothers decide whether or not to breastfeed. We inferred from the many positive responses from participants that a majority of the mothers enjoyed breastfeeding. Some mothers even reported that the best way to avert the obesity pandemic is for mothers to nurse their children.

Although some mothers indicated that falling asleep together with their child while nursing in a chair made them happy, caution should be taken because this could lead to a baby falling out of the mother's arms while both mother and baby are asleep and possibly hurting herself/himself.

Additionally, our data indicate that some African-American mothers indicated that breastfeeding was not encouraged enough at the time of having their babies. This lack of information thus contributed, in part, to the situation whereby some of them did not consider breastfeeding as an option. The findings of this study show how crucial it is for healthcare professionals to inform mothers and families about breastfeeding and about the differences between breast milk and milk substitutes for infants.

The findings in this study offer information about the positive attributes of breastfeeding and incentives that might encourage mothers to breastfeed their children. The kinds of incentives that mothers need to encourage them to breastfeed should be investigated along with how these incentives will reach mothers. This study could also be replicated, using equal number of mothers from diverse backgrounds and ethnicities to enable a better understanding of the situation and to subsequently learn about the positive attributes of breastfeeding. A quantitative and qualitative study to examine mothers' knowledge of nutrition and their views on the differences between breast milk, cow's milk, and formula could also be done.

The fact that there were only 26 participants in this study and that the study was done in only one state in the United States prevents the study from being a true representation of the whole country. In addition, there were not many participants from the Hispanic and Native American communities. Having participants from different states and more participants from the Hispanic and Native American communities will be needed in order to reveal the more accurate nature and extent of positive attributes that encourage mothers to nurse. Based on the findings in this study, the following recommendations are made:

- Healthcare professionals should teach mothers the differences between breast milk and other infant foods right from the beginning at their first visit to doctor's office and when their babies are born.
- Insurance companies should be encouraged (or even required) to pay for breast pumps and to give incentives (e.g., provide diapers, reduce insurance premiums) to encourage mothers to breastfeed, given the fact that research shows that breastfeeding helps to reduce the incidence of many childhood diseases and consequently helps to reduce healthcare costs.

REFERENCES

[1]   MacDorman MF, Mathews TJ. Behind international rankings of infant mortality: how the United States compares with Europe. Int J Health Serv 2010;40(4):577-88.

[2]   Center for Disease Control and Prevention. Accessed 2012 Apr 15. URL: http://www.cdc.gov/mmwr /preview/mmwrhtml/mm5642a8.htm

[3]   American Academy of Pediatrics (AAP). Policy statement. Accessed 2012 Apr 15. URL: http://pediatrics.aappublications.org/content/early/2012/02/22/peds.2011-3552

[4]   World Health Organization. Infant and young child feeding. Accessed 2012 Apr 15. URL: http://www.who.int/child_adolescent_health/documents/9789241597494/en/index.html

[5]   Bartick M, Reinhold A. The burden of suboptimal breastfeeding in the United States: A pediatric cost analysis. Pediatrics 2010;125(5):1048–56.

[6]   Williams JD. Early childhood obesity: A call for early surveillance and preventive measures. Can Med Assoc J 2004;171:243-4.

[7]   Lobstein T, Baur L, Uauy R. Obesity in children and young people: A crisis in public health. Report to the World Health Organization by the International Obesity Task Force. Obes Rev 2004;5(1):5– 104.

[8]   Strauss AL, Corbin J. Grounded theory research: Procedures, canons and evaluative criteria. J Sociol1990;19:418-32.

In: Food, Nutrition and Eating Behavior
Editors: Joav Merrick and Sigal Israeli

ISBN: 978-1-62948-233-0
© 2014 Nova Science Publishers, Inc.

Chapter 2

ROLE OF BREASTFEEDING IN PRIMARY PREVENTION OF BONE AND JOINT DISEASES IN CHILDREN: CURRENT CONCEPTS

Angelos Kaspiris, MD, MPhil, Efstathios Chronopoulos, MD, Chrisi Zaphiropoulou, MD and Elias Vasiliadis, MD*

Department of Trauma and Orthopedics, "Thriasio" General Hospital-NHS, Attica and Department of Orthopaedics, Laboratory for Research of the Musculoskeletal System, School of Medicine, University of Athens, Athens, Greece

ABSTRACT

Breastfeeding is beneficial and recommended for more than six months. According to a WHO analysis, its extensive use would result in the reduction of child mortality in countries where it is high. There are many studies on its positive impact on the pediatric immune system, both as regards cellular immunity and immunity through the production of immunoglobulins, and its anti-inflammatory action, which are all important for the protection of children from different infectious agents and inflammatory diseases. Therefore, although few studies have been conducted in this field, its link to diseases involving the bones and joints is established. Inflammatory diseases that affect the joints, such as SLE or Juvenile Rheumatoid Arthritis (JRA) are deemed to occur less frequently in individuals who have been breastfeed. Although the exact mechanism remains unclear, the observation that other autoimmune disorders, such as inflammatory bowel disease, Diabetes Mellitus and Multiple Sclerosis appear less frequently in children who are breastfeeding leads to the conclusion that the anti-inflammatory action of breast milk exercises a regulatory action on their emergence. In addition, we may observe beneficial effects directly on the bones. It is observed that a breast milk diet may lead to increased bone mass in early childhood. This chapter is a review of the current literature.

* Correspondence: Angelos Kaspiris, MD, MPhil, Department of Trauma and Orthopedics, "Thriasio" General Hospital – NHS, G Gennimata Avenue, Magoula 19600, Attica, Greece. E-mail: angkaspiris@hotmail.com.

INTRODUCTION

In recent decades, numerous studies have shown the beneficial properties of breastfeeding for children, not only during the neonatal period and childhood, but throughout adult life. Epidemiological studies and research in the field of molecular medicine have supported the Barker hypothesis, according to which exposures during the neonatal period are involved in the pathophysiology of diseases not only in this period, but in adult life as well, relating to chronic diseases (1, 2). This hypothesis is also applicable to breastfeeding, where a large number of diseases seem to occur less frequently epidemiologically in breastfed children. Such diseases include obesity, diabetes mellitus type I and II, and diseases related to the functioning of the immune system, such as allergies and asthma, celiac disease, inflammatory bowel disease, Helicabacter pylori and various forms of cancer.

Maternal milk provides children with a significant number of quality nutritional substances, important for the child's growth and development, the strengthening of the immune system and protection from pathogens. It also contains biological macromolecules involved in the biochemical pathways of the body and, obviously, in signal transduction to the cells. For this reason, breastfeeding is recommended for longer than six months. Inadequate breast-feeding has been incriminated by the WHO as a critical risk factor for infant mortality. Specifically, it is estimated that in 42 countries with high infant mortality, an adequate breast milk diet could prevent more than 1.3 million deaths (3, 4).

This article examines the protective role of breastfeeding for children in cases of bone- and joint-related diseases. Particular reference is made to its contribution in the development and activation of the pediatric immune system, as it plays a regulatory role in the occurrence of arthropathies, such as Juvenile Rheumatoid Arthritis, or malignant bone diseases. Moreover, we look at its influence on metabolic disorders associated with bone mass in children and vitamin D deficiency, or diseases of unknown etiology with musculoskeletal symptomatology (Growing pains). Of course, it must be stressed that few studies have been published in international literature concerning this field, but it seems that its beneficial effect is significant and important. For this reason, we would like to provide a stimulus for further research in this area that will lead, we feel, to even more documented results.

BREASTFEEDING AND THE IMMUNE SYSTEM

Newborns have an underdeveloped immune system, equaling only one percent that of an adult. The main cause for its development after birth is its exposure to microbes that colonize the intestine. Thus, staphylococcus aureus appears early in the feces and is found in the majority of infants at the age of 2-6 months while Gram negative microbes appear later (6). Therefore, sufficient time is needed for specific types of immunological reactions to develop, directly after an infection or after vaccination.

Breast milk appears to play an important role in the defense of the newborn's immune system, exercising a regulatory action and supporting its protection, both passively and actively. The main protein of colostrums and mature milk is secretory sIgA. This is produced in the mammary glands after exposure of antigens to the mother's Payer's patches. These immunoglobulins seem to protect children from many microbes, including E coli, V cholera, giardia lamblia and campylobacter (6). Moreover, IgM and IgG immunoglobulins are also transferred from the mother to the infant (7, 8).

The most important protein in breast milk is lactoferrin, which acts in a variety of ways, such as by destroying bacteria, viruses (such as Rotavirus), fungi and cancer cells. In addition, it blocks the production of cytokines such as IL - 1b, IL - 6 and TNF. Other major proteins with bioactive action found in breast milk include lysozyme, casein and alpha-Lactalbumin. Lysozyme leads to the disruption of bacterial cell walls, links to endotoxins reducing their harmful effect, leads to increased production of IgA and contributes to the activation of macrophages. Casein, finally, inhibits the adhesion of different bacteria to epithelial cells (7, 8). In addition, it contains soluble receptors (IL-1Ra, s-TNF a R1 and R2) for various cytokines, minimizing their inflammatory activity (8).

Another protective mechanism of breast milk relates to its content in antioxidant substances. These include alpha-tocopherol, b-carotene, ascorbic acid and L-histidine, which bind oxygen free radicals. Furthermore, the prostaglandins PGE1 and PGE2 minimize the production of peroxide (8). Apart from the above, breast milk also includes a large number of other substances, such as the AF peptide (Anti-secretory Factor), 90 - K and Mac - 2 binding glycoprotein which helps to prevent infections of the upper respiratory tract (6).

Many of the beneficial effects that have been reported epidemiologically are attributed to the significant anti-inflammatory and immunomodulatory properties of breast milk. Many such studies have shown that breast-feeding for 3 to 4 months and can exert long-term protection against infections such as otitis media, diarrhea, or infections of the upper respiratory tract (6, 7). In addition, it can exercise a regulatory role in vaccination effects. After the MMR, children who breast-feed show significant changes in CD8 + T cells and natural killer cells compared to formula-fed children aged 1 year. Also, serum antibodies after use of an oral polio vaccine are higher in children who breast-feed (6, 7).

It also appears that infections of the bones and joints in the neonatal period are limited by breastfeeding. The organisms that lead to osteomyelitis and septic arthritis include staphylococcus aureus, the group B streptococci and gram negative bacteria that colonize the intestine of newborns (9-12). These microbes can be inoculated in bones through hematogenic transport; the main risk factors are premature birth, critical illness and a formula diet (13). Studies in animal models have shown that the use of formula feeding dramatically increases the translocation of bacteria from the intestine (S aureus, proteus, enterobacter, E coli) and their entry in the bloodstream (13, 14). This is an important factor in the initiation of hematogenous osteomyelitis and septic arthritis, infections that can lead to destruction of children's growth plates.

BREASTFEEDING AND JUVENILE RHEUMATIC ARTHRITIS

The regulatory role of breast milk in the growth and maturation of the pediatric immune system is also directly linked to its influence on the emergence of various autoimmune diseases. Since 1984, when Borch-Johnsen reported that insulin-dependent diabetes mellitus (IDDM) occurs at a higher rate in children who do not breastfeed for at least 3 months (15, 16) numerous studies have investigated not only the above hypothesis, but also its correlation with other immune-system diseases, such as Multiple Sclerosis, Henoch-Schonlein purpura, inflammatory bowel disease and others (15). A disease with a predominantly immune basis, localized in the bones, which has been associated with breastfeeding is juvenile rheumatoid arthritis (JRA).

JRA is a relatively common childhood disease with an incidence of almost 1 in 1,000 children. It is classified into three sub-types, based on the symptoms occurring during the first semester of the disease. Pauciarticular, when 4 or fewer joints are affected, polyarticular when 5 or more are affected and systematic when extra-osseous symptoms such as fever or rashes, occur (17). Epidemiological studies reveal the involvement of breastfeeding in preventing the disease. Furthermore, there seems to be a statistically lower risk of the disease's occurrence in breast-feeding children, which mainly concerns its pauciarticular, and not polyarticular, form. In addition, the period of breast-feeding plays an important role. According to a study by Mason et al. (17) in children who were breast-fed for more than 3 months, the risk of disease decreased even more, compared with children who were breast-fed for a shorter period.

The mechanisms that have been proposed to explain the above analysis are based on the immunological properties of breast milk. One hypothesis is that breast milk protects children from exposure to an antigenic peptide that is likely to be involved in the pathogenesis of the disease. Another hypothesis is based on the mechanism of immune desensitization. Breast milk's content of autoantigens in small quantities, which come in contact with the immune system of the newborn, lead to its gradual desensitization. This mechanism has been reported and compared with other clinical studies (17, 18). Finally, another proposed mechanism is the significant protection afforded against infectious agents, such as viruses, which have common antigens with our body, eliminating the stimulation of autoimmune mechanisms. These are reinforced by the fact that breastfed individuals are less likely to be ANA or RF seropositive (17).

Despite the fact that other studies (19-20) showed no strong correlation of breastfeeding with the prevention of this disease, this - strong or less evident - protection from JRA is a fact, and a further beneficial property associated with the protection affords in arthropathies, mainly based on its immunological properties.

BREASTFEEDING AND MUSCULOSKELETAL CANCER

The causes that may lead to cancer in childhood vary and are still under investigation. Both genetic and environmental factors have been incriminated in their pathology. Exposure to ionizing radiation, strong electromagnetic fields, chemicals or toxins, infectious agents, dietary substances are some of the causes that have been experimentally investigated or verified for their involvement in the creation of childhood tumors. Many studies have investigated the possible protective role of breastfeeding in their development.

Developing the above hypothesis, Greaves suggested that breast milk plays an important role in protection against childhood ALL, either through the direct activation of the immune system, or by playing a regulatory role in this, to allow it to sufficiently respond adequately to inflammatory factors at a later age ("Greaves delayed hypothesis") (21). Breast-feeding has antimicrobial properties, but also activates the immune system sooner in these children, compared with children who are not breastfed (22). Until now many essays have investigated the relationship of breast milk with cancer in childhood. In their vast majority, they agree that children fed exclusively on breast milk present a lower risk of developing acute leukemia, particularly ALL, and Acute Myeloid Leukemia, Non-Hodgkin Lymphomas, Hodgkin Lymphomas, Wilm's Tumors and tumors of the sympathetic nervous system. Additionally, this did not concern a specific subtype, but all histological types of tumors, suggesting a common mechanism of protection against cancer (23). The risk reduction percentages reported differ depending on the study and the period of breast feeding and the method of assessing infant feeding, ranging from 2 to 16% for ALL and nonlymphoblastic leukemia, 3 - 40% for Hodgkin's disease and 22 -56% for neuroblastomas (23).

Moreover, the overall rate of childhood tumors is lower in breastfed children, including malignant osseous tumors and soft tissue sarcomas (24). Concerning childhood malignant osseous tumors, these represent 6 to 7% of all pediatric tumors; the most common types are osteosarcomas and Ewing sarcomas, with a frequency of 56% and 34% respectively. Apart from genetic diseases involved in their pathophysiology, such as hereditary retinoblastoma, Bloom syndrome, Blackfan-Diamond anemia, environmental factors are also involved in their creation (25). According to a study by Frentzel-Beyme et al. (26), one such factor is breastfeeding. In particular, breastfeeding for more than two months was linked to a lower statistical risk of these bone tumors in boys. Girls do not seem to be affected in this way; here, the most important risk factor was the age of the father.

A molecular-level mechanism that has been proposed is through a multimeric form of alpha-lactalbumin found in abundance in human milk that leads to the apoptosis of tumor cells. This form of lactalbumin is described as "potent Ca 2 + - elevating- and apoptosis-inducing agent with broad, selective cytotoxic activity" (27, 28) and seems to have a selective capacity, as normal cells are unaffected. The authors named this isomorph HAMLET (human a-lactalbumin made lethal to tumor cells); it seems to appear in the acidic environment of the gastrointestinal system, leading cancer and potentially malignant cells to apoptosis (27, 28). The conversion of the a – lactalbumin at low pH requires unfolding of the protein and the addition of a lipid cofactor identified as oleic acid (C18:1, 9 cis), which is released form milk oligosaccharides. Moreover, due to the stabilizing fatty acid in the HAMLET complex, it is resistant to proteolysis and may survive the passage through intestinal canal (29, 30). HAMLET - induced cell death differs from most classical apoptotic system and is independent of p53 (30). The main question would be how could HAMLET influence tumor development later in life. This can be explained by the molecular level of the infant. Cell proliferation is extremely rapid during the first month of life and high division rates increase the risk of mutation and malignant malformation. Cells with a premalignant genotype may then act as founders for future tumor development. HAMLET targets these cells leading them to apoptosis exerting a long –term protective effect (31).

BREASTFEEDING AND BONE MASS

Bone mass in adult life is a key element in public health and a key factor for the time of appearance and severity of osteoporosis. A large number of fractures are attributed to reduced bone density. It is believed that bone density reaches its maximum before the age of 14 years. Various factors, such as physical exercise, the chronic use of steroids and diet-especially calcium uptake - in early childhood and adolescence contribute to its optimization.

Breastfed infants absorb about 200 mg of calcium daily, a sufficient quantity for their development (32). In a 2000 longitudinal study (2) it seems that a long-term diet with breast milk leads to increased bone mass in later childhood. According to a study by Jones et al. (2), there is a beneficial relationship between breast feeding and bone mass at age 8 years. The measurement was conducted in the femoral neck, lumbar spine and total body (gr/cm2) and with the exception of BMD (Bone Mass Density) the femoral neck presented a statistically significant difference compared with bottle-fed children. The result seems to be more pronounced in children who breastfed for longer than 3 months. This is in agreement with the hypothesis that early exposure to breast milk, even just for 4 weeks, may lead to changes in the cycle of bone cells that lead to increased bone mass in later life (2). In a recent study by Foley et al., using a DXA method, breastfeeding was an important factor for positive spine aBMD activity compared with bottle-fed children. In light of the above, it seems that these children follow a different course of bone formation resulting in greater long term protection (33) and a reduced risk of fractures in the prepubertal period (34). In addition, breastfeeding is linked with the prevention of fall fractures in children even with the same BMD, which is attributed to additional non-BMD-related factors, such as the qualitative superiority, due to mineralization differences, of the bones in particular children (34). Indeed, a European study reported that the bones of infants who are formula-fed have slightly lower bone mineral mass in relation to breast-fed infants (35, 36). This, however, does not seem to occur in children younger than 4 years, when bone mineral content and bone mineral density among children who have breastfed for at least four months and in children who have not breastfed was studied (37).

Furthermore, several studies have shown that duration of breastfeeding influences bone mass beyond infancy. In Fewtrell's et al. study, breast – milk consumption was found to result in higher adult BMD, despite the milk being unfortified and having a lower mineral content than formula. This suggests a possible role for beneficial non – nutrient componenets such as growth factors or hormones (38). In another study, bone mass at follow – up age of approximately ten years, was positively associated with the duration of breastfeeding (39). Other studies have not demonstrated an ongoing relationship an adulthood between breastfeeding and Bone mass (40, 41).

Given the high calcium content of breast milk, a sufficient duration of breastfeeding appears to have a long-term effect on bone mass in relation to reducing the incidence of fractures in childhood, a possible regulatory action on the time of appearance and severity of osteoporosis in adult life and preventing fractures resulting from it. Nevertheless it is clear that further investigations will be needed to confirm the contribution of breastfeeding in preventing the occurrence and minimizing the severity of osteoporosis.

BREASTFEEDING AND GROWING PAIN

Recurrent pain in the legs (or "growing pain") constitutes the most frequent cause of musculoskeletal pain in childhood, with a frequency that can reach 49.4% (42). Although first mentioned in 1823 by the French physician Duchamp (43), their patho-physiological mechanisms are still under investigation. They appear more frequently at ages 4 to 6 years, but may be seen until adolescence. Their diagnosis is mainly based on their clinical picture, using Petersen's criteria, which are pain in both legs for less than 72 hours, especially late in the afternoon or evening, without bone localization and restriction of the joint's mobility and without the presence of redness, swelling or signs of inflammation and infection (44). Breast-feeding appears to significantly reduce their incidence. According to a study by Kaspiris et al. (45), children who are breast-feed have a statistically significant lower incidence of growing pains (19.6%) compared with those who are not breastfed (32.5%) (Fisher's Exact Test p value = 0.001 <0,005). Furthermore, the period of breastfeeding seems to play a very important role. When it lasted for less than 40 days, growing pains occurred in 29.8% of children, whereas in children breastfed for over 40 days, they reduced to 16.2% (Fisher's Exact Test p value = 0.001 <0.005).

$\Omega - 3$ fatty acid content is a main difference between breast and artificial milk. Data indicate that $\omega - 3$ fatty acids may reduce pain in joint and muscle and may have role in regulating bone growth (46). However, the study of Golding et al. found no evidence that $\omega - 3$ fatty acid status protects against the development of growing pains in childhood (47).

Certainly, further investigations to determine whether this mode of action is due to metabolic or immunological factors could be very important to explore the unknown, so far, pathophysiology of the disease.

BREASTFEEDING AND VITAMIN D DEFICIENCY

Despite the observed apparent benefits of breast-feeding in preventing bone disorders, there is a significant risk that mainly concerns children fed exclusively with breast milk. The concept that it is an excellent diet for children and the widespread view that 'breast is best' can lead to a reduced intake of vitamin D, necessary for bone metabolism (2, 48, 49).

Vitamin D (ergosterol) is absorbed from milk products and then synthesized in the skin after direct exposure to UV light at wavelengths of 295 - 310 nm (50, 51). This product, known as vitamin D2 or ergocalciferol, is converted to 25-hydroxyvitamin D in the liver and 1-25 hydroxyvitamin D in the kidneys. In people with dark skin, melanin competes with the skin's 7- dehydrocholesterol in the uptake of UV-B photons (50, 51).

Lack of vitamin D leads to reduced absorption of calcium by the intestine with subsequent hypocalcaemia and rachitis (rickets). It has been verified that the frequency of its deficiency increases with the frequency of breast-feeding (51). Indeed, its frequency can reach from 82% and 52% to 20% as it ensue of data come from the UAE, Pakistan, China and India respectively (4, 52, 53). In addition, studies have been published for the U.S. in the period from 2000 to 2003 with references to the occurrence of rachitis due to reduced dietary vitamin D intake in children in North Carolina, Texas, Georgia and the mid-Atlantic region (54-58).

Apart from biochemical disorders, rachitis is linked to clinical bone disorders (craniotabes, rickety rosary of the rib cage, bone swelling and epiphyseal enlargement, frontal bossing of the skull), convulsions, tetanus, and development and psychomotor delay (59-61). Its high-risk for group comprises infants from the lower socioeconomic classes with a poor education, probably because they spend prolonged periods in their houses (62, 63), as well as dark-skinned children, especially those residing in northernmost latitudes.

For this reason, in 2003 the American Academy of Pediatrics (AAP) issued new guidelines for the supplement of vitamin D. As breast milk contains between 20 and 60 iu/l of vitamin D, which is unsatisfactory, the AAR recommended that all newborns, including those fed exclusively on breast milk, take a minimum amount of 200 iu of Vitamin D per day during the first two months of life. In addition, all breast-feeding infants should be given a vitamin D supplement during the first two months of life unless they consume at least 500 mL of a Vitamin D-fortified milk formula (64).

An important factor in preventing rachitis is adequate sun exposure, which may be reduced either in the autumn and winter months, either due to air pollution or the coverage of large parts of the body with clothing for cultural reasons. It is recommended that infants be exposed to sunlight for a minimum two hours per week, if only the face is exposed and for 30 minutes when the upper and lower extremities are exposed, always taking the necessary measures to protect against melanoma (i.e., avoiding the sun between 10.00 - 16.00, using sunscreen etc.) (65).

CONCLUSION

Breastfeeding is a natural source of quality nutritious substances for infants, which may determine their healthy development not only in later childhood, but also in adult life. Both immunological and metabolic factors have been investigated for their participation in its beneficial effect. It seems that these play an important role in the healthy musculoskeletal development of children. Bone and joint diseases occur less frequently in individuals who have been breastfed. Breast-feeding reduces the occurrence of osteomyelitis and septic arthritis in both human infants and animal models, limits the appearance of autoimmune etiology arthritis and contributes to a reduced incidence of osteosarcomas or Ewing sarcomas. Moreover, it structures a healthy skeleton by increasing bone mass that leads to a reduced rate of fractures in childhood and the decreased severity of osteoporosis in later life. Even with diseases of unknown pathophysiology that have musculoskeletal manifestations, such as growing pains, these appear modified in breastfed individuals and are linked, like all the above diseases, with the duration of breastfeeding. The lack of vitamin D in children fed exclusively with milk, which can lead to rachitis, requires, however, attention. A combination of vitamin D supplements and adequate sun exposure manage this disease.

REFERENCES

[1]   Barker DJP, ed. Fetal and infant origins of adult disease. London: BMJ Press, 1993.
[2]   Jones G, Riley M, Dwyer T. Breastfeeding in early life and bone mass in prepubertal children: a longitudinal study. Osteoporos Int 2000;11: 146-52.
[3]   Lauer JA, Betran AP, Barros AJ, De Onis M. Deaths and years of life lost due to suboptimal breast feeding among children in the developing world: a global ecological risk assessment. Public Health Nutr 2006;9:673-85.
[4]   Balasubramanian S, Ganesh R. Vitamin D deficiency in exclusively breast – fed infants. Indian J Med Res 2008;127:250-5.
[5]   Nielsen LS, Michaelson KF. Breast feeding and future health. Curr Opin Clin Nutr Metab Care 2006;9:289-96.

[6]   Hanson LA, Sifverdal SA, Stomback L, Erling V, Zaman S, Olcen P, Telemo E. The immunological role of breast feeding. Pediatr Allergy Immunol 2001;12(suppl 14):15-9.

[7]   M'Rabet L, Vos AP, Boehm G, Garssen J. Breast – feeding and its role in early development of the immune system in infants: consequences for health later in life. J Nutr 2008;138:1782S-90S.

[8]   Lawrence RM, Pane CA. Human breast milk: current concepts of immunology and infectious diseases. Curr Probl Pediatr Adolesc Health Care 2007;37:7-36.

[9]   Bergdahl S, Ekengren K, Eriksson M. Neonatal hematogenous osteomyelitis: risk factors for long term sequelae. J Pediatr Orthop 1985;5:564-8.

[10]   Edwards MS, Baker CJ, Wagner ML, Taber LH, Barrett FF. An etiologic shift in infantile osteomyelitis: the emergence of group B streptococcus. J Pediatr 1978;93:578-83.

[11]   Dan M. Neonatal septic arthritis. Isr J Med Sci 1983;19:967-71.

[12]   Fox L, Sprunt K. Neonatal osteomyelitis. Pediatrics 1978;62:535-42.

[13]   Steinwender G, Schimpl G, Sixl B, Kerbler S, Ratschek M, Kilzer S, Hollwarth ME, Wenzl HH. Effect of early nutritional deprivation and diet on translocation of bacteria from the gastrointestinal tract in the newborn rat. Pediatr Res 1996;39:415-20.

[14]   Steinwender G, Schimpl G, Sixl B, Wenzl HH. Gut – derived bone infection in the neonatal rat. Pediatr Res 2001;50(6):767-71.

[15]   Davis MK. Breastfeeding and chronic disease in childhood and adolescence. Pediatric clinics of North America 2001;48(1):125-41.

[16]   Borch-Johnsen K, Joner G, Mandrup-Poulsen T, Christy M, Zachau-Christiansen B, Kastrup K, Nerup J. Relation between breastfeeding and incidence rates of insulin-dependent diabetes mellitus: a hypothesis. Lancet 1984;2(8411):1983-6.

[17]   Mason T, Rabinovich CE, Fredrickson DD, Amoroso K, Reed AM, Stein LD, Kredich DW. Breastfeeding and the development of Juvenile Rheumatoid Arthritis. J Rheumatol 1995;22:1166-70.

[18]   Trentham DE, Dynesius-Trentham RA, Orav EJ. Effects of oral administration of type II collagen on rheumatoid arthritis. Science 1993;261:1727-30.

[19]   Rosenberg AM. Evaluation of associations between breast feeding and subsequent development of Juvenile Rheumatoid Arthritis. J Rheumatol 1996;23:1080-2.

[20]   Kasapcopur O, Tasdan Y, Apelyan M, Akkus S, Caliskan S, Sever L, Arisoy N. Does breastfeeding prevent the development of Juvenile Rheumatoid Arthritis? J Rheumatol 1998;25:2286-7.

[21]   Greaves MF. Etiology of acute leukemia. Lancet 1997;349:344-9.

[22]   Pabst HF. Immunomodulation by breastfeeding. Pediatr Inf Dis J 1997;16:991-5.

[23]   Ortega-Garcia JA, Ferris-Tortajada J, Torres-Cantero AM, Soldin OP, Torres EP, Fuster-Soler JL, Lopez-Ibor B, Madero-Lopez L. Full breastfeeding and paediatric cancer. J Paediatr Child Health 2008;44: 10-3.

[24]   Martin RM, Gunnell D, Owen CG, Smith GD. Breast-feeding and childhood cancer: a systematic review with metaanalysis. Int J Cancer 2005;117:1020-31.

[25]   Ferris I, Tortajada J, Tornero B, Ortega Garcia JA, et al. Risk factors for pediatric malignant bone tumors. An Pediatr (Barc) 2005;63(6): 537-47.

[26]   Frentzel-Beyeme R, Becher H, Salzer-Kuntschik M, Kotz R, Salzer M. Factors affecting the incident juvenile bone tumors in an Austrian case - control study. Cancer Detect Prev 2004;28:159-69.

[27]   Hakansson A, Zhivotovsky B, Orrenius S, Sabharwal H, Svanborg C. Apoptosis induced by a human milk protein. Proc Natl Acad Sci 1995;92(17):8064-8.

[28]   Svensson M, Hakansson A, Mossberg AK, Linse S, Svanborg C.. Conversion of a- lactalbumin to a protein inducing apoptosis. Proc Natl Acad Sci 2000;97(8):4221-6.

[29]   Hallgren O, Aits S, Brest P, Gustafsson L, Mossberg AK, WuLLT b, Svanborg C. Apoptosis and tumor cell death in response to HAMLET (human alpha – lactalbumin made lethal to tumor cells). Adv Exp Med Biol 2008;606:217-40.

[30]   Gustafsson L, Hallgren O, Mossberg AK, Pettersson J, Fischer W, Aronsson A, Svanborg C. HAMLET kills tumor cells by apoptosis: Structure, cellular mechanisms and therapy. J Nutr 2005;135:1299-1303.

[31]   Svanborg C, Aderstam H, Aronson A, Bjerkvig R, Duringer C, et al. HAMLET kilss tumor cells by an apoptosis - like mechanism – cellular, molecular, and therapeutic aspects. Adv Cancer Res 2003; 88:1-29.

[32]   Sabatier JP, Guaydier-Souquieres, Laroche D. Bone mineral acquisition during adolescence and early adulthood: a study in 574 healthy females 10 – 24 years of age. Osteoporos Int 1996;6:141-8.

[33]   Foley S, Quinn S, Jones G. Tracking of bone mass from children to adolescence and factors that predict deviation from tracking. Bone 2009;44:752-7.

[34]   Ma DG, Jones G. Clinical risk factors but not bone density are associated with prevalent fractures in pre-pubertal children. J Paediatr Child Health 2002;32(5):497-500.

[35]   Kennedy K, Fewtrell MS, Morley R. Double – blind, randomized trial of a synthetic triacylglycerol in formula – fed term infants: effects on stool biochemistry, stool characteristics, and bone mineralization. Am J Clin Nutr 1999;70:920-7.

[36]   Abrams SA. Building bones in babies: Can and should we exceed the human milk – fed infant's rate of bone calcium accretion? Nutr Rev 2006;64(11):487-94.

[37]   Harvey NC, Robinson SM, Crozier SR, Marriott LD, Gale CR, Cole ZA, Inskip HM, Godfrey KM, Cooper C, the Southampton Women's Survey Study Group. Breast – feeding and adherence to infant guidelines do not influence bone mass at age 4 years. Br J Nutr 2009; 2:1-6.

[38]   Fewtrell MS, Williams JE, Singhal A, Murgatroyd PR, Fuller N, Lucas A. Early diet and peak bone mass: 20 year follow-up of a randomized trial of early diet in infants born preterm. Bone 2009; 45(1): 142 – 149.

[39]   Jones G, Riley M, Dwyer T. Breastfeeding in early life andbone mass in prepubertal children: a longitudinal study. Osteoporos Int 2000; 11(2): 146 – 152.

[40]   Kalkwarf HJ, Zemel BS, Yolton K, Heubi JE. Bone mineral content and density of the lumbar spine of infants and toddlers: influence of age, sex, race, growth and human milk feeding. J Bone Miner Res 2013; 28(1): 206 – 212.

[41]   Pirila S, Taskinen M, Vijakainen H, Kajosaari M, Turanlanti M, Saarinen – Pihkala UM, Makitie O. Infant milk feeding influences adult bone health: a prospective study from birth to 32 years. PLoS One 2011; 6(4): 1 – 8.

[42]   Evans AM, Scutter SD. Prevalence of "Growing pains" in young children. J Pediatr 2004;145(2):255-8.

[43]   Duchamp M. Maladies de la croissance. In: Levralt FG, ed. Memoires de Medecine Practique. Paris: Jean-Frederic Lobstein, 1823. [French]

[44]   Petersen H. Growing pains. Pediatr Clin North Am 1986;33(6):1365-72.

[45]   Kaspiris A, Zafiropoulou C, Tsadira O, Petropoulos C. Can breastfeeding avert the appearance of growth pains during childhood? Clin Rheumatol 2007; 26:1909-12.

[46]   Goldberg RJ, Katz J. A meta – analysis of the analgesic effects of ω – 3 polysaturated fatty acid supplementation for inflammatory joint pain. Pain 2007; 129: 210 – 223.

[47]   Golding J, Northstone K, Emmett P, Steer C, Hibben JR. Do ω – 3 or other fatty acids influence the development of "growing pains"? A prebirth cohort study. BMJ open 2012;2 (4): 1 – 6.

[48]   Morley R, Lucas A. Influence of early diet on outcome in preterm infants. Acta Paediatr Suppl 1994;405:123-6.

[49]   Henderson A. Vitamin D and breast – fed infant. J Obstet Gynecol Neonatal Nurs 2005;34:367-72.

[50]   Holick MF, McLaughlin JA, Clark MB. Photosynthesis of previtamin D3 in human skin and physiologic consequences. Science 1980;210: 203-5.

[51]   Holick MF, McLaughlin JA, Doppelt SJ. Regulation of cutaneous previtamin D photosynthesis in man: skin pigment is not an essential regulator. Science 1981;211:590.

[52]   Atiq M, Suria A, Nizami SQ. Vitamin D status of breastfed Pakistani infants. Acta Paediatr Scand 1998;87:737-40.

[53]   Ho ML, Yen HC, Tsang RC, Specker BL, Chen XC, Nichols BL. Randomized study of sunshine exposure and serum 25 – OHD in breast fed infants in Beijing, China. J Pediatr 1985;107:928-31.

[54]   Simon SR, ed. Orthopedic basic science. American Academy of Orthopedic Surgeons. Columbus, OH: Ohio State Univ Press 1994: 168-9.

[55] Weisberg P, Scanlon KS, Li R, Cogswell ME. Nutritional rickets among children in United States: review of cases reported between 1986 and 2003. Am J Clin Nutr 2004;80(suppl):1697S-1705S.

[56] Kreiter SR, Schwartz RP, Kirkman HN Jr, Charlton PA, Calikoglu AS, Davenport ML. Nutritional rickets in African American breast fed infants. J Pediatr 2000;137:153-7.

[57] Shah M, Salhab N, Patterson D, Seikaly MG. Nutritional rickets still afflicting children in North Texas. Texas Med 2000;96:64-8.

[58] Tomashek KM, Nesby S, Scanlon KS. Nutritional rickets in Georgia. Pediatrics 2001;107: e45.

[59] O'Riordan JLH. Rickets, from history to molecular biology, from monkeys to YACS. J Endocrinol 1997;154:S3-13.

[60] Carvalho NF, Kenney RD, Carrington PH, Hall DE. Severe nutritional deficiencies in toddlers resulting from health food milk alternatives. Paediatrics 2001;107: e51.

[61] Biser-Rohrbaugh A, Hadley-Miller N. Vitamin D Deficiency in breast fed toddlers. J Pediatr Orthopedics 2001;21:508-11.

[62] Dawodu A, Agarwal M, Hossain M, Kochiyil J, Zayed R. Hypovitaminosis D and vitamin D deficiency in exclusively breast – feeding infants and their mother in summer: a justification for vitamin D supplementation of breast – feeding infants. J Pediatr 2003;142: 169-73.

[63] Ferguson M. A study of social and economic factors in the causation of rickets. London: HMSO Med Res Community, Spec Report 20; 1917.

[64] Gartner LM, Greer FR, American Academy of Pediatrics, Section on Breastfeeding and Committee on Nutrition. Prevention of rickets and vitamin D deficiency: new guidelines for vitamin D intake. Pediatrics 2003;111:908-10.

[65] Specker BL, Valanis B, Hertzberg V, Edwards N, Tsang RC. Sunlight exposure and serum 25 – hydroxyvitamin D concentrations in exclusively breast-fed infants. J Pediatr 1985;107:372-6.

Section 2:
Nutrition and malnutrition

In: Food, Nutrition and Eating Behavior   ISBN: 978-1-62948-233-0
Editors: Joav Merrick and Sigal Israeli   © 2014 Nova Science Publishers, Inc.

Chapter 3

LOW-FAT, NO-FAT, AND SUGAR-FREE

Kim Bissell, PhD

Department of Journalism, University of Alabama, Tuscaloosa, Alabama, US

ABSTRACT

The prevalence of childhood obesity remains a critical issue as the number of children being diagnosed as overweight or obese is continuing to rise. This chapter examines 601 3rd-6th grade children's time spent viewing television, their nutritional knowledge, their nutritional reasoning, their food preferences, and their dietary behavior at home and at school to determine which factors were stronger predictors of children's nutritional knowledge. Using a survey, students were presented with food pairs increasing in difficulty and asked to select the food they thought was most capable of helping them grow up to be healthy and strong. A nutritional knowledge scale was constructed and then compared with other predictor variables to identify the factors related to higher or lower knowledge scores. Regression analysis indicates that television viewing was related to increased levels of nutritional knowledge. Television viewing was also related to a stronger preference for unhealthy foods across the sample. Children in the sample further perceived the food they consumed at school to be significantly healthier than the food they consumed at home. Demographic variables proved to be strong predictors of students' nutritional knowledge and also proved to be a significant predictor of students' preferences toward healthy food. Children across demographic groups believed the foods they received in school lunch and breakfast programs were healthy and high in nutritional value even though the actual food consumed was similar to what was consumed at home.

* Correspondence: Professor Kim Bissell, Ph.D., Associate Dean for Research, College of Communication and Information Sciences, University of Alabama, Box 870172, Tuscaloosa, AL 35487 United States. E-mail: kbissell@ua.edu.

INTRODUCTION

Recent reports from the International Obesity Task Force indicated that in 2006, 22 million children worldwide under the age of five years were classified as obese or overweight. Furthermore, results from the 2003-2004 National Health and Nutrition Examination Survey indicated that an estimated 17% of children in the US between 2-19 years were overweight. What is known from empirical studies across disciplines is that multiple factors may be related to the likelihood of a child to be overweight or obese: genetics, lack of physical activity, and increased consumption of high-calorie, low-nutrition foods and beverages (1). Of importance here are factors that children cannot control—access or encouragement to participate in physical activities, access to healthy or unhealthy foods at home or at school, and a social or home environment that either promotes or discourages healthy eating and exercise. Along these lines, children and adolescents may presume that their parents are making responsible and healthy choices for them as it relates to food and physical activity (2), and probably will not spend a great deal of time analyzing the nutritional attributes of a specific food item (3). Children will either rely on parents to make good choices for them, or respond to terms on the products such as "low fat" or "low sugar", and they may not examine the actual nutritional content of the products themselves. A recent study published by the Institute of Medicine of the National Academies (IOM report) indicated that the current practices for food marketing put children at a health risk because dietary patterns begin early in childhood and are shaped by social, cultural and mediated factors, including television advertising. Furthermore, children may presume that the foods they receive at school in lunch or breakfast programs are also healthy and may not critically consider the nutritional attributes of the foods being served. Accordingly, this study examined 3rd-6th graders' television use, their knowledge of nutrition, their food preferences, and their food intake at home and at school in order to better assess which factors may prove more influential in shaping their overall knowledge about nutrition and health.

Even though parents are responsible for the food children consume at home, many researchers suggest the media, especially advertising, influence children's purchasing behavior and food purchase requests (4). Certainly, as studies over the last decade have illustrated, food ads targeted toward children have often emphasized unhealthy options versus healthy options (5). They further report that in the ads targeted toward children, few health-related messages were found, but of the ones with some mention of health, the message was related to the food containing natural ingredients or that the food was low in calories.

Studies more recently have examined the nutritional value of food served in public schools, suggesting that the school environment may be one source of a child's higher calorie diet. With the introduction of vending machines in schools and the shift to cheaper foods in bulk, the nutritional value of food served during the school day is questionable at best. Children, however, may not recognize the poor nutritional value of the foods they are consuming, especially if the food is coming from home or school. Children may further lack the awareness or understanding related to nutritional guidelines and may simply assume what they are eating is healthy. More sedentary lifestyles and changes in the home environment have also contributed to a shift in eating habits and behavior in the last few decades, especially in the foods children eat on a daily basis and their daily media diet.

Roberts and Foehr report that the average child spends up to five hours a day with various media (6), and as reported in a more recent study, elementary aged children spent several hours a day watching television programs on the Disney Channel, Nickelodeon, and the Cartoon Network and spent additional time on the websites associated with those channels as well as websites targeted toward children (webkins.com, neopets.com, and playhousedisney.com) (7). Harrison (8) and Peterson, Jeffrey, Bridgewater, and Dawson (9) argue that the way food products are advertised on television does affect children's understanding of nutrition and further influences the choices they make about food and the amount of food they consume. Brownell and Horgen (10) further suggest that food products that are associated with a media tie-in and that have a corresponding "toy" make resisting the food even more difficult.

Empirical studies examining children's overall knowledge of nutrition are scant at best, but a few studies have examined nutritional knowledge as it relates to media exposure. Signorielli and Staples (11) found that children who spent more time watching television were more likely to select a food that was unhealthy and this was found across gender, race, or reading ability. In a similar study, Harrison (12) examined adolescents' television viewing with their knowledge of nutrition using similar measures for the dependent variable. Harrison also examined nutritional reasoning, which was defined as the child's rationale for selecting the specific food from the food pairing as being the healthier or more nutritionally sound choice. Harrison found that heavier television viewing was related to lower levels of nutritional knowledge and nutritional reasoning, but this relationship was only found for food that were marketed as weight-loss products.

The media are often blamed for the increases in childhood obesity, but beyond articulating that children spend too much time with the media, very little is known about how the specific content children are exposed to may influence their thoughts and decisions about the foods they consume. Lowry, Wechsler, Galuska, Fulton, and Kann (13) report in their study of high school students' media use and their rates of sedentary lifestyles and obesity that one in three White students, one in two Hispanic students, and three in four Black students watched more television per day than what is recommended by the American Academy of Pediatrics (two hours per day). Most importantly, the authors report that in their sample, television viewing was found to be positively related to the consumption of high-fat foods and those participants who were overweight were also more likely to spend more time with television.

The general conclusion from these studies is that television viewing may be negatively related to children's food preferences, food intake and nutritional knowledge because it may not only shape what they view to be healthy and good for them, but it may also shape their preferences for specific foods and affect how much food they eat while watching television.

Hammermeister, Brock, Winterstein, and Page (14) found in their analysis of psychosocial health characteristics in television-free and television-viewing individuals that those who viewed moderate amounts of television were more likely to display a negative psychosocial health profile compared to their non-viewing counterparts. Based on the literature reviewed, the following research questions were posed:

- RQ1: How is television viewing related to children's nutritional knowledge?
- RQ2: How is television viewing related to children's food preferences?

- RQ3: How do food preferences and the home dieting environment relate to nutritional knowledge?

THE PRESENT STUDY

In order to examine the relationship between media consumption, food preferences, knowledge of nutrition, and the home and social eating environment, a survey was administered to children in grades 3-6 in several counties in a state in the South. Of the 601 participants, 45% were boys and 55% were girls with an ethnic representation that was closely matched to that of the counties where data was collected: Eighty percent of the sample was Caucasian, 16% was African American, and the remaining 4% reported to be Hispanic, Asian or "other."

Children were asked to list the television shows they watched "yesterday before school," "yesterday after school but before dinner," and "yesterday after dinner but before bed." This measure of television viewing was used in place of the traditional items that ask participants to report the average number of minutes per day spent viewing television and has been validated in studies using similar samples (16).

Throughout the instrument, children in this sample were shown pictures of three different foods and were asked the following question: Which of the foods above would you most like to eat right now? This item was not designed to measure purchase intent nor was it designed as a measure of nutritional knowledge; rather, it was designed to measure the preferences toward specific types of foods and potentially tap into participants' gut-reactions or instinctual responses to food preferences. Options for the food choices were as follows: Reese's Peanut Butter Cup, Doritos, carrots; McDonald's French Fries, M&Ms, grapes; Subway sandwich, Pizza Hut pizza, watermelon. For each of the three questions, responses were recoded as healthy or unhealthy, resulting in a recoded, additive scale representing food preferences. For this scale, unhealthy food choices (Reese's, Doritos, fries, M&Ms, pizza) were recoded as a 0 and healthy food choices (carrots, grapes, sandwich, and watermelon) were recoded as a 1. Results from responses to all three items were combined with a mean score of 1.27 (sd=.97). The scale ranged from a low of 0, meaning a participant chose all unhealthy foods to a high of 3, meaning a participant chose all healthy food options. In the sample of 601 3rd-6th graders, 24% had a score of 0, 37% had a score of 1, 25% had a score of 2, and 13% had a score of 3. The scale used to measure food preferences simply represents an additive scale of responses recoded as either healthy or non-healthy choices on food preferences. Cronbach's alpha on this scale was .70.

Finally, children were asked a series of questions about their eating habits and patterns, the source of the foods they consumed, and how nutritious they felt their food was. Participants were asked to indicate their frequency of consuming a long list of food items ranging from healthy to unhealthy choices each day at home and at school. Responses to these items were used to create a daily food intake index, which had secondary component to it related to the child's perceived nutritional value of his/her daily diet. As expected, daily food intake varied across the sample, but the following patterns were observed. When asked about the frequency of consuming foods such as fruits, vegetables, milk, or other dairy products, children indicated consuming these foods an average 3.67 (sd=1.78) days per week at school and 2.78 days per week at home (sd=2.01). When asked about the consumption of eating foods such as potato chips, candy, or soda, participants reported eating these foods an average of .91 (sd=1.32) days per week at school and 5.74 (sd=1.79) days per week at home. Participants perceived the food they consumed at school, including food brought in a lunch box, to be significantly more healthy than the foods they consumed at home (school mean=3.79, sd=2.21, home mean=2.24, sd=1.89, on a scale ranging from 1-5 with 5 representing the most nutritious).

Dependent variables

To measure knowledge of nutrition, participants were shown four pairs of foods (fat-free ice cream/yogurt, orange juice/Diet Coke, white bread/wheat bread, fruit snack/granola bar) and were asked the following question: which of the two items above is better to help you grow up healthy and strong? Respondents could only select one answer. These specific food pairings were selected because they represented a range of foods and because they represented varying degrees of difficulty in terms of assessing which would be more nutritional. All responses were recoded as being correct or incorrect. Each response option was recoded as a healthy or unhealthy choice and those four responses were added together for the final nutritional knowledge scale with a Cronbach's alpha of .64. Participants' responses were added together to create a final scale ranging from 0 (all incorrect answers) to 4 (all correct answers). The mean nutritional knowledge score was 2.62 (sd=1.09, N=560).

Table 1. Independent t-tests for television exposure and Internet use by gender

Minutes during the day	Boys Mean SD N	Girls Mean SD N	F	df	p value
TV before school	36.46 (28.27) 246	39.00 (32.96) 300	6.07	544	n.s.
TV after school	40.24 (27.46) 246	45.67 (28.59) 305	5.28	549	*p<.05*
TV before bed	48.10 (26.16)	51.74 (29.54)	2.10	550	n.s.
Weekly minutes viewing	874.17 (450.89) 246	955.03 (482.14) 300	3.45	544	*p<.05*
Internet usage*	3.68 (1.59) 244	3.58 (1.66) 302	1.85	500	n.s.

* Internet usage was measured using the following responses (0=never, 1=once a week, 2=a few days a week, 3=almost every day of the week, 4=every day of the week, 5=an hour or more each day).

Participants were also asked about their reasoning behind making the above choices. After indicating which food they thought was better to help them grow up healthy and strong, they were then asked why. Responses for this item were as follows: it is good for you; it tastes good; it will keep you healthy; my mom says it is good for me; it is nutritious. Answers were then recoded in terms of whether the child's response reflected nutritional reasoning (it is good for you, it will keep you healthy, my mom says it is good for me, it is nutritious) or non-nutritional reasoning (it tastes good). Responses for all four items were then combined to create a single score representing each child's nutritional reasoning. Each non-nutritional reasoning response was recoded as 0, and each nutritional reasoning response was recoded as 1, and when the responses for all four items were added together, the nutritional reasoning scale had a mean score of 2.92 (sd=1.19, N=554). Reliability analysis on the 4-item scale was .69 using Cronbach's alpha.

FINDINGS

The first research question addressed the relationship between television viewing and participants' knowledge of nutrition. Regression analysis indicated a significant relationship between television viewing and knowledge of nutrition; however, the results indicate that children who watched more television had higher scores on the nutritional knowledge scale than those who watched less television. When the television viewing variable was recoded into low, medium and high groups, one-way ANOVA tests indicated that those in the high viewing group had a mean nutritional knowledge score of 2.80 (sd=1.06, on a scale ranging from 0-4, with 4 representing the greatest nutritional knowledge) compared to those in the low viewing group who had a mean nutritional knowledge score of 2.56 (sd=1.02). Post-hoc Tukey's tests indicate differences between the high and low viewing groups were significant.

The second research question examined the relationship between television viewing and food preferences. As reported in findings from earlier studies, it was projected that children who spent more time watching television would be more inclined to prefer food that had less nutritional value than children who spent less time with television. While regression analysis indicated a significant relationship between the variables, the beta was very low, (.13), so additional tests were run to examine this relationship. One-way ANOVA tests were run again to examine the food preferences of high, medium and low television viewers, and in this case, those watching the most television were also the most likely to prefer non-nutritional foods. For example, those in the high viewing group (N=157) had a mean food preference score of 1.06 (sd=.95, on a scale of 0-3 with 0 representing the least nutritional choices of the food groups) whereas those in the low viewing group (N=182) had a mean food preference score of 1.34 (sd=.98). Participants in the medium viewing group (N=213) had a mean nutritional food preference score of 1.21 (sd=.97). Post-hoc Tukey's LSD tests indicated significant differences between the low and high television viewing groups. Thus, findings from this statistical test parallel what's been reported in other studies—television viewing was related to children's preferences for foods that have less nutritional value.

The third research question examined the relationship between food preferences, the home dieting environment, and nutritional knowledge. In this case, it was predicted that children who tended to prefer foods that were less nutritious would also exhibit an inability to make accurate choices about what foods would be healthier options for them. While preferences for specific foods could be related to a variety of social, environmental and media factors, as indicated from the descriptives reported earlier, only 13% of the sample of 601 children chose healthy options in all three cases and 24% chose the unhealthy option in all three cases. Regression analysis indicated a significant relationship between the two variables (β=.36, p<.001). One-way analysis of variance tests using the recoded food preference score (0-3 with 3 representing a stronger preference for healthier foods) indicated similar patterns in a very linear fashion. Children who preferred healthier foods (N=73) had the highest nutritional knowledge scores with a mean of 3.19 (sd=.81) compared to those who preferred the non-healthy foods (N=130) who had a mean nutritional knowledge score of 2.30 (sd=1.27). Post-hoc Tukey's tests indicated significant differences between all groups except the group scoring a 0 on the food preference score, meaning they chose no nutritional foods, and those scoring a 1, meaning 1 healthy food choice was made. When age, gender and race were considered as predictors in the regression model, the significant relationship held except for race. Regression analysis using age, gender, and food preferences as a predictor of nutritional knowledge resulted in a beta of .43 (p<.001), and regression tests using TV exposure, age, gender and food preferences also resulted in a significant, positive beta of .57 (p<.001, see Table 2).

Table 2. Summary of Multiple Hierarchical Regression Analyses Regressing Overall Nutritional Knowledge on Television Viewing, Age, Gender, and Food Preferences

Predictor Variable	β	R^2	F	df
Dependent Variable: Nutritional Knowledge Index				
Step 1				
Television Viewing	.07	.01	.37	458
Step 2				
Age	-.06	.05	2.15	456
Gender	.43***			
Step 3				
Food Preferences	.57***	.11	12.58	455

***p<.001.

A child's home and social eating environment was also significantly related to food preferences and nutritional knowledge. Children who reported eating unhealthy foods at home tended to select unhealthy foods as their preference and had significantly lower nutritional knowledge scores (β=.42, p<.001). When asked to indicate how healthy their food choices were in terms of their daily food intake, participants acknowledged that many of the foods they consumed at home (friend chicken, fast food, candy, and soda) were not the most healthy for them. When asked about the nutritional value of the foods consumed at school, participants were more likely to associate their school-consumed foods as healthy. When each index was compared with nutritional knowledge, the home eating index was a significant predictor of lower nutritional knowledge scores (r=.42, p<.01), but the school eating index was not statistically related to nutritional knowledge or nutritional reasoning.

DISCUSSION

This study of 601 3rd-6th grade boys and girls in a Southern state in the United States examined their time spent viewing television along with their knowledge of nutrition, their nutritional reasoning, their food preferences, and their home and school food intake. Results indicate that television viewing was not a strong predictor of decreased levels of nutritional knowledge but rather that television viewing was related to increased levels of nutritional knowledge. However, television viewing was also related to a stronger preference for unhealthy foods across the sample.

When television viewing was examined with the individual nutritional knowledge items, results indicate that as the nutritional knowledge items became more difficult, television viewing was a stronger predictor of participants making an incorrect choice. For example, when television viewing was grouped into high, medium and low groups, participants across the groups had roughly equal numbers of correct or incorrect answers when asked to select between fat free ice cream or yogurt. When participants were asked to choose between orange juice and Diet Coke, children in the low and medium viewing groups were more likely to get the answer correct when compared to those in the high viewing group. But, when examining responses to the question related to fruit snacks or granola bars, the number of children getting the answer correct was roughly the same across viewing groups. Analysis of television viewing with the individual food preference items also proved interesting. For the first item (Reese's Peanut Butter Cup, Doritos, carrots), 38% of the sample chose Doritos, followed by 36% of the sample choosing the Reese's, and 26% choosing carrots. Children who spent the most time watching television were the least likely to select carrots as the food they would like to eat right now but were the most likely to select Doritos. Children who watched the least amount of television were also more likely to select Doritos, but a significantly higher number of them selected carrots than those in the high viewing category. While the role of television in this sample's decision-making with regard to food preferences and nutritional knowledge is still largely unclear, other variables examined remain important considerations.

One interesting finding from the study was participants' perceptions of the nutritional value of the foods they consumed at home and at school. Participants readily admitted some of the foods they consumed at home were unhealthy, and this could simply be because of the packaging of the food (frozen dinners or pre-packaged meals) or because they know the food came from a fast food restaurant. However, even though the actual food consumed (fried chicken or French fries) might have been the same at home and at school, the perceived nutritional value of it was higher when consumed at school. As Harrison (12) reported in an earlier study, the way foods are presented in a mediated context will influence the way they subsequently think about the nutritional value of food.

Even though the findings of this study contribute to knowledge in the area of health communication and media, this study is not without its limitations. One important limitation was the exclusion of exposure to media other than television. It is possible that children learn about food and nutrition from media sources other than television, but given the large amount of evidence documenting the frequency of food ads on television, it was thought appropriate to only include television exposure in this study. These other possible predictor variables include measures related to the child's social and home environment. An important missing variable from this study was a measure of each child's daily dietary intake and the environment in which food is consumed.

Findings from this study suggest that it is quite possible the media may serve a role in educating children about diet, nutrition, and overall health. The key to this is in finding a way to get children's attention in this area so they can start playing a role in decision-making as it relates to their own health.

Table 3. Exploratory factor analysis of four food choices with varimax rotation

	Rotated loadings		
	Factor 1	Factor 2	Factor 3
Food choices			
Choice 1 (*orange juice* vs. diet coke)	.74	.03	.03
Choice 2 (fat-free ice cream vs. *yogurt*)	.58	.24	.24
Choice 3 (white bread vs. *wheat bread*)	.70	.06	.21
Choice 4 (fruit snack vs. *granola bar*)	.09	.16	.90

*The three factors reported in this table were those with eigenvalues over 1.00. Factor 1 explained 27% of the variance; Factor 2 explained 14% of the variance; Factor 3 explained 13% of the variance. Food choices that were considered the more nutritious of the two are noted in italics.

REFERENCES

[1]   Warren R, Wicks RH, Wicks JL, Fosu I, Chung D. Food and beverage advertising on U.S. television: A comparison of child-targeted versus general audience commercials. J Broadcasting Electronic Media 2008;52:231-46.

[2]   Campbell KJ, Crawford DA, Ball K. Family food environment and dietary behaviors likely to promote fatness in 5-6 year-old children. Int J Obesity 2006;30:1272-1280.

[3]   Gibson EL, Wardle J, Watts CJ. Fruit and vegetable consumption, nutritional knowledge and beliefs in mothers and children. Appetite 1998; 31:205-228.

[4]   Donkin AJ, Neale RJ, Tilston C. Children's food purchase requests. Appetite 1993;21:291-294.

[5]   Strasburger VC. Children and TV advertising: Nowhere to run, nowhere to hide. J Dev Behav Pediatr 2001;22:185-7.

[6]   Roberts DF, Foehr UG. Kids and media in America. New York: Cambridge University Press, 2004.

[7]   Bissell K, Hays H. Understanding anti-fat bias in children: Television exposure and demographic variables in 3rd-6th graders' implicit and explicit attitudes toward obesity. Mass Commun Society 2011;14(1):113-40.

[8]   Harrison K. Fast and sweet: Nutritional attributes of television food advertisements with and without Black characters. Howard J Commun 2006;17:249-64.

[9]   Peterson PE, Jeffrey DB, Bridgwater CA, Dawson, B. How pro-nutritional television programming affects children's dietary habits. Dev Psychol 1984;20:55-63.

[10]   Brownell KD, Horgen KB. Food fight: The inside story of the food industry, America's obesity crisis, and what we can do about it. New York: McGraw-Hill, 2004.

[11]   Signorielli N, Staples J. Television and children's conceptions of nutrition. Health Commun 1997;9:289-301.

[12]   Harrison K. Is "fat free" good for me? A panel study of television viewing and children's nutritional knowledge and reasoning. Health Commun 2005;17:117-32.

[13]   Lowry R, Wechsler H, Galuska DA, Fulton JE, Kann L. Television viewing and its association with overweight, sedentary lifestyle, and insufficient consumption of fruits and vegetables among US high school students: Differences by race, ethnicity and gender. J Sch Health 2002;72:413-21.

[14]   Hammermeister J, Brock B, Winterstein D, Page R. Life without TV? Cultivation theory and psychosocial health characteristics of television-free individuals and their television-viewing counterparts. Health Commun 2005;17:253-64.

In: Food, Nutrition and Eating Behavior
Editors: Joav Merrick and Sigal Israeli

ISBN: 978-1-62948-233-0
© 2014 Nova Science Publishers, Inc.

Chapter 4

Nutritional status of Nigerian children with sickle cell anaemia

Barakat A Animasahun[*], *MBBS, MPH, FACC, FWACP, FMCPaed,*
Urowoli P Nwodo, MBBS, DPH, MWACP,
Adaobi N Izuora, MBBS, MPH, FMCPaed
and Olisamedua F Njokanma, MBBS, FWACP, FMCPaed

Department of Paediatrics and Child Health, Lagos State University College of Medicine, Ikeja, Lagos, Department of Paediatrics and Child Health, Premier Specialist Hospital, Ikeja, Lagos, Department of Paediatrics and Child health, Isolo General Hospital, Isolo, Lagos and Department of Paediatrics and Child Health, Lagos State University College of Medicine, Ikeja, Lagos

Abstract

Sickle cell anaemia has multi-systemic manifestations and is associated with severe morbidity and high mortality. It commonly affects growth leading to wasting and stunting. In this chapter we aim to determine the nutritional status using anthropometry, of children with homozygous sickle cell anaemia (SCA), aged one year to ten years in steady state at the Lagos University Teaching Hospital (LUTH). Methods: A cross-sectional study involving 100 children with sickle cell anaemia and 100 age, sex, and social class matched controls that fulfilled the inclusion criteria. Height and weight were measured while Weight-for- age, Height- for- age and Weight-for-height and their z scores were derived from NCHS standard while Body mass index was calculated using the formula Weight in kg/ Height in m^2 in Kg/m^2 . Results: The study demonstrated a significantly lower mean weight and weight-for-height in the SCA patients than those of controls ($p < 0.001$) irrespective of gender, however, female SCA patients were shorter than their healthy controls. There was no significant difference with respect to BMI. The z score analysis revealed that SCA patients had significantly lower z scores for height-

[*] Correspondence: Barakat A Animasahun, MBBS, MPH, FACC, FWACP, FMCPaed, Senior lecturer, Department of Paediatrics and Child Health, Lagos State University College of Medicine, Ikeja, Lagos, Nigeria. E-mail: deoladebo@yahoo.com.

for-age, and weight-for-age compared with controls (p< 0.02). Further analysis by sex revealed that the difference was more marked in males than in the females. Conclusion: The study revealed age related poor nutritional status in children with sickle cell anaemia compared with contemporary healthy controls and there was no association between anthropometry of subjects and haemoglobin concentration.

INTRODUCTION

Sickle cell anaemia (SCA) is a chronic haemolytic disorder caused by homozygous inheritance of abnormal haemoglobin called 'haemoglobin S' (HbS). It is an example of a single point mutation resulting in a qualitative defect in haemoglobin synthesis (1). It is structurally different from the normal haemoglobin, due to replacement of the glutamic acid by valine in the sixth position of the β Globin.[2]

About 25% of Nigerians are heterozygous carriers of genes for sickle haemoglobin while the incidence of its homozygous state is about 2 - 3% (1).

Sickle cell anaemia is the commonest haemoglobinopathy affecting people of the Negroid race (3, 4). It has multisystemic manifestations and commonly affects growth leading to wasting and stunting (5). Assessment of the growth and nutritional status can be done using anthropometry (6). The present chapter aim to determine the nutritional status using anthropometry, of children with homozygous sickle cell anaemia (SCA), aged one year to ten years in steady state at the Lagos University Teaching Hospital.

OUR STUDY

This was a prospective, cross sectional and analytical study carried out at the Lagos University Teaching Hospital (LUTH) in Idi-Araba as part of a large study between October 2005 and January 2006. The subjects were 100 paediatric patients attending the Thursday LUTH sickle cell anaemia clinic who were consecutively recruited. They had haemoglobin genotype 'SS' on haemoglobin electrophoresis and were aged one to ten years. They were in steady state at the time of recruitment.

Steady state was defined as absence of any crisis in the preceeding four weeks no recent drop in the haemoglobin level and absence of any symptoms or sign attributable an acute illness (7). Patients with any form of acute illness, congenital heart disease or acquired heart disease, renal disease and hypertension were excluded from the study. Healthy controls were of genotype "AA," from the Community Health Outpatient and Well baby clinics and healthy children attending other clinics at the POP department and were matched for age and sex, one for every sickle cell anaemia patient.

Height was measured to the nearest centimeter with the aid of a graduated wooden panel fixed to a vertical wall with the child barefooted, standing erect with the heels together against the wall, and looking straight ahead with the back against the wall. The head was held in such a way that the subject was looking forward with the lower border of the eye sockets in the same horizontal plane as the external auditory meatus. The wooden panel had a perpendicular (horizontal) projection built in to slide up and down which rested on the head of the subject (8). Subjects were weighed to the nearest 0.1kg using a Seca® scale or basinet scale as appropriate for the patients age with the subject standing or sitting respectively, barefoot wearing only their under-wear. The scales were checked for accuracy with standard weights after every 10th measurement, or whenever it was moved from place to place (8). Weight-for- age, Height- for- age and Weight-for-height were derived from NCHS standard while Body mass index was calculated using the formula Weight in kg/ Height in m^2 in Kg/m.^{2} Derived measurements were expressed as centiles using NCHS (9) standards and z scores were generated for each measurement (10).

Haemoglobin concentration was determined using the oxy-haemoglobin method. The data were recorded on standard questionnaires and later entered into a standard IBM compatible computer. The data were analyzed using Microsoft Excel Statistical Software supplemented by Mega Stat Statistical Package. The mean, median, standard deviation and other parameters of statistical location were generated as necessary for continuous data. Tests of statistical significance between subjects and controls included Student t-test for continuous data and chi-square analysis for discrete data. Regression and correlation models were set up and analyzed as necessary. Level of significance was set at $p < 0.05$.

The Research and Ethical Committee of the Lagos University Teaching Hospital approved this study. Informed consent was sought from parents or caregivers of potential subjects and the controls before enrolment into the study.

FINDINGS

A total of 200 children were recruited into the study, this comprise of 100 test subjects in the 12 month to 10 year age bracket confirmed to have haemoglobin genotype SS who were all in steady state and receiving routine drugs consisting of folic acid, Proguanil and multivitamins. The control group consisted of 100 children within the same age bracket who had haemoglobin genotype AA.

Table 1. Gender-specific comparison of anthropometry between subjects and controls

	Males			Females		
	Subjects n =65 Mean± (SD)	Controls n =65 Mean± (SD)	p	Subjects n =35 Mean ±(SD)	Controls n =35 Mean±(SD)	p
Variables						
Height (m)	1.11±1.0	1.28±0.12	0.17	1.16±0.09	1.20±0.01	0.02*
Weight (Kg)	18.3±4.5	20.9±0.6	0.001*	19.8±6.6	22.1±1.1	0.04*
Wt for ht in (kg/m)	15.4±3.3	16.2±0.4	0.049*	18.3±4.13	20.4±0.7	0.002*
BMI (Kg/m^2)	14.8±3.5	15.1±0.4	0.43	14.3±2.6	15.1±0.4	0.06

* Statistically significant.

m = meters.

Kg = Kilograms.

Wt for Ht = Weight- for -height in Kilograms per meter.

BMI = body mass index.

Kg/m^2 = Kilogram per meter squared.

Table 2. Comparison of anthropometry between under-5 subjects and controls

	Males			Females		
	Subjects n=27 Mean±(SD)	Controls n=27 Mean±(SD)	p	Subjects n=8 Mean±(SD)	Controls n=8 Mean±(SD)	p
Variables						
Height (m)	0.94±1.6	1.26±0.3	0.3	0.98±0.1	0.98±0.0	0.87
Weight (Kg)	13.79±3.4	14.92±0.7	0.08	14.13±2.9	15.00±1.0	0.4
Wt for Ht	14.24±3.9	14.42±0.8	0.81	16.04±2.9	17.84±1.0	0.08
BMI	15.67±4.5	15.42±0.86	0.78	13.03±1.8	14.03±0.6	0.11

m = meters.
Kg = Kilograms.
Wt for Ht = Weight- for -height in Kilograms per meter.
BMI = body mass index.
Kg/m^2 = Kilogram per meter squared.

The mean age was comparable between subjects and controls (75.1± 30.3 Vs 74.8± 29.4: t = 1.02, p =0.15). The male: female ratio in both subjects and controls was 1.9:1. The mean height and body mass index of the subjects were comparable with those of the controls. Controls however were significantly heavier and also had significantly higher mean weight-for-height. (p = 0.0001).

Further analysis (see table 1) showed that irrespective of gender, subjects were smaller than controls in terms of weight and weight-for-height. Female sickle cell anaemia patients were also significantly shorter than their healthy controls. There was no significant difference with respect to BMI. When the analysis was repeated for under-5 children (see table 2), subjects showed a fairly consistent trend of being smaller but no significant difference was observed with respect to any of the selected anthropometric values. A similar trend was observed in children older than five years but this time, subjects were significantly smaller than controls in all parameters except BMI (see table 3).

Table 3. Comparison of Anthropometry between subjects and controls older than five years

	Males			Females		
	Subjects n=38 Mean±(SD)	Controls n=38 Mean±(SD)	p	Subjects n=27 Mean±(SD)	Controls n=27 Mean±(SD)	p
Variables						
Height (m)	1.22±0.11	1.29±0.01	0.002*	1.22±0.1	1.26±0.01	0.003*
Weight (Kg)	21.5±5.7	25.2±0.9	0.001*	21.42±6.7	24.16±1.3	0.03*
Wt for Ht	16.23±2.8	17.5±0.5	0.007*	19.0±4.5	21.2±0.9	0.009*
BMI	14.2±2.6	14.9±0.4	0.08	14.8±2.8	15.5±0.6	0.17

* Statistically significant.
m = meters.
Kg = Kilograms.
Wt for Ht = Weight- for -height in Kilograms per meter.
BMI = body mass index.
Kg/m^2 = Kilogram per meter squared.

Table 4. Comparison of weight-for-age z scores, height-for-age z scores and body mass indices-for-age z scores of subjects and controls

Variables	Subjects n = 100 Mean ±SD	Controls n =100 Mean ±SD	t	p
Height-for-age z scores	-0.46 ± 0.96	-0.11± 0.1	-3.59	0.001*
Weight-for-age z scores	-0.56 ± 0.63	-0.29± 0.1	-4.35	0.001*
BMI z scores	-0.50± 0.79	-0.33± 0.1	-2.02	0.04 *

* Statistically significant.
BMI =Body mass index.

Table 5. Gender-specific comparison of weight-for-age z scores, height-for-age z scores and body mass indices-for-age z scores of subjects and controls

	Males			Females		
	Subjects n =65 Mean SD	Controls n =65 Mean SD	p p	Subjects n =27 Mean SD	Controls n= 27 Mean SD	p
Height-for-age z scores	-0.47±1.0	-0.11± 0.1	0.005*	-0.44± 0.8	-0.12± 0.1	0.03*
Weight-for-age z scores	-0.55± 0.6	-0.25± 0.1	0.001*	-0.58± 0.6	-0.36± 0.1	0.03*
BMI z scores	-0.52± 0.9	-0.31± 0.1	0.17	-0.44± 0.5	-0.37± 0.1	0.36

Figures shown are mean ± one standard deviation of the mean.
*Statistically significant.
BMI =Body mass index.

Tables 4 and 5 show the comparison of weight-for-age z scores, height-for-age z scores and body mass index z scores of subjects and controls. They revealed that sickle cell anaemia patients had significantly lower z scores for height-for-age, and weight-for-age compared with controls (p< 0.02). Further analysis by sex revealed that the difference was more marked in males than in the females. There was no statistically significant correlation between nutritional status and haemoglobin concentration in both subjects and controls.

DISCUSSION

Our study was designed to determine the relationship between the steady state haemoglobin, nutritional status using anthropometry measurements of SCA aged one year to ten years at the LUTH. It was partly based on the premise that repeated and/or severe illness may manifest as sub-optimal growth detectable by anthropometry. Also, steady state haemoglobin level of any index patient may potentially impact on growth because of its direct relationship with oxygen delivery to tissues.

The study revealed poor nutritional status in children with sickle cell anaemia compared with contemporary healthy controls. Sickle cell anemia patients had a significantly smaller mean weight compared with controls ($p<0.001$). A similar finding was recorded by earlier authors (11-14). This is because weight can be affected by acute and chronic stress (15) like sickle cell anaemia which is a chronic disease. On the other hand, in the present study there was no statistically significant difference between the mean heights of sickle cell anemia patients and controls. This agrees with the findings of Scott et al. (16) in a study with a similar age cohort. Deficiency in height is a reflection of chronicity and severity of nutritional insult. It is plausible that the degree of nutritional insult in the sickle cell anaemia subjects was not severe enough to produce a significant difference. On the other hand, some workers demonstrated significant reduction in height among patient with sickle cell anaemia compared to healthy controls (12-14, 16, 17). The explanation for the discrepancy in findings is not immediately clear. Whitten (13) and Ebomoyi et al. (14) studied children of comparable age (2 years to 13 years) so it is not easy to explain the difference in findings on the grounds of age alone. It may be speculated that other factors like severity of illness, which may not be readily comparable across studies might account for the disparity. However, some of the cited studies (12, 17, 18) included much older subjects (16 to 20 years) than the current one. It is attractive to argue that the height of older patients would be more adversely affected because they have had the disease for a longer period. This may not be entirely applicable as some other report (19) observed that sickle cell anaemia patients tend to catch up in height in late adolescence. Unfortunately, the studies referred to earlier (12, 17, 18) did not stratify subjects by age to enable further comments. On the contrary, when height was related to age using z scores, subjects were found to be significantly further away from the mean than the controls.

The Z score is a more specific way of commenting on the anthropometry. Most other studies (12-14, 17, 18) did not reduce anthropometry to z scores and so it was not possible to make comparisons and draw conclusions. The significantly lower height-for-age z score obtained in the subjects can be explained by chronic ill-health, increased susceptibility to infections, high metabolic rate leading to energy wastage, chronic anaemia and relative tissue hypoxia that characterize sickle cell anaemia. The same explanation can be offered for the significantly lower z scores for weight-for-age found among sickle cell anaemia patients. The trend was worse among the males who also had significantly lower BMI z scores.

The weight-for-height of patients with sickle cell anaemia was significantly lower than the controls in this study ($p<0.001$). This is in agreement with the findings of Ebomoyi et al. (14) in Ilorin. Weight-for-height is an index of wasting. Thus, the difference observed reflects some degree of wasting among patient with sickle cell anaemia. This may be due to the elevated resting energy expenditure and elevated protein turnover in these patients (20).

In our study there were no statistically significant difference between the body mass indices of subjects and controls. This is contrary to the findings of Emodi and Kaine (8) in Enugu. The differences in the findings might be due to differences in the age groups studied. While the current study involved children aged one to ten years, the Enugu study (8) excluded under-fives and included adolescents up to 16 years old and found a statistically significant difference between the body mass indices of subjects and controls. Another plausible reason for similarity in BMI among subjects and controls in the present study may be that subjects and controls were matched for social class. The potential effects of social class may be indirect to the extent that people in the same social class are likely to have comparable health seeking behavior or access to quality health care.

The subjects had a mean steady state haemoglobin concentration of 76.9±19.5g/l, which was significantly lower than that (118.1±2.0) obtained for the controls (t=-21.1, p=0.000). This is in agreement with the findings in other report (5) and is probably as a result of premature haemolysis and reduced red blood cell lifespan in the subjects. Females subjects were observed to have higher haemoglobin level compared with controls, although this did not reach a level of statistical significance. The reasons advanced for this gender difference include hormonal problems secondary to severe hypogonadism in male sickle cell anaemia subjects, which leads to reduced androgen levels and hence poor growth. Females have also been found to have higher oxygen delivery to the tissues (21) and hence vaso-occlusive destruction of tissues is usually comparatively minimal compared with what happens in males. This has been attributed to the transcription factor for haemoglobin F which has been linked to X chromosome, therefore female sickle cell anaemia patient tend to have a higher mean haemoglobin F value and hence less vaso-occlusion, less destruction of RBC, higher haemoglobin and higher packed cell volume (21).

It was also observed that the mean steady state haemoglobin concentration obtained in the current study was somewhat lower than (78.7g/l to 96g/l) reported in some other studies (5, 22-23). There is no obvious reason for the observed difference.

Our study also attempted to establish an association between anthropometry of subjects and haemoglobin concentration, but no such association was found except with height for age. This observation suggests that haemoglobin concentration is not a reliable index of nutritional status, with specific reference to the sickle cell anaemia subject. This is because steady state haemoglobin does not depend on the nutritional status, but on the severity of the disease which depends on genetic factors (1).

In conclusion this study revealed age related poor nutritional status in children with sickle cell anaemia compared with contemporary healthy controls; the mean steady state haemoglobin concentration of subjects with sickle cell anaemia was 76. 9 (SD 19.5) g/l which was significantly lower than 118.1 (SD 2.0) g/l obtained in the controls and there was no association between anthropometry of subjects and haemoglobin concentration.

There is a need for another to verify the claims in this study that prolong frequent crises has effect on the nutritional status of SCA patients and growth monitoring should extend beyond five years of age for SCA patients.

ACKNOWLEDGEMENTS

We specially acknowledge the subjects and controls who participated in this study, including their parents.

REFERENCES

[1]   Adekile AD. Haemoglobinopathies. In: Azubuike JC, Nkanginieme KEO, eds. Paediatrics and child health in a tropical region. Owerri: African Educational Services, 1999;194-213.

[2]   Ingram VM. Abnormal haemoglobins. The difference between normal and sickle cell haemoglobins. Biochem Biophys Acta 1959;36:402-11.

[3]   Omotade OO, Kayode CM, Falade SL, Ikpeme S. Routine screening for sickle cell haemoglobinopathy by electrophoresis in an infant welfare clinic. West Afr J Med 1998;17:91.

[4]   Attah EB, Ekere MC. Death pattern in sickle cell anaemia. JAMA 1975;233:889-90.

[5]   Konotey-Ahulu FID. The sickle cell diseases, Clinical manifestations including the "Sickle Crisis". Arch Intern Med 1974;133:611-9.

[6]   Francis JRB, Johnson CS. Vascular occlusion in sickle diseases: Current concepts and unanswered questions. Blood 1991;77:1405-14.

[7]   Anotia-Egebo O, Alikor EAO, Nkanginieme KEO. Malaria parasite density and splenic status by ultrasonography in stable sickle cell anaemia (HbSS) children. Nig J Med 2004;13:40-3.

[8]   Emodi KJ, Kaine WN. Weights, heights and Quetelet's indices of children with sickle cell anaemia. Nig J Paediatr 1996;23:37-41.

[9]   US Department of Health and Human Services. Atlanta, GA: National Centre for Health Statistics, 2000.

[10]   Dibley MJ, Staehling N, Nieburg P, Trowbridge FL, Interpretation of z-scores anthropometric indicators derived from international growth reference. Am J Clin Nutr 1987;46:749-62.

[11]   Lesi FEA. Anthropometric status of sickle cell anaemia patients in Lagos. Nig Med J 1979;9:337-42.

[12]   Olanrewaju DM, Adekile AD. Anthropometry status of sickle cell anaemia patients in Ile-Ife, Nigeria. Nigerian Medical Practitioner 1989:18;63-66.

[13]   Whitten CF. Growth status of children with sickle cell anaemia. Am J Dis Child 1961;102:355-64.

[14]   Ebomoyi E, Adedoyin MA, Ogunlesi FO. A comparative study of the growth status of children with or without sickle cell disease at Ilorin, Kwara State, Nigeria. Afr J Med Sci 1989:18;69-74

[15]   Tanner JM. Physical growth and development. In: Forfar JC and Arneil GC, eds. Textbook of Paediatrics. London: Churchill Livingstone,1984:26-56.

[16]   Scott RB, Ferguson AD, Jerkins ME, and Clarke HM. Studies in sickle cell anaemia. VIII. Further observation on the clinical manifestation of sickle cell anaemia in children. Am J Dis Child 1965;90:683-91.

[17]   Osinusi K, Oyejide CO. Secular trends in Nutritional status of children from a low socio-economic background. Nig J Paediatr 1987;14(1):7-12.

[18]   Phebus CK, Gloninger MF, Maciak BJ. Growth pattern by age and sex in children with sickle cell disease. J Pediatr 1984;105:28-33.

[19]   Henry HB, Kenneth K, Mary EF, Ronald LN. The percentage of dense red cell does not predict incidence of sickle cell painful crisis. Blood 1985;68:301-3.

[20]   Barden EM, Kawchak DA, Ohene-Frempong K, Starlings VA, and Zemel BS. Body composition in children with sickle cell disease. Am J Nutr 2002;76:218-25.

[21]   Wang WC. Sickle cell anaemia and other sickling syndromes. In: Green JP, Forester J, Lukens JN, et al., eds. Wintrobes clinical haematology. Philadelphia, PA: Lippinkott William Wilkison 2004;1263-1311.

[22]   Ozigbo CJ, Nkanginieme KEO. Body mass index and sexual maturation in adolescent patients with sickle cell anaemia. Nig J Paediatr 2003;30:39-44.

[23]   Batra AS, Acherman RJ, Wong W, Wood JC, Chan LS, Ramicone E, et al. Cardiac abnormalities in children with sickle cell anaemia. Am J Haematol 2002;70:306-12.

In: Food, Nutrition and Eating Behavior   ISBN: 978-1-62948-233-0
Editors: Joav Merrick and Sigal Israeli   © 2014 Nova Science Publishers, Inc.

Chapter 5

NUTRITION AMONG SAHARAWI CHILDREN HOSTED IN SPAIN

Gloria Domènech, BSND, Sabina Escortell, BSND, Rosa Gilabert, BSND, Manuel Lucena, BSND, Ma C Martínez, BSND, Jordi Mañes, PhD and Jose M Soriano, PhD*

Observatory of Nutrition and Food Safety in Developing Countries, Faculty of Pharmacy,
University of Valencia, Burjassot, Spain

ABSTRACT

In this chapter we examine anthropometric measurements and evaluate the daily energy and nutrient intakes of Saharawi children of Tindouf (Algeria) hosted in Spain. To date, it is the first report about energy and nutrient intakes in these hosted children. Study group: Saharawi children of refugees camp in Tindouf (Algeria) aged 4-13 years (n =270), hosting in Spanish families during summertime. Methods: Anthropometric measures and energy and nutrient intakes for a 7-day periods using the weighed food intake method were evaluated in these children and compared with the values of Institute of Medicine. Results: The highest value of BMI was obtained for girls aged from 9 to 13 (20.2 kg m-2). Mean energy intake was ranged from 8.0 to 9.0 MJ day-1 for girls aged from 4 to 8, and for boys aged from 9 and 13, respectively. The highest value of the carbohydrate and fat intakes were for Saharawi boys aged from 9 to 13, but the highest value of protein intake were Saharawi girls aged from 9 to 13. The PUFA/SFA ratio is lower than 0.5 and the (PUFA+MUFA)/SFA values are <2 for studied Saharawi children. Five (vitamin D and E, potassium, calcium and iodine) out of twenty-three micronutrients intakes below than the recommended values, being the low value of iodine an advantage for these children due to that suffer goitre for excessive intake of iodine in their refugee camps. Conclusions: Our study reflected in some nutrients an inadequately intakes for these hosted children.

---

* Correspondnece: Jose M Soriano, PhD, Observatory of Nutrition and Food Safety in Developing Countries, Faculty of Pharmacy, University of Valencia, Burjassot, Spain. E-mail: jose.soriano@uv.es.

INTRODUCTION

The Saharawi refugee camps is located in four remotely camps (Dakhla, Smara, Al-'Uyun and Awsard), since 1976, in a territorial zone set up in the harsh Algerian desert 30 km from the westernmost town of Tindouf (1). There are also some smaller satellite camps, called the "February 27", serving as a boarding school for women. The headquarters of Polisario Front, which is a Saharawi rebel movement working for the independence of Western Sahara from Morocco, with the government in exile of the Saharawi Arab Democratic Republic (SADR), are headquartered in Rabouni, a camp dedicated to administration (2). According to the United Nations High Commission for Refugees (3), approximately estimated 165.000 Saharawi refugees currently live in a hostile environment that make difficult to deliver and impede refugee self-sufficiency. International aid groups provide most of the consumed food, medicine and other basic supplies by camp residents (4, 5) and around 2.987 children attend school in the camps around Tindouf, supported by 78 education personnel, mostly volunteers, working in 40 educational units, including 28 primary schools (1, 2). Today, nearly 90% of Saharawi refugees are able to read and write, the number having been less than 10% in 1975, and several thousands have received university educations in foreign countries as part of aid packages (mainly Algeria, Cuba and Spain). Some of these Saharawi children between the ages of eight and thirteen are hosted by Spanish families in their homes for a two-month period during the summer according to the "Holidays in Peace" program organized by a national Spanish Non Governmental Organization. As part of this action, between 7.000 and 10.000 Saharawi children arrives in Spain to spend the summer with host families and allows receive medical examinations and treatment, as well as gifts of clothes, toys, and money which they take back with them to the camps and many of them return year after year to the same host homes. Additionally, Spanish host families often visit the camps, buying local products or leaving similar cash gifts. The relationships established during the program often endure beyond the summer months, as strong proto-familial relationships form between the children and their Spanish host families, and return trips reinforce such cross-border bonds (2, 3, 6).

The aims of this study are to examine anthropometric measurements and to evaluate the daily energy and nutrient intakes of Saharawi children of Tindouf (Algeria) hosted in Spain during the summer. To date, it is the first report about energy and nutrient intakes in these hosted children.

OUR STUDY

Research was conducted in Spain in collaboration with a local nongovernmental organization (NGO) for a two-month period during the summer in 2007 according to the "Holidays in Peace" program. This study was approved by the Human Subjects Committee of the University of Valencia (Spain), and informed consent was obtained from parents. The sample was 270 Saharawi children (130 boys and 140 girls), which were grouped from 4 to 8 years and from 9 to 13 years. These ranges were used according to the Dietary Reference Intakes (DRIs), Recommended Dietary Allowances (RDAs) or Adequate Intakes (AIs) of the Institute of Medicine (7-12). The study protocol was approved by the Ethical Committee of University of Valencia and each head of household gave their verbal consent after the study had been fully explained to them.

All the anthropometric measurements were performed in triplicate accordingly to the Anthropometric Standardization Reference Manual (13) with the subjects wearing light clothing and barefoot, by the same trained anthropometrist. A Plenna scale (model MEA 07 400, USA; accuracy of 100 g) was used to determine weight and a Seca stadiometer (model 208, Germany; accuracy of 0.5 cm) was used to determine height. Body mass index (BMI) was calculated as body weight divided by the square of the height (kg/m2).

Several dieticians recorded from food preparer daily dietary intake for a 7-day periods using the weighed food intake method (14), being the method that provides the most accurate estimation of usual individual intake (15). Furthermore, data about all foods and beverages consumed since the previous day, including methods of food preparation, description of ingredients and condiments consumed were compiled from the food preparer. The study was carried out from the stayed third week in Spain because these children in the first two weeks eat little. The daily average quantities are converted into energy and nutrient through the DIAL program, version 1.02 for Windows XP (Alceingenieria, Madrid, Spain). Dietary intakes of nutrients were compared with reference values reported by the DRIs, RDAs or AIs of the IOM (7-12).

Table 1. Mean values and standard deviations of the physical characteristics of the Saharawi children hosted in Spain

	4-8 years (n=140)		9-13 years (n=130)	
	Boys (n=70)	Girls (n=70)	Boys (n=60)	Girls (n=70)
Age (years)	8.9±0.9	9.0±0.7	12.4±1.4	12.9±2.1
Height (cm)	135.0±10.1	136.1±14.1	144.0±10.8	141.2±23.1
Weight (kg)	31.5±4.8	26.7±3.1	39.4±7.2	40.2±8.9
BMI (kg m^{-2})	17.3±3.1	14.4±2.8	19.1±1.2	20.2±3.1

Table 2. Mean values and standard deviations of the daily energy, macronutrients, fibre, water and profile of fat intake of the Saharawi children hosted in Spain

	4-8 years (n=140)		9-13 years (n=130)	
	Boys (n=70)	Girls (n=70)	Boys (n=60)	Girls (n=70)
Energy (MJ)	8.3±2.2	8.0±3.4	9.0±2.9	8.9±2.8
Protein (g)	60.9±10.8	60.7±8.9	73.2±25.5	74.1±34.2
Carbohydrate (g)	222.1±48.3	212.4±87.9	251.4±84.1	248.4±98.7
Fat (g)	79.9±14.4	78.9±23.4	89.9±29.9	88.8±21.4
MUFA (g)	39.7±6.6	36.5±5.8	40.5±15.4	42.9±23.4
PUFA (g)	9.9±1.6	9.1±2.3	8.7±3.4	8.1±4.5
SFA (g)	23.4±3.6	20.2±2.4	24.6±9.2	25.4±11.1
PUFA/SFA	0.42±0.05	0.45±0.07	0.35±0.09	0.31±0.04
(PUFA+MUFA)/SFA	2.11±0.14	2.26±0.20	2.00±0.15	2.00±0.16
Cholesterol (mg)	248.0±114.2	238.7±108.1	352.5±130.5	324.2±110.1
Dietary fibre (g)	20.8±5.2	23.2±5.4	22.9±8.5	22.5±9.1
Water (g)	1322.4±144.7	1345.4±234.0	1564.1±477.5	1687.2±267.1

Anthropometric, energy and nutrient intake values are presented as means and standard deviations (SD) grouped by group of age and by sex. A Kolmogorov–Smirnov test was used to test for normality. To compare the means of boys and girls, the Independent-Samples T-Test was used in case of a normal distribution, otherwise the Mann–Whitney U test was used. Statistical significance was established at a P-value<0.05. All statistical analyses were performed using the SPSS Statistics 19.0 (SPSS Inc., Chicago, IL, USA).

OUR FINDINGS

Table 1 shows the mean physical characteristics of the studied Saharawi children hosted in Spain. No significant differences were found in studied children in mean of height, weight and BMI. The highest value of BMI is obtained for girls aged from 9 to 13 (20.2 kg m-2). For the study of energy and nutrient intakes, dates are shown in Table 2, 3 and 4. Mean energy intake was 8.3, 8.0, 9.0 and 8.9 MJ day-1 for boys and girls aged from 4 to 8, and for boys and girls aged from 9 and 13, respectively. The highest value of the carbohydrate and fat intakes were for Saharawi boys aged from 9 to 13, but the highest value of protein intake were Saharawi girls aged from 9 to 13. No significant differences in profile of fat intake were detected among studied Saharawi children (see table 2). The PUFA/SFA ratio is lower than 0.5 and the (PUFA+MUFA)/SFA values are <2 for studied Saharawi children. The highest value of daily cholesterol intake is obtained for boys aged from 9 to 13 (352.5 mg day-1). No significant differences were found in studied children in mean dietary fibre. The intake of water was significantly higher in boys aged from 9 to 13 than boys aged from 4 to 8.

Table 3. Mean values and standard deviations of vitamin intake of the Saharawi children hosted in Spain

	4-8 years (n=140)		9-13 years (n=130)	
	Boys (n=70)	Girls (n=70)	Boys (n=60)	Girls (n=70)
Thiamin (mg)	2.2±0.6	2.4±1.4	2.2±0.8	3.1±1.1
Riboflavin (mg)	1.4±1.1	1.2±1.0	1.9±0.9	2.1±0.7
Niacin (mg)	22.6±7.2	23.4±8.9	27.8±11.1	30.1±10.8
Panthotenic acid (mg)	4.1±0.5	5.1±0.8	4.9±1.6	4.9±1.3
Vitamin B6 (mg)	2.2±0.7	3.1±1.8	2.5±0.9	3.2±1.2
Biotin (µg)	24.6±8.6	22.7±9.1	32.5±11.5	33.4±21.3
Folate (µg)	294.2±88.5	280.5±78.5	311.1±143.7	333.4±190.2
Vitamin B12 (µg)	4.7±4.1	4.1±3.8	4.2±2.8	4.6±3.6
Vitamin C (mg)	150.3±17.5	160.8±28.2	177.9±67.8	176.4±56.7
Vitamin A (µg)	1148.0±368.7	1054.2±468.7	970.5±489.1	1111.4±678.3
Vitamin D (µg)	3.4±2.1	2.8±2.2	2.9±2.6	3.3±3.0
Vitamin E (mg)	10.2±1.1	10.5±2.4	8.9±3.5	11.3±5.6
Vitamin K (µg)	121.4±86.5	130.4±90.1	111.1±104.5	143.6±88.9

Table 3 reflects the values of vitamin intakes being the intake of thiamin was higher in girls aged from 9 to 13 than boys aged from 4 to 8. Vitamin B6 intake is higher in girls than boys aged from 4 to 8. Furthermore, non significant differences in panthotenic acid were found between boys aged from 4 to 8 and the remainder of the children. The mineral intake is demonstrated in the Table 4 and potassium was found significant differences between boys and girls aged from 4 to 8 (p<0.05). Furthermore, significantly differences between the iron intake of boys aged from 4 to 8 and girls from 9 to 13.

Table 4. Mean values and standard deviations of mineral intake of the Saharawi children hosted in Spain

	4-8 years		9-13 years	
	Boys (n=70)	Girls (n=70)	Boys (n=60)	Girls (n=70)
Sodium (mg)	3385.4±747.3	3200.5±890.5	3496.0±1311.3	3679.7±1777.7
Potassium (mg)	3045.6±469.9[*]	2300.2±540.6[*]	2349.5±1224.3	2567.8±1165.8
Calcium (mg)	785.4±178.7	810.4±156.4	844.2±290.3	898.5±313.2
Fluoride (mg)	2.2±0.6	2.0±0.9	2.4±1.0	2.6±1.1
Magnesium (mg)	267.4±33.6	288.9±43.6	302.3±107.4	319.2±110.8
Phosphorus (mg)	1200.1±225.4	1122.4±333.3	1357.2±491.4	1209.5±651.3
Iron (mg)	14.1±3.2	14.5±6.5	16.7±5.8	17.2±4.1
Zinc (mg)	6.8±2.9	5.3±2.2	9.0±3.4	8.8±4.5
Selenium (µg)	55.3±26.7	51.2±36.5	55.1±29.9	56.7±31.1
Iodine (µg)	53.6±23.1	54.1±34.3	64.3±25.5	62.4±33.3

* Mean value was significantly different between boys and girls.

DISCUSSION

In our study, the lowest and highest values of energy intake are obtained by the girls aged from 4 to 8 and boys aged from 9 to 13, respectively (Table 2). Compared to DRIs (12), energy intakes appeared to be generally satisfactory. The DRIs (12) recommended 10-30% of daily energy intake for protein being this value obtained in all studied groups. However, our values of carbohydrate and lipids are lower (44.4-46.7%) and higher (36.2-37.6%) than DRIs (12), which 45-65% and 25-35% of daily energy intake, respectively. For the cholesterol, the DRIs (12) suggest a range from 205 to 259 mg/day being these values exceed for children aged from 4 to 13 (Table 2). In the other hand, a deficiency in total fiber and water intakes is reflected in our study in comparison with AIs (12); 1.7, 2.1 and 2.4 litre of water/day and 25, 26 and 31 g of fiber /day from children (4-8 y), males (9-13 y) and females (9-13 y), respectively. The intake of water was significantly higher in boys aged from 9 to 13 than boys aged from 4 to 8 (p<0.05).

Tables 3 and 4 reflected the analyzed micronutrients. Vitamin values are adequate, except in boys aged from 9 to 13 which have a quantity ingested for vitamin E (8.9 mg day-1) lower than the DRIs (9 mg day-1) (9). Furthermore, the intake of vitamin D is below for all studied children (Table 3) according to the AIs (7) (5 µg day-1 for all studied children). The intake of calcium is inadequate for all studied children (800 and 1300 mg day-1 for children aged from 4 to 8 and from 9 to 13, respectively) except for females aged from 4 to 8 (Table 4) according to the AIs (7) being the calcium/phosphorus ratio ranged between 1 and 0.5. It is due to the increased intake of beverages like colas and other soft drinks, especially those that use phosphoric acid as acidifier, among the studied children. In our study, they have iodine intakes (Table 4) below than the RDAs (10) (90 and 120 µg day-1 for children aged from 4 to 8 and from 9 to 13, respectively). In our view, this last micronutrient is very important in the Saharawi children because several studies (5, 16-18) reflected a high urinary iodine levels (965±348 µg/l) and high iodine concentration (180-400 µg/l) in drinking water in refugee camps in Tindouf (Algeria), which is related with clinical observation of goitre. Goitre is common around the world because many regions have inadequate iodine intake; however the situation is "slightly" different because in Saharawi refugee camps, there is an excessive intake of iodine (19), this situation has been cited in other places in the world; Central China (20) and Hokkaido (Japan) (21) that have an endemic goitre caused by excessive iodine intake. Díaz-Cadórniga et al. (16) reflected that the goiter was found in 58.1% of the school children placed in Tindouf (Algeria). Our recommendation2 for host families is not given iodized salt from these children during the summer holidays. In the other hand, our values reflected that the iron is adequately intake in all groups being this date important due to that iron deficiency anaemia can lead to several health consequences, including impaired cognitive and physical development. According to the World Health Organization (22), these children have iron deficiency anaemia, according to the rutinary analysis carried out when they arrived to Spain, reflected in low iron values in conjunction with elevated iron-binding capacity values, yielding less than 16 percent transferrin saturation. Lopriere et al. (23) suggested in a personal communication of one of authors indicated a 70% of Saharawi children were anaemic.

In conclusion, our study reflected in some nutrients an inadequately intakes for these hosted children, although it should be better, with nutritional counselling from dietitians, to increase the nutritional and health benefits when these children returning to their refugee camps.

ACKNOWLEDGMENTS

We are especially grateful to hosted families, Federació d´Associacions de Solidaritat amb el Poble Saharaui Pais Valencià and Conselleria de Inmigración y Ciudadanía of the Generalitat Valenciana (3014/2007). J.M. Soriano thanks to the European Union for the grant Long Life Learning Programme.

REFERENCES

[1]   Spiegel PB. Forgotten refugees and other displaced populations. Lancet 2003;362:72-4.
[2]   Soriano JM. Niños y niñas Saharauis: Guía alimentaria para las familias de acogida. Servei de Publicacions. Universitat de València, 2008. [Spanish]
[3]   United Nations High Commissioner for Refugees (UNHCR)/World Food Programme (WFP)/Institute of Child Health (ICH). Anthropometric and micronutrient nutrition survey. Saharawi Refugee Camps. Tindouf. Geneva: United Nations High Commissioner for Refugees, 2007. Accessed 2013 Jul 12. URL: www.unhcr.org/publ/PUBL/45fa67bf2.pdf.
[4]   Dukic N, Thierry A. Saharawi refugees: life after the camps. Forced Migration Rev 1998;2:18-21.
[5]   Soriano JM, Domènech G, Mañes J, Catalá-Gregori AI, Barikmo IE. Disorders of malnutrition among the Saharawi children. Rev Esp Nutr Hum Diet 2011;15:10-9.

[6]   Refugee Studies Centre. The transnationalisation of care: Sahrawi refugee children in a Spanish host programme. Lessons Learned Report. Oxford: University Oxford, 2005.

[7]   Institute of Medicine. Dietary Reference Intakes for calcium, phosphorus, magnesium, vitamin D and fluoride. Washington DC: National Academies Press, 1997.

[8]   Institute of Medicine. Dietary Reference Intakes for thiamin, riboflavin, niacin, vitamin B6, folate, vitamin B12, pantothenic acid, biotin, and choline. Washington DC: National Academies Press, 1998.

[9]   Institute of Medicine. Dietary Reference Intakes for vitamin C, vitamin E, selenium, and carotenoids. Washington DC: National Academies Press, 2000.

[10]   Institute of Medicine. Dietary Reference Intakes for vitamin A, vitamin K, arsenic, boron, chromium, copper, iodine, iron, manganese, molybdenum, nickel, silicon, vanadium, and zinc. Washington DC: National Academies Press, 2001.

[11]   Institute of Medicine. Dietary Reference Intakes for water, potassium, sodium, chloride, and sulfate. Washington DC: National Academies Press, 2004.

[12]   Institute of Medicine Dietary Reference Intakes for energy, carbohydrate, fiber, fat, fatty acids, cholesterol, protein, and amino acids (macronutrients). Washington DC: National Academies Press, 2005.

[13]   Lohman TG, Roche AF, Martorell R. Anthropometric Standardization Reference Manual. Champaign, IL: Human Kinetics Publishers, 1988.

[14]   Bingham SA. The dietary assessment of individuals; methods, accuracy, new techniques and recommendations. Nutr Abstr Rev (Series A) 1987;57: 705-42.

[15]   Buzzard M. 24-hour recall and food record methods. In: Willett, WC, ed. Nutritional Epidemiology. New York: Oxford University Press, 1998:50-73.

[16]   Díaz-Cadórniga FJ, Delgado E, Tartón T. Endemic goitre associated with high iodine intake in primary school children in the Saharawi Arab Democratic Republic. Endocrinol Nutr 2003;50:357-62.

[17]   Domènech G, Escortell S, Gilabert R, Lara M, Martínez MªC, Soriano, JM. Dietary intake and food pattern of Saharawi refugee children in Tindouf (Algeria). Proc Nutr Soc 2008; 67:E174.

[18]   Paricio Talayero JM, Santos Serrano L, Fernández Feijoo A. Health examination of children from the Democratic Sahara Republic (North West Africa) on vacation in Spain. An Esp Pediatr 1998;49:33-8.

[19]   Pezzino V, Padova G, Vigneri R. Iodine-independent endemic goiter in Saharawi refugee camps in Southwestern Algeria. IDD Newsletter 1998;14:1-3.

[20]   Li M, Liu DR, Qu CY Endemic goitre in Central China caused by excessive iodine intake. Lancet 1987;2:257-9.

[21]   Suzuki H, Higuchi T, Sawa K. Endemic coast goitre in Hokkaido, Japan. Acta Endocrinol (Copenh) 1965;50:161-76.

[22]   World Health Organization (WHO). Iron deficiency anaemia–Assessment, prevention, and control. A guide for programme managers. Geneva: World Health Organization; 2001. Accessed 2012 Jan 12. URL: www.who.int/nutrition/publications/en/ida_assessment_prevention_control.pdf

[23]   Lopriore C, Guidom Y, Briend A. Spread fortified with vitamins and minerals induces catch-up growth and eradicates severe anemia in stunted refugee children aged 3-6 y. Am J Clin Nutr 2004;80:973-80.

In: Food, Nutrition and Eating Behavior   ISBN: 978-1-62948-233-0
Editors: Joav Merrick and Sigal Israeli   © 2014 Nova Science Publishers, Inc.

Chapter 6

SODIUM INTAKE AND HYPERTENSION IN CANADA

Frank Mo[*], *MD, PhD*[1,2], *Bernard CK Choi, PhD*[3,4,5] *and Howard Morrison, PhD*[1,4]

[1]Social Determinants and Science Integration Directorate, Public Health Agency of
Canada, Ottawa, Ontario, Canada,[2]The R Samuel McLaughlin Centre, Institute of
Population Health, University of Ottawa, Ottawa, Ontario, Canada, [3]Dalla Lana School of
Public Health, University of Toronto, Toronto, Ontario, Canada, [4]Department of
Epidemiology and Community Medicine, University of Ottawa, Ottawa, Ontario,
Canada, [5]Centre for Chronic Disease Prevention, Public Health Agency of Canada,
Ottawa, Ontario, Canada

ABSTRACT

How does dietary sodium intake in relation to hypertension differ by ethnicity in Canada? To
answer this question, we used the health and nutrition survey component of the Canadian
Community Health Survey (CCHS 2.2), conducted in 2004 and Proportional Hazard Regression
(PHREG) models to analyze the percentages and the potential associations between dietary sodium
intakes in relation to hypertension in different ethnic groups in Canada. Our results showed that
adult Caucasian Canadians (9.10%) and Black Canadians (9.02%) were more likely to have high
level of sodium (>2,300mg/day) consumption compared to other ethnic groups. Females consumed
more than males in total sodium intake; the ratios for female/male are from 1.01 to 1.41. However,
a higher proportion of males consumed high levels of sodium (>2,300mg/day) in all ethnic groups
except East Asian Canadians and Other Canadians. The adjusted hazard ratios in the PHREG
multivariate analysis of adult high blood pressure (HBP)related to high (more than 2,300mg/day)
sodium intake compared to low (Less than 1,500mg/day) controlled for age, sex, body mass index
(BMI),and total energy intake in different ethnicities. All ethnic groups significantly exceeded
those of the Caucasian group (HR, from 1.19 to 1.41) except other Canadians group. In conclusion,
when confounding factors are considered and controlled, males consumed more high level sodium

---

[*]   Correspondence: Frank Mo, PhD, MD, Research Scientist, Science Integration Division,
Social Determinants and Science Integration Directorate, Health Promotion and Chronic Disease Prevention
Branch, Public Health Agency of Canada, 785 Carling Avenue, Ottawa, Ontario K1A 0K9, Canada. E-mail:
Frank.Mo@phac-aspc.gc.ca.

than females in all ethnicities except East-Asian Canadians and Other Canadians. Overweight/obesity and corresponding high sodium intake is strongly associated with an increased risk of hypertension. Native Canadians, East-Asian Canadians, Black Canadians, and South-Asian Canadians exceeded those of the Caucasian subjects at a significantly statistical difference when compared people with high blood pressure (HBP) by those without HBP.

INTRODUCTION

With a disease attributable risk of 35% for the development of atherosclerotic cardiovascular events, 69% for stroke, 49% for congestive heart failure, and 24% for premature death (1-5), high blood pressure is one of the most important risk factors for cardiovascular mortality and morbidity. The raise in blood pressure with age has been associated with high sodium intake, independent of weight, physically activity, alcohol consumption and metabolic status (6). More than 90% of individuals with normal blood pressure will develop hypertension over their lifetime (7).

Sodium reduction is one of the most cost-effective public health strategies to prevent cardiovascular disease, reduction in sodium intake with an 1,840mg/day would reduce blood pressure by 5.1/2.7mmHg, and could prevent 1 in 6 cases of hypertension, 1 in 7 stroke deaths, 1 in 11 coronary heart disease deaths, and 1 in 14 deaths from any cause (8-10). These reductions could be even greater in specific ethnic and age groups as a result of salt sensitivity and over-consumption (11-16).

Many studies reported that high sodium intake is a major factor increasing blood pressure at the population level. The effect of sodium intake on hypertension is much stronger than the effect of other lifestyle factors, such as weight gain, lack of fruit and vegetable consumption and lack of physical exercise. Many studies suggested that evidence linking sodium to high blood pressure is as strong as those linking cigarette smoking to cancer and heart disease (17-28).

In Canada, hypertension affects nearly one in four people and it is the most common reason for a Canadian to visit a physician. Over 4 million prescriptions for antihypertensive medications are written every month (29, 30), and almost 46% of women and 38% of men aged 60 or over are on drug therapy for hypertension (31). In average adult Canadians consume approximately 3500mg of sodium per day, more than double the intake level of 1,500 recommended by the National Academies of Science (32).

In this chapter we study the potential associations of high sodium intake in relation to high blood pressure in different ethnicity groups in Canada, whether reduced sodium intake can reduce the risk of hypertension or suffering from subsequent cardiovascular complications in hypertensive patients, and to evaluate the recommendations that sodium intake be reduced to less than 2,300 mg/day in normotensive adults, and no more than 1,500 mg/day for people with hypertension of the Canadian hypertension education program (33), in different ethnicity groups.

OUR STUDY

The health and nutrition component of the Canadian Community Health Survey (CCHS 2.2) in 2004 was developed by Statistics Canada in consultation with an expert advisory group, with data collected between January 2004 and January 2005. This component focused on general health and nutrition. Individuals' daily sodium intake was estimated from 24-hour recall of food and beverage consumption. Daily sodium intake was averaged and compared by hypertension status (34). This study was conducted according to the guidelines laid down in the Declaration of Helsinki and all procedures involving human subjects/patients were approved by the Canadian ethics committee; and there is no conflict of the ethics in this study.

The CCHS 2.2 survey targeted a sample size of 30,000respondents from all age groups (aged 12 and older) living in privately occupied dwellings in all ten provinces of Canada. Excluded from the sampling frame were residents of the three territories, persons living on Indian reserves or Crown Lands, persons living in institutions, full-time members of the Canadian Forces and residents of some remote regions (Table 1). We selected all adults aged 18 and over in this study. The overall household-level response rate in this survey was 84.4%.

Table 1. Targeted sample sizes by province, CCHS 2.2, 2004, Canada

Province	Total Sample
Newfoundland & Labrador	1,662
Prince Edward Island	1,120
Nova Scotia	1,957
New Brunswick	1,833
Quebec	4,864
Ontario	6,740
Manitoba	2,170
Saskatchewan	1,976
Alberta	3,116
British Columbia	3,562
Canada	29,000

Source: Statistics Canada, 2004.

The information collected included two distinct and complementary parts: the general health and the 24-hour dietary recall component. The general health status, including chronic conditions, health-related behaviours in food, vegetable and fruit, vitamin and mineral consumption, physical and sedentary activities, measured height and weight and smoking and alcohol consumption. Socio-demographic characteristics were also collected as part of the general health component.

The 24-hour dietary recall component was designed to collect information on all the foods and beverages consumed during the previous day's 24 hours from midnight to midnight. Respondents were asked to provide information on the time the food was consumed, the occasion (e.g., breakfast, lunch), additions to foods (e.g., butter on toast), detailed food descriptions, amounts consumed, and whether the meal was prepared at home or elsewhere.

In the first phase of data analysis, cross-tables method was used to analyze the different percentages between sodium intake and occurrences of high blood pressure by sex and ethnicity. In the second phase, the Proportional Hazard Regression (PHREG) multivariate models were used to estimate the potential associations between dietary sodium intakes related to the occurrence of hypertension in the different ethnicities in Canada by two levels (less than 1,500mg/day and more than 2,300mg/day) of sodium consumption, by sex and ethnicity. The Hazard Ratios (HR) were calculated adjusted for age, sex, BMI, lifestyle (e.g., cigarette smoking and physical inactivity), socioeconomic status (e.g., family income and education level), and total energy intake.

For the purpose of this chapter, hypertension is defined as systolic blood pressure greater than or equal to 140 mmHg or diastolic blood pressure greater than or equal to 90 mmHg. But if people have diabetes or chronic kidney disease, 130/80 mmHg is considered high blood pressure (35).

Table 2. Weighted percentages of adult sodium intake (mg) by level of sodium consumption with high blood pressure (HBP) by sex in different ethnicity groups, CCHS 2.2, 2004, Canada

Levels of Sodium	Male				Female				Ratio for female/male
	<1500mg /day(%)*	1500-2300mg /day(%)*	>2300mg /day (%)*	Total	<1500mg Day(%)*	1500-2300mg /day(%)*	>2300mg/ Day(%)*	Total	
Caucasian Canadians	1.50	3.26	10.77	15.53	3.42	4.66	7.53	15.60	1.01
Black Canadians	1.54	1.98	10.37	13.89	8.32	1.53	7.52	17.37	1.25
East-Asian Canadians	2.92	3.35	2.67	8.94	0.65	1.53	9.14	11.32	1.27
South-Asian Canadians	2.01	0.18	4.31	6.50	1.97	4.15	2.18	8.30	1.28
Native Canadians	1.62	3.59	6.33	11.54	3.59	8.00	4.58	16.16	1.40
Other Canadians	0.43	0.16	3.58	4.01	1.80	0.11	3.84	5.64	1.41

* Weighted based on total Canadian population in 2004.

FINDINGS

The age-adjusted percentages of two levels of sodium consumption by ethnicity and by gender showed that male adult Caucasian Canadians(10.77%), male adult Black Canadians (10.37%), and male adult Native Canadians (6.33%) with HBP had a higher percentage of high level (>2,300mg/day) consumption of sodium than other ethnicity groups (Table 2). On the other hand, female adult East-Asian Canadians (9.14%), female adult Caucasian Canadians (7.53%), and female adult Native Canadians (1.62%) with HBP had a higher percentage of high level (>2,300mg/day) consumption of sodium. Females consumed more than males in all three levels of sodium (from <1,500mg to >2,300mg/day) in all ethnicities, the (female/male) ratios are from 1.01 to 1.41 (Table 2).

Table 3 showed the differences in consumption of sodium, physical activity, and BMI categories between ethnicity groups. We found that Caucasian Canadians (15.57%), Black Canadians (15.54%), and Native Canadians (14.05%) who had higher percentages in total sodium consumption, also had higher percentages in the inactive physical activity (Native Canadians (11.88%), Black Canadians (11.55%), and Caucasian Canadians (10.14%)). In the same time, the corresponding Native Canadians (4.76%), Caucasian Canadians (3.96%), and Black Canadians (1.89%) had a higher percentage of high BMI level (BMI $\geq$31) than other ethnicities.

Table 3. Weighted percentages from cross-table analysis of adult sodium intake (mg) by level of sodium consumption with high blood pressure (HBP) status and related to physical activity, Body Mass Index (BMI) in different ethnicity groups, CCHS 2.2, 2004, Canada

Ethnicity	Caucasian Canadians	Black Canadians	East-Asian Canadians	South-Asian Canadians	Native Canadians	Other Canadians
Sodium (%)						
< 1500 mg/day	2.49	4.75	1.92	1.99	2.69	1.27
1500-2300mg/day	3.98	1.77	2.55	1.95	5.99	2.36
>2300mg/day	9.10	9.02	5.51	3.37	5.38	3.74
Total	15.57	15.54	9.99	7.30	14.05	7.37
Physical activity (%)						
Active	1.98	2.52	1.63	0.95	1.06	0.24
Moderate	3.44	1.47	1.81	2.31	2.45	1.02
Inactive	10.14	11.55	6.78	4.03	11.88	3.75
BMI (%)						
$\leq$25	8.18	11.24	7.01	5.28	6.62	4.23
26 – 30	3.42	2.40	1.80	1.32	2.67	0.57
>30	3.96	1.89	1.17	0.70	4.76	0.20

* Weighted based on total Canadian population in 2004.

In PHREG models, adjusted by age, sex, lifestyle (e.g., cigarette smoking and physical inactivity), socioeconomic status (e.g., family income and education level), and total energy intake, the Hazard Ratio (HR) and 95% confidential interval (95% C.I.) in the high level (>2,300mg/day) sodium consumption with HBP, all ethnicity subjects exceeded those of the Caucasian subjects at a statistical significant level (HR, from 1.19 to 1.41). East-Asian Canadians (HR, 1.41, 95% CI, 1.19-1.68; P<0.0001), Black Canadians (HR, 1.35,95% CI, 1.06-1.65; P=0.0046), South-Asian Canadians (HR, 1.29, 95% CI, 1.03-1.63; P=0.00301), Native Canadians (HR, 1.19, 95% CI, 1.01-1.59; P=0.0055), except other Canadians (HR, 1.24, 95% CI, 0.95-1.61; P=0.1140) (Table 4).

Table 4. Adjusted hazard ratios in PHREG multivariate analysis of adult high blood pressure (HBP)related to high (more than 2,300mg) sodium intake compared to low (Less than 1,500mg) in different ethnicities, CCHS 2.2, 2004, Canada

Ethnicity	Hazard Ratio (HR)	95% confidence interval(95% C.I)$^{\pm}$	P-Values
	HR	95% C.I	
Caucasian Canadians	1.00	---	---
Black Canadians	1.35	1.06 – 1.65	P=0.0046
East-Asian Canadians	1.41	1.19 – 1.68	P<0.0001
South-Asian Canadians	1.29	1.03 – 1.63	P=0.0301
Native Canadians	1.19	1.01 – 1.59	P=0.0055
Other Canadians	1.24	0.95 – 1.61	P=0.1140

$^{\pm}$ Hazard Ratios were compared to Caucasian ethnicity, and adjusted by age, sex, BMI and total energy intake.

DISCUSSION

Sodium, like most other micronutrients, plays an important role in normal physiological process of human body. Adequate dietary intake not only helps maintain physical metabolism and normal blood pressure levels, it's also indirectly involved in the anatomic and physiologic function of left ventricle and kidney. Excessive consumption gives rise to elevated blood pressure and believed to be an independent risk factor of cardiovascular disease (36). Experimental and population-based observational studies have established the role of dietary factors on the differences of blood pressure in various ethnic populations.

There is little or no hypertension or rise of blood pressure with age in populations with habitual low sodium diet (37). Population level decline of sodium consumption was accompanied by falls in the blood pressure levels, in the prevalence of hypertension and also in stroke mortality (38). The Intersalt study established a linear relationship between the median 24-hour urinary sodium excretion and the slope of systolic blood pressure with age (39). A Japanese trial was successful in reducing salt intake of average from13.5 grams to 12.1 grams per day, and in the north areas from 18 grams to 14 grams per day. The results showed that there was an evident fall in blood pressure both in adults and children, and an 80% reduction in stroke mortality at the same time (40) in Japan. All these studies supported the fact that dietary sodium positively related to human blood pressure through a long and continuous process, to various degrees affecting a large percentage of population. Our result in this study is consistent with these studies conducted on other populations indicating that dietary sodium intake increases risk of hypertension independent of other risk factors examined in this study including age, gender, body mass index (BMI), physical activity, smoking, ethnicity, socioeconomic status, and major contributing comorbidity--diabetes (41-42).

Our findings, based on the most recent Canadian nationally representative CCHS-2.4 data, revealed a significant difference between higher dietary consumption of sodium, for the individuals with hypertension and higher BMI related to different ethnicities in Canada. For example, the HRs between Caucasian Canadians and other ethnicities were from HR, 1.41,

95% CI, 1.19-1.68; P<0.0001 for the East Asian Canadians, HR,1.35,95% CI, 1.06-1.65; P=0.0046 for the Black Canadians, HR, 1.29, 95% CI, 1.03-1.63; P=0.00301 for the South Asian Canadians, and HR, 1.19, 95% CI, 1.01-1.59; P=0.0055 for the Native Canadians respectively.

Although the mechanism of reduction in sodium intake lowers blood pressure (BP) is not fully clear, many previous studies (43-45) have shown that the fall in BP with sodium restriction is significantly related to the responsiveness of the renin-angiotensin-aldosterone system (RAAS). RAAS responsiveness has been shown to be lower in different populations, possibly constituting a physiological basis for salt sensitivity (46-49). Specific genetic susceptibilities that tend to associate with specific races have been identified (e.g., some First Nations and Inuit peoples) (50, 51), while observational studies showed that African Americans are more likely to develop high blood pressure than Caucasians and other ethnic groups. At least 40 percent of African Americans over age 40 have high blood pressure (52). The DASH (Dietary Approaches to Stop Hypertension) sodium trial also confirmed that sodium restriction lowers BP to a greater extent in blacks compared with non-blacks, and in hypertensives compared with normotensives (53).

Salt sensitivity (SS) has been examined to link to human hypertension and ethnic differences in the relation between erythrocytesodium (Na^+_i), calcium (Ca^{2+}_i), potassium (K^+_i), and magnesium (Mg^{2+}_i); In hypertensives, increase in mean arterial pressure was 12.6 vs 8.2 mmHg in African-Americans vs whites, respectively ($P<0.01$), and for systolic BP, it was 23 vs 14.8 mmHg ($P<0.01$). In the investigation, researchers found that higher level of Na^+_i and Ca^{2+}_i were noted in the African-Americans than in the corresponding white subjects when SS and salt-intermediate were tested (54). African descent who excrete sodium less efficiently and have an associated increase in systolic blood pressure during the daytime and blunted nocturnal systolic blood pressure dipping response. Clinical research found that changing renal handling function of calcium and magnesium suggestive of increased activity of the sodium-potassium-chloridecotransporter (NKCC2) were also found in Black, but not White, subjects (55-57). Another study reported that by segmental controlling of sodium along the proximal (RNa_{prox}) and distal (RNa_{dist}) nephron might be heritable and different between black and white individuals. From independent of urinary sodium excretion, South Africans had higher RNa_{prox} ($P<0.001$) than Belgians. Of the filtered sodium load, black reabsorb more than white in the proximal nephron and less postproximally (58).

There are different hypotensinogenic correlates for race vs. ethnicity; as well there is some interplay between the racial and ethnic correlates. Some of the associations between blood pressure and race have been identified at a genetic level. Sex differences involving hormones (estrogen, testosterone) and physiology (menopause) have been cited in association with hypertension (50, 51, 59). Gender differences, however, may have much additional explanatory power. Men have a greater overall risk; however, female's risk equals that of men. Women who are 75 and older have a higher risk (60-63). Females in our study consumed more than males in all three levels of sodium (from <1,500mg to >2,300mg/day) in all ethnicities, this also relates to higher prevalence in females than in males in this study.

Our study confirmed some interesting findings regarding the effects of dietary sodium intake related to overweight or obesity. Our results also revealed the associations between excess sodium intake and obesity and hypertension outcomes between Canadian ethnicities. For example, the results from the PHREG models, adjusted for age and sex, and other potential confounding factors such as lifestyle, socioeconomics, and total energy intake variables showed that East Asian Canadians, Black Canadians, South Asian Canadians, and Native Canadians consumed more sodium and positively associated with high blood pressure than Caucasian Canadians. Reduction of body weight can reduce the risk of hypertension and cardiovascular disease (CVD), and a corresponding daily sodium reduction was also associated with reduction in the risk of hypertension and CVD (64-65).

The Canadian Community Health Survey (CCHS) cycle 2.2 self-reported data can be used to provide information on reliable, timely information about dietary intake, nutritional well-being and health-related issues. Important strengths include the large amount of data available on a population representative of all Canadians. The presence of questions on various chronic diseases as reported to have been diagnosed by a physician allowed the estimation of chronic disease in the population. There are also limitations. The accuracy of the dietary data may vary by ethnicity, with the dietary question doing a better job with the western diet than with an ethnic one. Self-reported information may be influenced by factors such as a respondent's socio-demographic characteristics, cognitive ability or memory, stigma related to health care utilization, questionnaire design and/or the mode of data collection (66-67).

The 24-hour dietary recall is a main component in the CCHS 2.2 survey, which uses an innovative computer-assisted interviewing instrument called the Automated Multiple-Pass Method (AMPM), and helps respondents remember and report the foods they consumed during the 24-hour period prior to the interview, from midnight to midnight of the CCHS 2.2 survey.

The AMPM, which was used in the 24-hour dietary recall component of the CCHS 2.2, was composed of five steps (Quick List, Forgotten Foods, Time and Occasion, Detail Cycle, and Final Reviews). Each step was designed in order to help keeping respondents interested and engaged during interview process, and to help them to remember all the foods and beverages they consumed during the previous 24-hour period (68). This method might help to reduce some non-responses and selection bias in the data analysis and result evaluations.

When all confounding factors are considered and controlled, males consumed more high level sodium than females in all ethnic groups. Overweight/obesity and corresponding high sodium intake is strongly associated with an increased risk of hypertension. Native Canadians, East Asian Canadians, Black Canadians, and South Asian Canadians exceeded those of the Caucasian Canadians at a significant difference when we compared people with HBP by those without HBP.

REFERENCES

[1]   World Health Organization. The World Health Report. Geneva: World Health Organization, 2002.
[2]   O'Donnell C, Kannel W. Cardiovascular risks of hypertension: lessons from observational studies. J Hypertens 1998; 16 (suppl 6):S3-7.
[3]   Levy D, Larson M, Vasan R, et al. The Progression From Hypertension to Congestive Heart Failure. JAMA 1996; 275:1557-62.
[4]   Kannel WB. Blood Pressure as a Cardiovascular Risk Factor. JAMA 1996; 275:1571-6.
[5]   Wolf-Maier K, Cooper RS, Banegas JR, et al. Hypertension Prevalence and Blood Pressure Levels in 6 European Countries, Canada, and the United States. JAMA 2003; 289:2363-69.
[6]   National Institutes of Health. The Seventh Report of the Joint National Committee on Detection, Evaluation, and Treatment of High Blood Pressure. Bethesda, MD: NIH, 2003.

[7] Vasan R, Beiser A, Seshadri S, et al. Residual Lifetime Risk for Developing Hypertension in Middle-aged Women and Men. JAMA 2002; 287:1003-10.

[8] He FJ, MacGregor GA. Effect of longer-term modest salt reduction on blood pressure. Cochrane Database Syst Rev 2004; (3):CD004937.

[9] He FJ, MacGregor GA. How Far Should Salt Intake Be Reduced? Hypertension 2003; 42:1093-99.

[10] Whelton PK, He J, Appel LJ, et al. Primary Prevention of Hypertension. Clinical and Public Health Advisory from the National High Blood Pressure Education Program. JAMA 2002; 288:1882-8.

[11] Madhavan S, Alderman MH. Ethnicity and the relationship of sodium intake to blood pressure. J Hypertens 1994; 12(1):97-103.

[12] Charlton KE, Steyn K, Levitt NS, et al. Ethnic differences in intake and excretion of sodium, potassium, calcium and magnesium in South Africans. Eur J Cardiovasc Prev Rehabil 2005;12(4):355-62.

[13] Somova L, Mufunda J. Ethnic differences of renin-sodium profile and renal prostaglandins in the pathogenesis of systemic arterial hypertension. Cent Afr J Med 1996; 42(6):170-5.

[14] Levy SB, Lilley JJ, Frigon RP, et al. Urinary kallikrein and plasma renin activity as determinants of renal blood flow. The influence of race and dietary sodium intake. J Clin Invest 1997; 60(1):129-38.

[15] Harshfield GA, Alpert BS, Pulliam DA, et al. Sodium excretion and racial differences in ambulatory blood pressure patterns. Hypertension 1991;18(6):813-8.

[16] Ajani S, Dunbar E, Ford A, et al. Sodium Intake Among People with Normal and High Blood Pressure. American Journal of Preventive Medicine 2005; 29(5):63-7.

[17] Page LB, Damon A, Moellering RC, Jr. Antecedents of cardiovascular disease in six Solomon Islands societies. Circulation 1974; 49:1132-46.

[18] Page LB, Vandevert DE, Nader K, et al. Blood pressure of Qash'qai pastoral nomads in Iran in relation to culture, diet, and body form. Am J ClinNutr1981; 34:527-38.

[19] INTERSALT. Intersalt: an international study of electrolyte excretion and blood pressure. Results for 24 hour urinary sodium and potassium excretion. Intersalt Cooperative Research Group. BMJ 1998; 297:319-28.

[20] Elliott P, Stamler J, Nichols R, et al. Intersalt revisited: further analyses of 24 hour sodium excretion and blood pressure within and across populations. Intersalt Cooperative Research Group. BMJ 1996; 312:1249-53.

[21] Trials of Hypertension Prevention Collaborative Research Group. Effects of weight loss and sodium reduction intervention on blood pressure and hypertension incidence in overweight people with highnormal blood pressure. The trials of hypertension prevention, phase II. The trials of hypertension prevention collaborative research group. Arch Intern Med 1997; 157:657-67.

[22] Cook NR, Cutler JA, Obarzanek E, et al. Long term effects of dietary sodium reduction on cardiovascular disease outcomes: observational follow-up of the trials of hypertension prevention (TOTP). BMJ 2007 334:885.

[23] Staessen J, Bulpitt CJ, Fagard R, et al. Salt intake and blood pressure in the general population: a controlled intervention trial in two towns. J Hypertens 1998; 6:965-73.

[24] Tuomilehto J, Puska P, Nissinen A, et al. Community-based prevention of hypertension in North Karelia, Finland. Ann Clin Res 16 Suppl 1984 43, S18-S27.

[25] Iso H, Shimamoto T, Yokota K, et al. Changes in 24-hour urinary excretion of sodium and potassium in a community-based health education program on salt reduction]. Nippon KoshuEiseiZasshi 1999; 46:894-903.

[26] Vartiainen E, Sarti C, Tuomilehto J, et al. Do changes in cardiovascular risk factors explain changes in mortality from stroke in Finland? BMJ 1995; 310:901-4.

[27] Alderman MH, Cohen H, Madhavan S. Dietary sodium intake and mortality: the National Health and Nutrition Examination Survey (NHANES I). Lancet 1998; 351:781-5.

[28] He FJ, Markandu ND, Sagnella GA, et al. Importance of the renin system in determining blood pressure fall with salt restriction in black and white hypertensives. Hypertension 1998; 32:820-4.

[29] Campbell NR, McAlister FA, Brant R, et al. Temporal trends in antihypertensive drug prescriptions in Canada before and after introduction of the Canadian Hypertension Education Program. Hypertension 2003; 21(8):1591-7.

[30] Campbell NR, Brant R, Johansen H, et al. Increases in antihypertensive prescriptions and reductions in cardiovascular events in Canada. Hypertension 2009; 53(2):128-34.

[31] Onysko J, Maxwell C, Eliasziw M, et al. Large Increases in Hypertension Diagnosis and Treatment in Canada Following a Health Care Professional Education Program. Hypertension 2006; 48:853-60.

[32] Lawes CMM, Vander Hoorn S, Law MR, et al. Blood pressure and the global burden of disease 2000. Part II: Estimates of attributable burden. J Hypertens 2006; 24:423-30.

[33] Canadian Hypertension Society. The Canadian hypertension education program. 2009; http//:www.hypertension.ca.

[34] Khan NA, Hemmelgarn B, et al. The Canadian hypertension education program recommendations for the management of hypertension: part2- therapy. Can J Cardiol 2008; 24(6):465-75.

[35] Statistics Canada. The Canadian Community Health Survey (CCHS-2.2). 2004; http://10.242.40.34:8080/displayPdf.jsp?url=L3BkZl9maWxlcy9jY2g0MnNkLnBkZg.

[36] Onysko J. A sociological diagnostic of hypertension in Canada: etiology, control and management. 2003; www.hypertension.ca/chep/wp-content/.../chep-business-plan.pdf.

[37] Intersalt Cooperative Research Group. Intersalt: an international study of electrolyte excretion and blood pressure: results for 24 hour urinary sodium and potassium excretion. BMJ 1988; 297(6644):319-28.

[38] Hashimoto T, and Fujita Y. Urinary sodium and potassium excretion, body mass index, alcohol intake and blood pressure in three Japanese populations.J Hum Hypertens 1989; (3): 315-21.

[39] Gleiberman L. Blood pressure and dietary salt in human populatios. Ecol Food Nutr 1973; 2:143-56.

[40] Iso H, Shimamoto T, Yokota K, et al. Changes in 24-hour urinary excretion of sodium and potassium in a community-based health education program on salt reduction. Nippon KoshuEiseiZasshi 1999; 46: 894-903.

[41] Carvalho JJ, Baruzzi RG, Howard PF et al. Blood pressure in four remote populations in the INTERSALT Study. Hypertension 1989; 14:238-46.

[42] British Columbia Ministry of Health Services. British Columbia Nutrition Survey. Report on energy and nutrient intakes. Victoria, BC: BC Min Health, 2004.

[43] Weinberger MH, Miller JZ, Luft FC, et al. Definitions and characteristics of sodium sensitivity and bloodpressure resistance. Hypertension 1986; 8Suppl 2, S127-S34.

[44] Cappuccio FP, Markandu ND, Sagnella GA, et al. Sodium restriction lowers high blood pressure through a decreased response of the renin system---Direct evidence using Saralasin. J Hypertens 1985; 3:243-7.

[45] He FJ, Markandu ND, Sagnella GA, et al. Importance of the renin system in determining blood pressure fall with salt restriction in black and white hypertensives. Hypertension 1998; 32:820-4.

[46] Falkner B. Differences in blacks and whites with essential hypertension: biochemistry and endocrine: state of the art lecture. Hypertension 1990; 15:681-6.

[47] Luft FC, Grim CE, Fineberg N, et al. Effects of volume expansion and contraction in normotensive whites, blacks, and subjects of different ages. Circulation 1979; 59:643-50.

[48] James GD, Sealey JE, Muller F, et al. Renin relationship to sex, race and age in a normotensive population. J Hypertens1986; 8(Suppl 4):S387-9.

[49] Fisher ND, Gleason RE, Moore TJ, et al. Regulation of aldosterone secretion in hypertensive blacks. Hypertension 1994; 23:179-84.

[50] Carriquiry, AL. Estimation of usual Intake distributions of nutrients and foods. J Nutr 2003; 133(2):601S-8.

[51] Kitler, ME. Difference in men and women in coronary artery disease, systemic hypertension and their treatment. Am J Cardiol 1992; 70:1077-80.

[52] Hughes GS, Cook NR, Oberman A, et al. Sex steroid hormones are altered in essential hypertension. J Hypertens 1989; 7:181-7.

[53] Sacks FM, SvetkeyLR, Vollmer WM et al. Effects on blood pressure of reduced dietary sodium and the dietary approaches to stop hypertension (DASH) diet. N Engl J Med 2001; 344:3-10.

[54] Wright JT Jr, Rahman M, Scarpa A, et al. Determinants of salt sensitivity in black and white normotensive and hypertensive women. Hypertension2003 Dec; 42(6):1087-92. Epub 2003 Nov 10.

[55]   Bankir L, Bochud M, Maillard M, et al. Nighttime blood pressure and nocturnal dipping are associated with daytime urinary sodium excretion in African subjects. Hypertension 2008;51:891–8.

[56]   Chun TY, Bankir L, Eckert GJ, et al. Ethnic differences in renal responses to furosemide. Hypertension 2008; 52:241–8.

[57]   Sanders PW. Dietary salt intake, salt sensitivity, and cardiovascular health. *Hypertension* 2009; 53:442.

[58]   Bochud, Murielle; Staessen, Jan A; Maillard, Marc; et al. Ethnic differences in proximal and distal tubular sodium reabsorption are heritable in black and white populations. J Hypertension 2009; 27(3):606-12.

[59]   The American Heart Association. African Americans at greater risk for stroke than other ethnic groups.J Natl Med Assoc 2004; 96(8):1019-23.

[60]   Messerli FH, Garavaglia GE, Schmieder RE, et al. Disparate cardiovascular findings in men and women with essential hypertension. Ann Int Med 1987; 107:158-161.

[61]   Dyer AR, Stamler R, Grimm R, et al. Do hypertensive patients have a different diurnal pattern of electrolyte excretion? Hypertens 1987; 10:417-24.

[62]   Adams-Campbell LL, Nwankwo MU, Ukoli FA, et al. Sex and ethnic differences associated with urinary sodiumand potassium in African-American US white and Nigerian college students. J Hum Hypertens 1993; 7:437-41.

[63]   Jurgita Grikinienė, Voldemaras Volbekas1, Donatas Stakišaitis. Gender differences of sodium metabolism and hyponatremia as an adverse drug effect. Medicina (Kaunas) 2004; 40(10):935-42.

[64]   He J, Whelton PK, Appel LJ, et al. Long-tern effects of weight loss and dietary sodium reduction on incidence of hypertension. Hypertension 2000; 35:544-9.

[65]   He J, Ogden LG, Vupputuri S, et al. Dietary sodium intake and subsequenct risk of cardiovascular disease in overweight adults. JAMA 1999; 282:2027-34.

[66]   Bhandari A, Wagner T. Self-reported utilization of health care services: Improving measurement and accuracy. Med Care Res Rev2006; 63(2):217–35.

[67]   Tjepkema M. Nutrition: Findings from the Canadian Community Health Survey—Adult obesity in Canada: Measured height and weight. Ottawa,Canada. CatalogueNo. 2005; 82-620-MWE2005001. URL: http://www.statcan.ca/english/research/82-620-MIE/2005001/pdf/aobesity.pdf.

[68]   Statistics Canada. *Canadian Community Health Survey (CCHS): Cycle 2.2, Nutrition: General Health Component Including Vitamin and Mineral Supplements, and 24-hour Dietary Recall Component, User Guide, 2008.* Available at: /imdb-bmdi/document/5049_D24_T9_V1-eng.pdf.

In: Food, Nutrition and Eating Behavior   ISBN: 978-1-62948-233-0
Editors: Joav Merrick and Sigal Israeli   © 2014 Nova Science Publishers, Inc.

Chapter 7

CHILD MALNUTRITION AND THE DEMOCRATIC PEOPLE'S REPUBLIC OF KOREA

Daniel Schwekendiek, PhD*
Faculty of Economics, University of Tuebingen, Tuebingen, Germany

ABSTRACT

This chapter provides evidence on the worldwide health status and North Korea's performance therein by looking at national child malnutrition rates found in one of the last surveys conducted around the year 2000. Child malnutrition classifications were based on low height-for-age z-scores as an indicator of chronic malnutrition, low weight-for-age as an indicator of acute malnutrition, and low-weight-for-age as an in-between indicator of the former and the latter. At the end of the second millennium, we find average world malnutrition rates of 25% based on the HAZ, 7% based on the WHZ, and 19% based on the WAZ. North Korea clearly shows higher malnutrition rates than the world average in terms of the HAZ (45%) and WHZ (9%). Looking at the world's nations classified by their economic development status, we find that North Korea can merely be described as a "least developed country". When looking at North Korea's international rank among 117 countries, stunting was found to be 12th highest, wasting 28th highest and underweight 30th highest. What also became clear is that North Korea represents an extreme outlier in both East Asia and the Eastern hemisphere in general.

INTRODUCTION

Totalitarian North Korea is a most ambiguous country. On the one hand, the country tested two nuclear bombs – one of the most advanced technical devices a nation can have. On the other hand, it is known that the North Korean people has been suffering from starvation and continuous deprivation (1-4). From a military-technological point of view, North Korea might

---

* Correspondence: Daniel Schwekendiek, Ph.D., Faculty of Economics, University of Tuebingen, Mohlstraße 36, 72074 Tuebingen, Germany. E-mail: daniel.schwekendiek@uni-tuebingen.de.

be on equal eye level with some developed nations. Yet in terms of human development, North Korea might reasonably be assumed to lag centuries behind.

We here want to take a closer look at a common indicator of the quality of life, namely child malnutrition. In research, malnutrition is commonly measured by standard anthropometric procedures. In other terms, by looking at the height and weight development of children, we can directly infer the health and wealth of a nation.

The aim of this chapter is to characterize the worldwide state of children in terms of the national prevalence of malnutrition. Based on anthropometry-related malnutrition indicators, we give a global overview of the magnitude of child malnutrition around the year 2000. We then specifically relate North Korea's rate of child malnutrition to global and regional averages in order to see the country's performance in living standards on a comparative and worldwide scale.

The remainder of this article is arranged as follows. In the next section, we explain the three commonly established indicators of child malnutrition: stunting, underweight and wasting. Afterwards, global data sources are introduced and discussed in terms of their statistical representativeness. Most importantly, we present the global prevalence of child malnutrition found around the year 2000 by making use of diagrams and cartographic illustrations. This section is followed by a discussion on North Korea's malnutrition rates vis-à-vis its neighbors in East-Asia and further developing countries throughout the world. The last section of this paper contains some concluding remarks.

ANTHROPOMETRIC INDICATORS OF MALNUTRITION

As recommended by the WHO (5), child malnutrition is commonly assessed by making use of z-score transformations of height and weight measurements. Let i indicate an individual examined in a sample or population. X denotes the primary indicator of concern, which is either height h or weight w. Y denotes a relative indicator referred to by X, and this is either age A, measured in months, or h. Z denotes the standardized z-score. The general equation for an anthropometric z-score transformation is given as:

$$XYZ_i = \frac{x_i^{Y_s} - \bar{x}_r^{Y_s}}{\sigma_{x_r^{Y_s}}}$$

(1.1)

where S represents the sex of the child and r indicates a healthy reference group which is classified by s and Y of i. If XYZi falls below −2, i would be classified as malnourished according to international conventions in research (6-8). Hence, the number of children falling below −2 is counted. These individuals are expressed in percent of the examined target group to reflect the magnitude of malnutrition within the observed sample or population.

Based on equation (1.1), these three indicators have been established in research: height for age z-scores (HAZi), weight for height z-scores (WHZi) and weight for age z-scores (WAZi). These are given as:

$$HAZ_i = \frac{h_i^{A_s} - \overline{h}_r^{A_s}}{\sigma_{h_r^{A_s}}}$$

(1.2)

$$WAZ_i = \frac{w_i^{A_s} - \overline{w}_r^{A_s}}{\sigma_{w_r^{A_s}}}$$

(1.3)

$$WHZ_i = \frac{w_i^{H_s} - \overline{w}_r^{H_s}}{\sigma_{w_r^{H_s}}}$$

(1.4)

Note that different terminologies exist in the literature, focusing either on the indicator itself or describing the process and outcomes involved in the specific anthropometric variable - for a brief overview, see table 3. Here, we follow the terminology given in the last column of table 3 by referring to "stunting" for HAZ<-2, "wasting" for WHZ<-2, and "underweight" for WAZ<-2 when specifying child malnutrition in this paper.

When should one select which indicator? First of all, it is important to bear in mind that none of the discussed indicators is perfect for all situations. The selection of a specific indicator depends highly on the research question. The two generally preferred indicators for a systematic distinction between chronic and acute malnutrition are height-for-age and weight-for-height (7).

Stunting is a residual of the past – it is a result of a cumulative process lasting from the early to current childhood. The most important advantage of height is certainly that it cannot decrease, unlike weight gains or losses, which can occur very fast. Moreover, specifically in the case of cross-sectional data which allow little control over food seasonality, diarrhoeal outbreaks and short-term macroeconomic shocks, height-for-age seems to measure human welfare more precisely. In this vein, height can be considered a standard of living indicator, as it clearly reflects the long-term conditions under which a child was raised: a high prevalence of stunting generally indicates poor overall socioeconomic conditions, continuous nutritional stress, and repeated outbreaks of diseases.

Weight-for-height is generally of interest when assessing the nutritional status of a population in the short run. For instance, after a natural disaster, wasting is of concern when distributing food aid in order to immediately identify - under conditions of fixed and limited resources - the most vulnerable regions in the country. Also on an individual level, a highly wasted child requires immediate nutritional and medical assistance to survive the next weeks, whereas short stature could likewise be the result of a genetic deficiency (10). A further advantage of the WHZ indicator is that it can be calculated without knowing the age of the child, which is frequently unknown or unreliable in many developing countries. Additionally, in developed countries, the WHZ can likewise indicate overnutrition (WHZ>2) as an additional health indicator, which the HAZ does not permit.

The WAZ indicator is a composite index of the WHZ and the HAZ. It is less frequently applied in research, although recommended to be reported whenever possible. It is between chronic and acute malnutrition and as it encompasses both the long-run component of age and the short-run component of weight, it is sometimes denoted as an indicator of "global malnutrition." However, the in-between indicator WAZ seems to be of less importance in practical research, as it particularly fails to differentiate between tall, thin, and short children with an appropriate weight.

From an empirical point of view, the HAZ and WHZ - thus chronic and acute malnutrition - are not strongly correlated (see table 1), as there is only a weak correlation between them (0.5). Hence, as noted above, one should have a clear study aim and interpret the respective indicators accordingly. What also becomes evident from table 1 is that the WAZ seems closely correlated to both the WHZ (0.8) and HAZ (0.9), as we would have expected from this in-between indicator.

Table 1. Correlations of anthropometric indicators of child malnutrition

		whz below -2 in %	haz below -2 in %	waz below -2 in %
whz below -2 in %	Correlation	1	.537	.785
	Sig.	.	.000	.000
haz below -2 in %	Correlation	.537	1	.860
	Sig.	.000	.	.000
waz below -2 in %	Correlation	.785	.860	1
	Sig.	.000	.000	.

** Correlation is significant at the 0.01 level.
Source: see text. Based on 117 countries around the year 2000.

In summary, the HAZ seems to be the preferable indicator for measuring the socioeconomic welfare of a nation. Additionally, in cross-sectional comparison, it also allows control over short-term macroeconomic biases. The WHZ seems to be more appropriate from a practical or medical point of view, as the measure of wasting can serve to immediately identify vulnerable groups and regions for the distribution of humanitarian aid in order to save the population or individuals from starvation. For a quick overview and as a combination of short- and long-term socioeconomic effects, the WAZ might be preferred, yet it does not have direct implications for theoretical or practical issues.

The use of -2 z-scores as a cut-off implies that 2.3% of the reference population will be classified as malnourished. Although there is discussion about this, we will only regard -2 z-score cut-offs in our study. Despite the fact that using -3 z-scores can yield information about severe malnutrition, we do not use them here to focus on just one analysis, and also because information might be lost on some countries for which no data on severe malnutrition was reported. In the same vein, the use of -1 z-scores as an indicator of mild malnutrition is sometimes recommended, for instance in the case of a number of Latin American countries. However, the global database does not include this kind of specific information. In conclusion, in this paper, we will provide evidence neither on severe nor on mild malnutrition, but limit ourselves to the -2 z-score cut-off points which are, by all means, standard in research and strongly recommend by the United Nations for assessing general nutritional stress within a population as well as for covering as many countries as possible.

OUR DATA SAMPLE

In this article, we make use of data collected and provided electronically by the United Nations. The Global Database on Child Growth and Malnutrition (hereafter referred to as 'the database') is maintained by the WHO. Initiated in 1986, the United Nations and the German government funded a three-year project to build up a worldwide nutritional surveillance database in order to characterize the nutritional status of children in different countries (11, 12). To the present, the database has been updated regularly - so far, over 800 anthropometric surveys have been included. Data were basically taken from three sources: published articles, governmental statistics, and reports by NGOs and UN agencies. To ensure the standardization of the huge variety of material available worldwide, each survey had to pass basic criteria such as population-based and probabilistic sampling, minimum sample size, standardized raw data based on the NCHS-reference population, and standardized measurement techniques for being included in the WHO database (12). Furthermore, to enforce quality control, all data were checked for inconsistencies and removed when necessary.

For our analysis, we first had to determine which surveys to select from the database. We primarily considered nationally representative surveys and discarded all sub-national surveys that were usually based on selected regions like provinces or districts. Even though these local surveys make up over 50% of the database, it does not make sense to use such information in a worldwide comparative study, as regional conditions will strongly bias anthropometric findings for a country.

On top of that, the main purpose of this paper is to paint with a broad brush rather than follow the development of specific countries over time, so that we had to limit ourselves to evidence on a single point in time: panel data would have been interesting for answering questions on dynamic developments, but for many countries in the world, information is available for only one year.

Therefore, we conducted a cross-sectional study with 2000 (end) as our reference year. There were two reasons for this: firstly, we realized that most surveys were completed by the year 2000 because in many countries, the United Nations carried out surveys under the World Summit Declaration's year-2000 goal of welfare for women and children. Secondly, from a historiographical point of view, we wanted to provide evidence on the worldwide health status at the end of the last millennium - as a quick and convenient cross-sectional yardstick for further studies. Hence, for every country for which data was available, we selected the survey closest to the reference year. As seen in figure 1, most of them were carried out in the late 1990s. Eventually, the data extracted from the database covered the time period 1995 to 2001, i.e., we likewise excluded surveys conducted before 1995. This left us with 117 countries for which information on overall child malnutrition could be found in the database.

Furthermore, the surveys in the WHO database generally target toddlers and children, and there are varying ranges the respondents had at the time of their measurement. As seen in equation (1.1) and discussed in WHO (1986, 1995), using z-score standardization based on a healthy reference group (usually the NCHS reference group which is based on the US population) makes it possible to compare these groups. However, comparing large differing age groups across surveys might induce certain distortions: the NCHS standardization implies that all children in the world follow the same genetic growth pattern, which might not be the case for all ethnic groups. However, Habicht et al. (13) have shown that different genetic growth potentials hardly matter, if at all, for young children under the age of five. Therefore, it should be mentioned that the dominant age group in the WHO surveys is 0-4.99 (i.e., children who completed 0-59 months). In our analysis, children under 5 years of age represent 97% of the measured individuals. Hence, the selection of sample age groups should not pose a problem here.

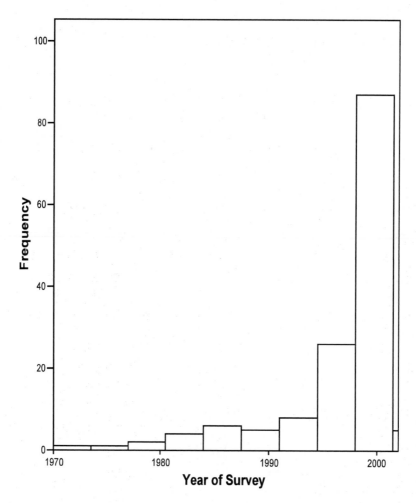

Figure 1. Frequencies of surveys by year.

GEOPOLITICAL PREPRESENTATIVENESS

In general, the WHO database is one of the most comprehensive information systems on nutritional indicators, as it covers a large number of countries and accounts for all world regions: the countries included represent 80-90% of the world's population and, most importantly, 99% of the under five-year-old children living in developing countries (12).

A complete list of our data, classified by country name, is given in Appendix 1. The reported years refer to the end of the year in which the respective survey was conducted. UN sub-regions are indicated in parentheses.

What is most striking is that few high-income countries are included in the database: for Europe, many EU countries are missing. Few of the North American countries are represented; and for East Asia, high-tech countries such as Japan and South Korea are excluded. Ironically, there is generally plenty of statistical information available on these countries, but specific data on child growth are lacking because for "most countries data is not available in the required standardized format" (11). We also had to reject a number of surveys mostly from high-income countries because they were conducted far before the 1990s (see figure 1). As a consequence, our dataset includes only two countries classified as developed by the UN: Australia and Gaza. Most of the countries represented in our dataset are developing (53%) and least developed countries (35%) countries, or countries in transition (10%). Thus, it should be mentioned that our cross-country study does not at all reflect the situation of high-income countries. However, the situation of most children in the world is quite well reflected, since more than 3/4 of the total world population are represented. Moreover, in most of the missing countries, child malnutrition is not really a problem of undernutrition, but of overnutrition which certainly has other causes and cures and would be far beyond the scope of this paper.

GLOBAL MALNUTRITION

Let us address the overall health status of children at the end of the millennium. Based on a country's level of development – UN classifications applied here - for least developed countries, we find a prevalence of child malnutrition of 37% in terms of stunting, 30% in terms of underweight and 9% if measured by wasting (see table 2). It is striking that countries which are classified as economies in transition and developing countries do not differ in stunting or wasting rates which are found to be 19% (HAZ<-2) and 5% (WHZ<-2). It is also important to note that even in the so-called developed countries, we find child malnutrition of 2-4%, suggesting that policies in developed areas must not neglect the poor.

Table 2. Worldwide malnutrition rates by development status

Level of development	N	Child malnutrition in %		
		HAZ<-2	WAZ<-2	WHZ<-2
Developed countries	2	4	2	2
Developing countries	63	19	14	5
Economies in transition	12	19	7	5
Least developed countries	41	37	30	9
North Korea	1	45	18	9

Table 3. Common terms for classifying malnutrition

Anthropometric indicator	Malnutrition indicator	Terms describing outcomes	Terms describing process	Frequently applied terms for malnutrition
height for age z-score (HAZ)	low HAZ	stunted, shortness	stunting (gaining insufficient height relative to age)	stunting
weight for height z-score (WHZ)	low WHZ	wasted, thinness	wasting (gaining insufficient weight relative to height, or losing weight)	wasting
weight for age z-score (HAZ)	low WAZ	underweight, lightness	gaining insufficient weight relative to age, or losing weight	underweight

Source: Based on WHO (1995).Table 4. Worldwide stunting, wasting and underweight ranks.

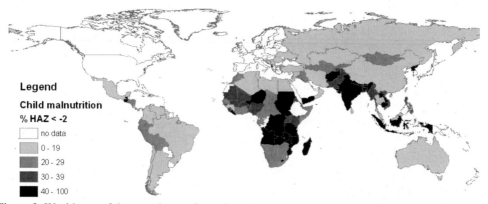

Figure 2. World map of the prevalence of stunting.

The regional prevalence of malnutrition in terms of stunting, underweight and wasting is shown in figures 2 to 4. For the world's total (represented by 117 countries), average stunting was found to be 25%. For wasting, the total average prevalence of malnutrition was found to be 7%, and 19% in terms of underweight. An inter-continental comparison clearly shows the net- nutritional gap between the geographical regions of the world. We find the highest rate of stunting, underweight and wasting on the African continent, with peaks of 32% (HAZ<-2), 23% (WAZ<-2) and 8% (WHZ <-2), followed by Asia which is likewise above world average. The healthiest children live in Oceania and on the European continent – the latter unfortunately only represented by Eastern and Southern Europe. LAC countries hold the middle position – with average chronic malnutrition rates of half of those found on the African continent. When comparing these findings to inter-continental malnutrition rates in terms of wasting, the rankings remain unchanged with one exception: more children in (Eastern and Southern) European countries seem to be wasted than in LAC countries (figure 3). Focusing on sub-regions, it becomes clear that a particularly large percentage of children in Eastern and Central Africa, as well as in South-Central and South-Eastern Asia suffer from malnutrition.

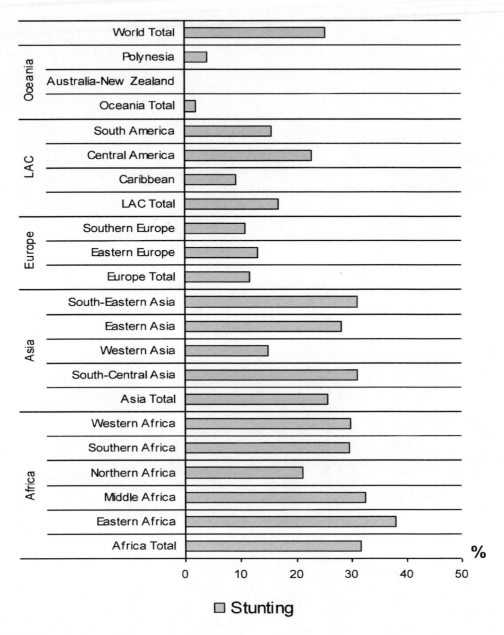

Figure 3. Worldwide prevalence of stunting by (sub-) continents.

For further illustration, consider figures 5 to 7 where we mapped malnutrition rates for each country. As proposed by the WHO as well as Gorstein et al. (7), we roughly classified the prevalence of malnutrition as low if stunting was 0-19%, medium if 20-29%, high if 30-39%, and very high if 40-100%. For wasting, the respective categories are 0-4%, 5-9%, 10-14% and 15-100%; for underweight, 0-9%, 10-19%, 20-29% and 30-100%. What can be seen in figures 5 to 7 is that there are indeed some clusters of countries where malnutrition is very high, like in certain Central African and South-East Asian regions; and clusters where malnutrition is generally rather low, like in Oceania, Eastern Europe, LAC, Northern Africa and China. By visual inspection, two regional outliers can be identified: North Korea in the East and Guatemala in the West show very high rates of malnutrition in otherwise rather healthy regions (figure 5). Until the late 1990s, the latter experienced several decades of civil war, and the former a famine which was perhaps the greatest humanitarian disaster of the 1990s (14).

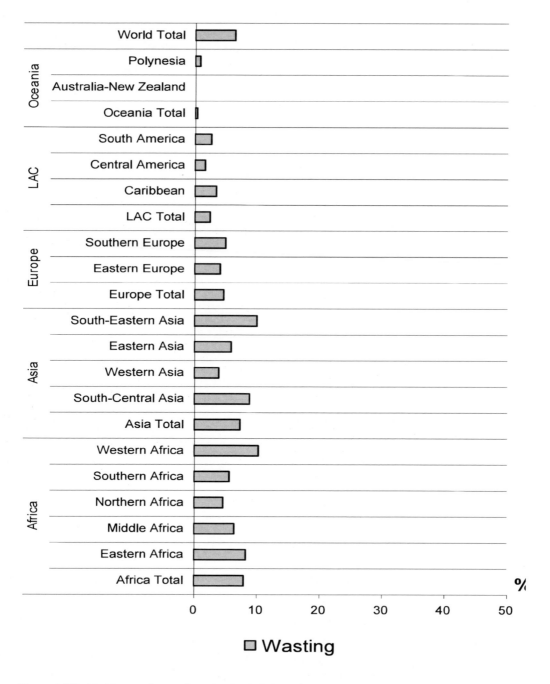

Figure 4. Worldwide prevalence of wasting by (sub-) continents.

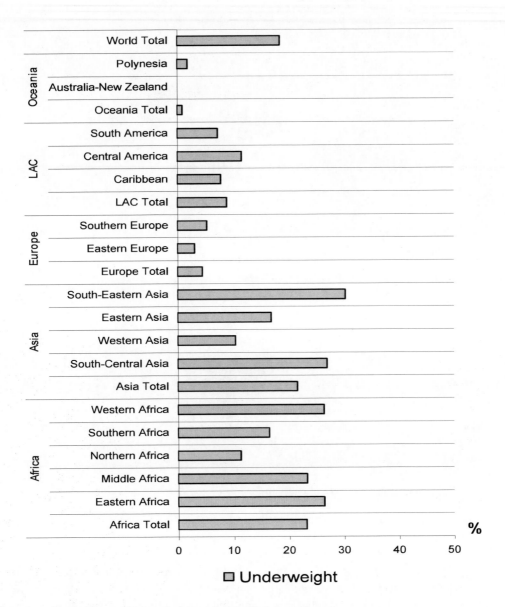

Figure 5. Worldwide prevalence of underweight by (sub-) continents.

KOREA

In figures 5 to 7, we have clearly identified North Korea as a regional outlier in the Far Eastern hemisphere in the year 2000 in terms of stunting, wasting and underweight. What is also quite striking is that North Korea is surrounded by very stable and prosperous economies like China, Taiwan and the two OECD members Japan and South Korea. Even though the WHO database did not include an anthropometric survey on North Korea's direct neighbor South Korea, it has been shown that heights and weights are drastically better in the southern part of the peninsula (1, 15, 16).

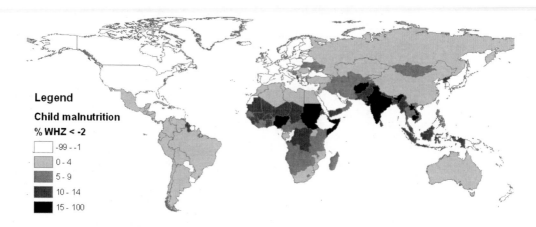

Figure 6. World map of the prevalence of wasting.

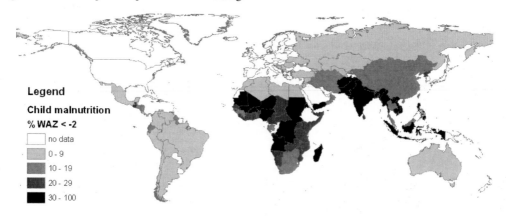

Figure 7. World map of the prevalence of underweight.

Why is North Korea such an obvious outlier in East Asia? Briefly, one of the main causes is certainly that the downfall of the communist regimes and the modernization of their economies - following the geopolitical collapse of the Eastern Bloc in the 1990s - did not take place in North Korea. Thus, Pyongyang became politically and ideologically deadlocked in the early 1990s. Because of North Korea's political and economic isolation – which prevails until today - we most likely see the last remaining Stalinist system on earth to be an extreme outlier in the East Asian region and, to a certain extent, in the world.

In North Korea, based on children below 5 years of age, the prevalence of stunting was found to be 45%, which is clearly above world average (figure 2). Wasting was found to be 9% in North Korea and likewise seems to be above world average (see figure 3). Only underweight, found to be 18% in North Korea, seems to be close to world average (see figure 4).

If we compare North Korea to all countries as classified by their development status, we get an even more exhaustive picture of the dire situation in North Korea around 2000. As seen in table 2, in terms of stunting, North Korea performs even worse than the average least developed country (35%). Yet in terms of wasting, North Korea seems to be on eye level with an average least developed country (9%). Underweight, found to be 18% in North Korea, corresponds to the averages of least developed countries (30%) and developing countries (14%). All in all, it seems to be safe to say that North Korea can even be classified as a least developed country in terms of both economic and human development. Specifically with regard to the living standard as reflected by stunting, it can be reasonably argued that North Korea is one of the poorest and most hostile places for children in the world.

This finding seems to be further corroborated by relative national malnutrition ranks. As seen in table 4, around the year 2000, North Korean stunting rates were the 12th highest in the world. Wasting and underweight were found to be on the 28th and 30th position among the 117 countries reviewed – revealing that North Korea clearly belongs to the poorest quarter of the world's nations. What can be also seen from table 4 is that the top positions in terms of the prevalence of child malnutrition are dominated by Sub-Saharan and South-East Asian countries – a finding already foreshadowed in figures 2 to 4. Because an extremely high prevalence of malnutrition is obviously clustered in these two world regions (figures 5 to 7), North Korea becomes even more a geographical outlier.

CONCLUSION

Above, we provided descriptive evidence on both the worldwide and North Korean health and wealth status by looking at national child malnutrition rates around the year 2000. Child malnutrition classifications were based on the standard anthropometric measurements height and weight, commonly used and recommended in research. In particular, low height-for-age z-scores as an indicator of chronic malnutrition, low weight-for-age as an indicator of acute malnutrition, and low-weight-for-age as an in-between indicator of both the former and the latter, were considered.

At the end of the second millennium, we find average world malnutrition rates of 25% based on the HAZ, 7% based on the WHZ, and 19% based on the WAZ. North Korea clearly shows higher malnutrition rates than the world average in terms of the HAZ (45%) and WHZ (9%). Looking at the world's nations classified by their (economic) development status, we find that North Korea can merely be described as a least developed country. When looking at North Korea's international rank among 117 countries, stunting was found to be 12th highest, wasting 28th highest and underweight 30th highest.

What was very striking throughout our analysis was that North Korea represents an extreme outlier in both East Asia and the Eastern hemisphere in general. This is due to North Korea's post-Cold War legacy of the last remaining wall on earth.

In conclusion, when comparing North Korea to the rest of the world, we can say that in terms of the human development of children below five years of age, North Korea is one of the poorest places on earth – a finding which reduces communism and the possession of high-tech weapons largely to absurdity.

Table 5. Worldwide stunting, wasting and underweight ranks

Rank	Stunting	Wasting	Underweight
1	Burundi	Somalia	Afghanistan
2	Yemen, Rep.	Afghanistan	Nepal
3	Nepal	India	Bangladesh
4	Malawi	Sudan	India
5	Madagascar	Nigeria	Yemen, Rep.
6	Afghanistan	Lao PDR	Cambodia
7	Zambia	Cambodia	Burundi
8	Timor-Leste	Sri Lanka	Timor-Leste
9	Lesotho	Mauritius	Sudan
10	Angola	Niger	Lao PDR
11	Congo, Dem. Rep.	Malaysia	Niger
12	*Korea, Dem. Rep.*	Burkina Faso	Madagascar
13	India	Pakistan	Eritrea
14	Bangladesh	Maldives	Myanmar
15	Cambodia	Yemen, Rep.	Pakistan
16	Guatemala	Indonesia	Congo, Dem. Rep.
17	Tanzania	Djibouti	Burkina Faso
18	Sudan	Mauritania	Indonesia
19	Rwanda	Eritrea	Vietnam
20	Lao PDR	Togo	Mali
21	Comoros	Timor-Leste	Mauritania
22	Indonesia	Comoros	Philippines
23	Mozambique	Chad	Nigeria
24	Bhutan	Albania	Angola
25	Niger	Mali	Maldives
26	Liberia	Guinea	Sri Lanka
27	Uganda	Guyana	Tanzania
28	Mali	*Korea, Dem. Rep.*	Zambia
29	Eritrea	Bangladesh	Chad
30	Tajikistan	Guinea-Bissau	*Korea, Dem. Rep.*
31	Burkina Faso	Sierra Leone	Sierra Leone
32	Pakistan	Nepal	Liberia
33	Vietnam	Congo, Dem. Rep.	Somalia
34	Kenya	Myanmar	Comoros
35	Mauritania	Ghana	Malawi
...	...	...	...
113	Lebanon	Colombia	Kuwait
114	Singapore	Croatia	Lebanon
115	Chile	Lebanon	Chile
116	Croatia	Chile	Croatia
117	Australia	Australia	Australia

Notes: ranks 1 to 117 denote highest to lowest prevalence of malnutrition.

APPENDIX

Appendix 1: Data coverage of surveys by country

Countries	Year	Continents and sub-continents
Afghanistan	1997	Asia (South-central Asia)
Albania	2000	Europe (Southern Europe)
Algeria	2000	Africa (Northern Africa)
Angola	2001	Africa (Middle Africa)
Argentina	1996	LAC (South America)
Armenia	2001	Asia (Western Asia)
Australia	1996	Oceania (Australia- New Zealand)
Azerbaijan	2000	Asia (Western Asia)
Bangladesh	2000	Asia (South-central Asia)
Benin	2001	Africa (Western Africa)
Bhutan	1999	Asia (South-central Asia)
Bolivia	1998	LAC (South America)
Bosnia and Herzegovina	2000	Europe (Southern Europe)
Botswana	2000	Africa (Southern Africa)
Brazil	1996	LAC (South America)
Burkina Faso	1999	Africa (Western Africa)
Burundi	2000	Africa (Eastern Africa)
Cambodia	2000	Asia (South-eastern Asia)
Cameroon	1998	Africa (Middle Africa)
Central African Republic	1995	Africa (Middle Africa)
Chad	2000	Africa (Middle Africa)
Chile	2001	LAC (South America)
China	2000	Asia (Eastern Asia)
Colombia	2000	LAC (South America)
Comoros	2000	Africa (Eastern Africa)
Congo, Dem. Rep.	1995	Africa (Middle Africa)
Costa Rica	1996	LAC (Central America)
Côte d'Ivoire	1999	Africa (Western Africa)
Croatia	1996	Europe (Southern Europe)
Djibouti	1996	Africa (Eastern Africa)
Dominican Republic	2000	LAC (Caribbean)
Ecuador	1998	LAC (South America)
Egypt, Arab Rep.	2000	Africa (Northern Africa)
El Salvador	1998	LAC (Central America)
Eritrea	2002	Africa (Eastern Africa)
Gabon	2001	Africa (Middle Africa)
Gambia, The	2000	Africa (Western Africa)
Georgia	1999	Asia (Western Asia)
Ghana	1999	Africa (Western Africa)
Guatemala	2000	LAC (Central America)
Guinea-Bissau	2000	Africa (Western Africa)

Appendix 1. (Continued)

Countries	Year	Continents and sub-continents
Guinea	2000	Africa (Western Africa)
Guyana	2000	LAC (South America)
Haiti	2000	LAC (Caribbean)
Honduras	2001	LAC (Central America)
India	1999	Asia (South-central Asia)
Indonesia	1995	Asia (South-eastern Asia)
Iran, Islamic Rep.	1998	Asia (South-central Asia)
Iraq	2000	Asia (Western Asia)
Jamaica	1999	LAC (Caribbean)
Jordan	2002	Asia (Western Asia)
Kazakhstan	1999	Asia (South-central Asia)
Kenya	2000	Africa (Eastern Africa)
Korea, Dem. Rep.	2000	Asia (Eastern Asia)
Kuwait	1997	Asia (Western Asia)
Kyrgyz Republic	1997	Asia (South-central Asia)
Lao PDR	2000	Asia (South-eastern Asia)
Lebanon	1997	Asia (Western Asia)
Lesotho	2000	Africa (Southern Africa)
Liberia	2000	Africa (Western Africa)
Libya	1995	Africa (Northern Africa)
Macedonia, FYR	1999	Europe (Southern Europe)
Madagascar	1997	Africa (Eastern Africa)
Malawi	2000	Africa (Eastern Africa)
Malaysia	1999	Asia (South-eastern Asia)
Maldives	2001	Asia (South-central Asia)
Mali	2001	Africa (Western Africa)
Mauritania	2001	Africa (Western Africa)
Mauritius	1995	Africa (Eastern Africa)
Mexico	1999	LAC (Central America)
Mongolia	2000	Asia (Eastern Asia)
Morocco	1997	Africa (Northern Africa)
Mozambique	1997	Africa (Eastern Africa)
Myanmar	2000	Asia (South-eastern Asia)
Namibia	2000	Africa (Southern Africa)
Nepal	2001	Asia (South-central Asia)
Nicaragua	2001	LAC (Central America)
Niger	2000	Africa (Western Africa)
Nigeria	1999	Africa (Western Africa)
Oman	1998	Asia (Western Asia)
Pakistan	2001	Asia (South-central Asia)
Panama	1997	LAC (Central America)
Peru	2000	LAC (South America)
Philippines	1998	Asia (South-eastern Asia)
Qatar	1995	Asia (Western Asia)
Romania	2000	Europe (Eastern Europe)

Countries	Year	Continents and sub-continents
Russian Federation	1995	Europe (Eastern Europe)
Rwanda	2000	Africa (Eastern Africa)
Samoa	1999	Oceania (Polynesia)
São Tomé and Principe	2000	Africa (Middle Africa)
Senegal	2000	Africa (Western Africa)
Serbia and Montenegro	2000	Europe (Southern Europe)
Sierra Leone	2000	Africa (Western Africa)
Singapore	2000	Asia (South-eastern Asia)
Somalia	2000	Africa (Eastern Africa)
South Africa	1999	Africa (Southern Africa)
Sri Lanka	2000	Asia (South-central Asia)
Sudan	2000	Africa (Northern Africa)
Syrian Arab Republic	2000	Asia (Western Asia)
Tajikistan	2000	Asia (South-central Asia)
Tanzania	1999	Africa (Eastern Africa)
Thailand	1995	Asia (South-eastern Asia)
Timor-Leste	2002	Asia (South-eastern Asia)
Togo	1998	Africa (Western Africa)
Trinidad and Tobago	2000	LAC (Caribbean)
Tunisia	1997	Africa (Northern Africa)
Turkey	1998	Asia (Western Asia)
Turkmenistan	2000	Asia (South-central Asia)
Uganda	2001	Africa (Eastern Africa)
Ukraine	2000	Europe (Eastern Europe)
Uzbekistan	2002	Asia (South-central Asia)
Venezuela, RB	2000	LAC (South America)
Vietnam	2000	Asia (South-eastern Asia)
West Bank and Gaza	1996	Asia (Western Asia)
Yemen, Rep.	1997	Asia (Western Asia)
Zambia	2002	Africa (Eastern Africa)
Zimbabwe	1999	Africa (Eastern Africa)

Notes: LAC = Latin America and the Caribbean; continents and sub-continents according to UN classifications.

Source: Guntupalli and Schwekendiek (17), data based on the WHO Global Database on Child Malnutrition.

REFERENCES

[1] Schwekendiek D. Height and weight differences between South and North Korea. Biosoc Sci 2009;41(1):51-7.

[2] Schwekendiek D. Regional variations in living standards during the North Korean food crisis of the 1990s. Asia-Pacific J Public Health, in press.

[3] Schwekendiek D. Determinants of well-being in North Korea: evidence from the post-famine period. Econ Hum Biol 2008;6(3):446-54.

[4] Schwekendiek D. The North Korean standard of living during the famine. Soc Sci Med 2008;66(3):596-608.

[5]   WHO. Use and Interpretation of Anthropometric Indicators of Nutritional Status. Bull World Health Org 1986;64(4):929-41.

[6]   WHO. Physical status: The use and interpretation of anthropometry. Geneva: WHO, 1995.

[7]   Gorstein J, Sullivan K, Yip R, de Onis M, Trowbridge F, Fajans P, et al. Issues in the assessment of nutritional status using anthropometry. Bull World Health Org 1994;72(2):273-83.

[8]   Waterlow J, Buzina R, Keller W, Lane J, Nichaman M, Tanner J. The presentation and use of height and weight data for comparing the nutritional status of groups of children under the age of 10 years. Bull World Health Org 1977;55(4):489-98.

[9]   Cogill B. Anthropometric indicators measurement guide. Washington, DC: Acad Educ Dev, 2003.

[10]   Tanner J. Foetus into man. Cambridge: Harvard Univ Press, 1990.

[11]   De Onis M, Blössner M. WHO global database on child growth and malnutrition. Geneva: WHO, 1997.

[12]   De Onis M, Blössner M. The World Health Organization global database on child growth and malnutrition: Methodology and applications. Int J Epidemiol 2003;32:518-26.

[13]   Habicht J-P, Martorell R, Yarbrough C, Malina R, Klein R. Height and weight standards for preschool children. How relevant are ethnic Differences in growth potential? Lancet 1974;1(7858):611-4.

[14]   Natsios A. The great North Korean famine. Washington DC: US Inst Peace Press; 2001.

[15]   Schwekendiek D, Pak S. Recent growth of children in the two Koreas: A meta-analysis. Econ Hum Biol 2009;7(1):109-12.

[16]   Pak S, Schwekendiek D, Kim HK. Height and living standards in North Korea, 1930s-1980s. Econ History Rev, in press.

[17]   Guntupalli A, Schwekendiek D. Is it better to live in urban areas? A worldwide study on the overall, rural and urban welfare of children. Paper presented at the 3rd Intl Conf Econ Hum Biol, Strasbourg 22-24 Jun 2006.

SECTION 3: DIABETES MELLITUS

In: Food, Nutrition and Eating Behavior
Editors: Joav Merrick and Sigal Israeli

ISBN: 978-1-62948-233-0
© 2014 Nova Science Publishers, Inc.

Chapter 8

ASYMPTOMATIC BACTERIURIA IN CHILDREN AND ADOLESCENTS WITH TYPE 1 DIABETES MELLITUS

Alphonsus N Onyiriuka, MD and Edirin O Yusuf, MD*

Department of Child Health and Department of Medical Microbiology,
University of Benin Teaching Hospital, Benin City, Nigeria

ABSTRACT

It is commonly believed that patients with diabetes mellitus are at increased risk of urinary tract infection compared with non-diabetic patients. Methods: Bacteriuria was screened for in 34 patients (17 with type 1 diabetes mellitus and 17 with non-diabetic endocrine disorders) at their regular follow-up visits using urine samples collected every three months for 12 months and cultured. The subjects were matched for age and sex. Results: Among the 34 patients screened, only two (one (5.9%) out of 17 diabetic and one (5.9%) out of 17 non-diabetic) had asymptomatic bacteriuria and the urine culture of each of them yielded a growth of Escherichia coli sensitive to gentamycin. The duration of diabetes in the girl with asymptomatic bacteriuria (ASB) was 7 years. She had a poor glycaemic control and some psychosocial challenges. Her pubertal maturation was delayed (Tanner Stage II at the age of 15 years and has not attained menarche). She weighed 29 Kg, with BMI of 16.0 kg/m^2 (< 5th percentile). In addition, she had vaginal candidiasis for which she was appropriately treated, using ketconazole. The other patient with ASB was a 7-year-old girl with precocious puberty due to congenital adrenal hyperplasia diagnosed at the age of 18 months. The two patients with ASB did not progress to symptomatic bacteriuria after a follow-up period of one year. Conclusion: The prevalence and incidence of asymptomatic bacteriuria in diabetic children and adolescents do not differ from those of their non-diabetic counterparts.

* Correspondence: Alphonsus N Onyiriuka, MD, Department of Child Health, University of Benin Teaching Hospital, PMB 1111, Benin City, Nigeria. E-mail: alpndiony@yahoo.com or didiruka@gmail.com.

INTRODUCTION

Asymptomatic bacteriuria refers to the presence of a positive urine culture in an asymptomatic person (1). It is commonly believed that individuals with diabetes mellitus are at increased risk of infection, particularly urinary tract infection (UTI) (2-4). Such an infection in diabetic patients may result in severe complications and death more frequently than would be anticipated among non-diabetics (2, 4). Most UTI in diabetic patients are relatively asymptomatic (4). Among diabetic patients, factors presumed to predispose to UTI include age, neurogenic bladder, duration of diabetes and degree of glycaemic control (2, 5). Some clinicians consider asymptomatic patients being screened for bacteriuria to be at risk of UTI if two or three consecutive cultures of freshly voided urine reveal more than 10^5 organisms/ml (6). Whether or not individuals with asymptomatic bacteriuria (ASB) should be treated with antibiotics remains debatable (4). It is recommended that ASB should be treated with antibiotics in pregnant women, children aged 5-6 years and prior to invasive genitourinary procedures (7).

It is not known with certainty whether individuals with diabetes mellitus are at a higher risk of bacteriuria than non-diabetics. Studies on this subject have yielded mixed results. For instance, Lindberg et al. (8) reported that three out of 304 (0.99%) girls and zero out of 337 boys with type 1 diabetes mellitus screened for bacteriuria were positive. They, therefore, concluded that the prevalence of ASB in diabetic children and adolescents did not differ from that of their non-diabetic peers. In contrast, a meta-analysis of published data involving 22 studies revealed that the prevalence of ASB was 12.2% in diabetic children compared with 4.5% in healthy controls (9). Point prevalence was also higher in children and adolescents with diabetes (12.9%) compared with their non-diabetic (2.7%) counterparts (9). A similar increased risk among diabetic children and adolescents was reported from Egypt (10). Some studies have concluded that screening for ASB in diabetic patients is warranted because it has been found to be a risk factor for developing symptomatic urinary tract infection (11). In a survey in Port Harcourt, Nigeria of secondary school students aged 10-17 years the prevalence of ASB was 6.5% and 4.5% in girls and boys respectively (12).

Despite the recognized potential of ASB in diabetic patients to cause renal damage and ultimately, chronic kidney disease, there is a general paucity of information in the literature on its incidence, particularly in developing countries. Besides, it is not known how often ASB progresses to symptomatic bacteriuria. In addition, infection itself can lead to poor diabetic control by increased secretion of counterregulatory hormones (glucagon, cortisol, growth hormone, catecholamines), inhibition of insulin secretion, and insulin resistance of peripheral tissues/increased cytokine secretion (13,14).

The purpose of the present chapter is to determine the incidence of ASB among children and adolescents with T1DM attending the Paediatric Endocrine-Metabolic Clinic, UBTH and compare the result with those of their non-diabetic peers.

OUR STUDY

The study was conducted in the Paediatric Endocrine-Metabolic Clinic of the University of Benin Teaching Hospital (UBTH), Benin City, Nigeria over a 12-month period for each of the subjects. The study was approved by UBTH Ethics and Research Committee. Consent was obtained from both the patient and their parents. Information sought from the subjects included age, sex, parents educational attainment, parents occupation, antibiotic use and duration of type 1 diabetes mellitus (T1DM). Patients with complaints suggestive of symptomatic urinary tract infection (such as dysuria, frequent micturiction, urgency, pain in the loin or suprapubic region) were excluded from the study. The socio-economic status of the parents of the subjects was determined using the classification suggested by Ogunlesi et al. (15). This was analyzed via combining the highest educational attainment, occupation and income of the parents (based on the mean income of each educational qualification and occupation). In this Social Classification System, classes I and II represent high social class, class III represents middle social class while classes IV and V represent low social class. In this way, the subjects were categorized into high, middle and low socio-economic groups.

A clean catch mid-stream urine specimen was obtained from each of the subjects every three months, over a total period of 12 months, amounting to four urine specimens per subject. In all the subjects, appropriate care was taken before collection of the urine specimen to avoid contamination. Each urine specimen was transported to the Research Laboratory, Department of Child Health, UBTH, where it was refrigerated immediately and cultured within two hours of collection. All the urine samples were cultured on Blood and MacConkey agar plates. The plates were incubated at 37 degree Celcius aerobically for 48 hours. Standard procedure was applied in the handling, staining, microscopy and culture of all the urine specimens (16). Full clinical examination was conducted on each of the patients at every visit. The presence of bacterial growth of 10^5 colony-forming units/ml was accepted as significant bacteriuria (17). Descriptive statistics such as frequencies, means, ratios, standard deviations, confidence intervals, percentages were used to describe all the variables.

FINDINGS

Two (one diabetic and one non-diabetic) out of the 34 patients screened for asymptomatic bacteriuria (ASB) had positive urine culture, giving a prevalence of 5.9% for diabetic and non-diabetic patients respectively. The urine culture of each case with significant asymptomatic yielded a growth of Escherichia coli sensitive to gentamycin. The diabetic patient was a 15-year-old girl diagnosed of type 1 diabetes mellitus 7 years ago. She had a poor glycaemic control and some psychosocial challenges. Her pubertal maturation was delayed (Tanner Stage II at the age of 15 years and has not attained menarche). She weighed 29 Kg, with BMI of 16.0 kg/m^2 (< 5th percentile). In addition, she had vaginal candidiasis for which she was appropriately treated, using ketoconazole. During the follow-up, appropriate urine samples were collected and screened every 3 months for 12 months for each of the patients but no other patient had significant asymptomatic bacteriuria. Neither of the two patients with significant asymptomatic bacteriuria progressed to symptomatic bacteriuria after one year of follow up. The mean age at presentation of the patients with diabetes was 11.0±4.2 years (95% Confidence Interval, CI=7.7-14.7) for boys; 13.5±1.6 years (95% CI=12.6-14.4) for girls; 12.8±2.9 years (95% CI=11.4-14.1) for both sexes combined. Mean age at presentation: boys versus girls t= 1.28 p>0.05. The age and gender distribution of the subjects is depicted in Table 1.The mean body mass index (BMI) was 18.6±2.5 kg/m^2 (95%

CI=17.4-19.8) with 6 (35.3%) having a BMI below 19.0 kg/m^2. None of the subjects had BMI > 25 kg/m^2. Over half of the families (52.9%) of the subjects were in the middle social class. Eleven point eight percent and 35.3% of the families of the subjects were in the high and low social classes respectively.

Table 1. Age and gender distribution of patients with diabetes mellitus

Age group at presentation	Gender		
	Male	Female	Both sexes
	No(%)	No(%)	No(%)
Below 10 years	2(33.3)	0(0)	2(11.8)
10-12 years	0(0)	3(27.3)	3(17.6)
13-15 years	3(50.0)	8(72.7)	11(64.7)
Above 15 years	(16.7)	0(0)	1(5.9)
Total	6(100.0)	11(100.0)	17(100.0)

DISCUSSION

The prevalence (5.9%) of asymptomatic bacteriuria (ASB) found in the present study is two- and five-fold lower than the 12.2% and 30.0% respectively reported from two different studies, one a meta-analysis of 22 studies and the other among diabetic Egyptian children and adolescents (9,10). Even, prevalence rates lower than that observed in the present study have been reported (8). All reflecting the reported mixed results of prevalence of ASB in children and adolescents, suggesting that some unidentified socio-demographic factors might influence the prevalence of ASB in these subjects. For instance, age, sex, glycaemic control, duration of diabetes and presence of long-term complications have all been variously reported as risk factors (2-4). The method of collection and processing of the urine specimens might have also influenced the different prevalence rates observed. The lower prevalence rate observed in the present study compared with the Egyptian study may partly be because of the differences in the age of the two study populations. Most of the subjects in the Egyptian study were older than 15 years while most the patient in the present study were below 15 years of age. This view is supported by the reports of two studies in Egypt and Hungary which separately showed the prevalence of ASB was higher in girls aged 15 years or older (10, 17). In consonance, the only diabetic patient with ASB in the present study was 15 years old. However, the prevalence from our data was within the range (4.5-6.5%) reported from Port Harcourt, Nigeria among non-diabetic secondary school students aged 6 to 15 years(11), suggesting that ASB is not commoner in diabetic compared with non-diabetic children and adolescents. This conclusion is reinforced by the results of the present study which showed that of the two patients with ASB one was diabetic and the other was non-diabetic. Furthermore, as reported by Rozsai et al. (14), the urinary cytokine response to pathogens in both diabetic and non-diabetic children with bacteriuria was comparable.

Consistent with previous reports, the most common bacterial agent in the present study was Escherichia coli (4, 10, 18). This finding is partly explained by the report of Geerlings et al. (19) which indicated that E coli expressing type 1 fimbrae adhere better to the uroepithelial cells of women with diabetes mellitus compared to the cells of women without diabetes mellitus. The girl with type 1 diabetes and ASB also had vaginal candidiasis which responded satisfactorily to treatment with ketoconazole. The finding of candidial infection in this adolescent with diabetes mellitus is not surprising as other investigators have reported a similar finding (20). The increased frequency of vaginal candidiasis in patients with diabetes mellitus is believed to be due to increase in ambient vaginal glycogen stores in them (20).

In conclusion, prevalence and incidence of asymptomatic bacteriuria do not differ between diabetic and non-diabetic children and adolescents.

REFERENCES

[1]   Ooi S, Frazee LA, Gardner WG. Management of asymptomatic bacteriuria in patients with diabetes mellitus. Ann Pharmacotherapy 2004;38(3):490-3.

[2]   Guillausseau PJ, Farah R, Laloi-Michelin M, Tielmans A, Rymer R, Warnet R. Urinary tract infections and diabetes mellitus. Rev Prat 2003;53(16):1790-6.

[3]   Funftuck R, Nicolle LE, Hanefeld M, Naser KG. Urinary tract infection in patients with diabetes mellitus. Clin Nephrol 2012;77(1):40-8.

[4]   Balachandar MS, Pavkovic P, Metelko Z. Kidney infections in diabetes mellitus. Diabetologia Croatica 2002;31(2):95-103.

[5]   Keane EH, Boyko EJ, Reller LB, Hamman RF. Prevalence of asymptomatic bacteriuria in subjects with NIDDM in San Luis Valley of Colorado. Diabetes Care 1988;11:708-12.

[6]   Rifkin RH. Urinary tract infection in childhood. Pediatrics 1977;60:508.

[7]   Raz R. Asymptomatic bacteriuria: Clinical significance and management. Int J Antimicrob Agents 2003;22(Suppl 2):45-7.

[8]   Lindberg U, Bergstrom AL, Carlsson E, Dahlquist G, Hermansson G, Larsson Y, et al. Urinary tract infection in children with type 1 diabetes. Acta Pediatr Scand 1985;74:85-8.

[9]   Renko M, Tapaainen P, Tossavainen P, Pokka T, Uhari M. Meta-analysis of the significance of asymptomatic bacteriuria in diabetes. Diabetes Care 2011;34(1):230-5.

[10]   Salem MA, Matler RM, Abdelmaksond AA, El Masry SA. Prevalence of asymptomatic bacteriuria in Egyptian children and adolescents with type 1 diabetes mellitus. J Egypt Soc Parasitol 2009;39(3):951-62.

[11]   Ribera MC, Pascual R, Barbar PC, Pederera V, Gil V. Incidence and risk factors associated with urinary tract infection in diabetic patients with or without asymptomatic bacteriuria. Eur J Clin Microbiol Infect Dis 2006;25:389-93.

[12]   Frank-Peterside N, Wokoma EC. Prevalence of asymptomatic bacteriuria in students of University of Port Harcourt Demonstration Secondary School. JASEM 2009;13:55-8.

[13]   Leibovici L, Yehehzkelli Y, Porter A et al. Influence of diabetes mellitus and glycaemic control on the characteristics and outcome of common infections. Diabet Med 1996;13:457-463.

[14]   Rozsai B, Lanyi E, Berki T, Soltesz G. Urinary cytokine response to asymptomatic bacteriuria in type 1 diabetic children and young adults. Pediatr Diabetes. 2006;7(3):153-8.

[15]   Ogunlesi TA, Dedeke IOF, Kuponiyi OT. Socio-economic classification of children attending Specialist Paediatric Centres in Ogun State, Nigeria. Nig Med Pract 2008; 54(1):21-5.

[16]   Collee JG, Duguid JP, Frasar AG. Laboratory strategy in the diagnosis of infective syndromes. In: Collee JG, Duguid JP, Frasar AG, Marmion DP, Simmon A eds. Mackie and McCarteney practical medical microbiology, 13 ed. Edinburgh: Churchill Livingstone, 1989:601-49.

[17]   Rozsai B, Lanyi E, Soltesz G. Asymptomatic bacteriuria and leucocytouria in type 1 diabetes children and young adults. Diabetes Care 2003;26(7):2209-10.

[18]   Makuyana D, Mhlabi D, Chipfupa M, Munyombwe T, Gwanzura L. Asymptomatic bacteriuria among outpatients with diabetes mellitus in urban black population. Cent Afr J Med 2002;48(7-8):78-82.

[19] Geerlings SE, Meiland R, Hoepelman AI. Pathogenesis of bacteriuria in women with diabetes mellitus. Int J Antimicrob Agents 2002;19(6):539-45.

[20] Rein MF, Holmes KK. Non-specific vaginitis, vulvovaginal candidiasis and trichomoniasis. Curr Clin Topics Infect Dis 1983;4:281.

In: Food, Nutrition and Eating Behavior
Editors: Joav Merrick and Sigal Israeli

ISBN: 978-1-62948-233-0
© 2014 Nova Science Publishers, Inc.

Chapter 9

THE EFFICACY, SAFETY AND TOLERABILITY OF DRUGS USED TO TREAT PAINFUL DIABETIC NEUROPATHY

John Edelsberg, MD, MPH, Claudia Lord, BA and Gerry Oster, PhD*

Policy Analysis Inc (PAI), Brookline, Massachusetts, US

Numerous drugs are used in clinical practice to treat patients with painful diabetic peripheral neuropathy (DPN). Their comparative efficacy, safety, and tolerability have not been well-documented. Objective. To evaluate systematically data from reports of placebo-controlled randomized trials (RCTs) on the efficacy, safety, and tolerability of drugs used to treat painful DPN. Methods. Using data from all published English-language reports of placebo-controlled RCTs of drugs for painful DPN, we compiled information on: 1) placebo-corrected % reduction in pain intensity from randomization to end of active treatment; 2) relative risk (RR) of withdrawal due to lack of efficacy; 3) RR of adverse events (AEs) and 4) RR of withdrawal due to AEs. When estimates were available from more than one trial for a given agent, we pooled data using meta-analysis. Significance of treatment effects versus placebo was based on Z scores. We identified 31 RCTs evaluating 14 different drugs in patients with painful DPN. Most trials were small (<200 patients). All agents were found to significantly reduce pain intensity (range: 8.0% [oxcarbazepine] to 26.4% [CR oxycodone]). RR of withdrawal due to lack of efficacy was significantly lower only for CR oxycodone and tramadol. Analysis of AEs was hampered by spotty and inconsistent reporting and wide variation in sample sizes. Conclusion. While all drugs that we examined were efficacious in painful DPN, available trial data provide only limited guidance regarding optimal therapy, due to small sample sizes, incomplete reporting of AEs, and no published reports of placebo-controlled RCTs of tricyclic antidepressants.

---

* Correspondence: Gerry Oster, PhD, Policy Analysis Inc (PAI), 4 Davis Court, Brookline, MA 02445 United States. E-mail: goster@pai2.com.

INTRODUCTION

Neuropathic pain is caused by dysfunction of the peripheral nerves or, less frequently, the central nervous system. Many neuropathic pain syndromes are recognized; most are named after the diseases with which they are associated (e.g., diabetic neuropathy, post-herpetic neuralgia). Different pain mechanisms may be involved in the different neuropathic pain syndromes, including peripheral sensitization, transcriptional and post-transcriptional regulation in sensory neurons (resulting in ectopic excitability), central sensitization, augmented facilitation, structural reorganization, and disinhibition (1). Multiple mechanisms appear to be at work in any given syndrome, and many mechanisms play important roles in several common syndromes (2).

Neuropathic pain is typically difficult to treat. Nonsteroidal anti-inflammatory drugs (NSAIDs) are generally ineffective (3). While opioids have demonstrated efficacy in clinical trials, they usually are not considered first-line therapy because of concerns about addiction and their relatively poor adverse-effect profiles. Even antidepressants and anticonvulsants, which have been the mainstays of pharmacologic treatment, have limited efficacy. Finding a satisfactory agent for the treatment of neuropathic pain can be a complex process, involving trials of several different agents and requiring dose titration to maximize analgesia while maintaining an acceptable level of adverse events. Patients not responding to pharmacotherapy may receive nontraditional therapy, such as acupuncture.

Most randomized controlled trials of agents used to treat neuropathic pain have been small (i.e., involving fewer than 100 patients), and only a handful have compared two active treatments, almost always with inconclusive results. Consequently, individual trials provide little evidence-based guidance as to the best medications for the treatment of neuropathic pain. To address this issue, several groups of investigators have conducted systematic reviews, in which the results of trials of the same agents (or groups of agents assumed to be essentially similar) have been combined using techniques of meta-analysis to yield overall estimates of efficacy. Most of these systematic reviews have been flawed because they have ignored the heterogeneity of both neuropathic pain syndromes and pharmacological mechanisms among the drugs studied (4), and hence combined data from trials involving patients with different neuropathic pain syndromes (e.g., all types of neuropathic pain, both peripheral and central) and across broad classes of drugs with different mechanisms of action (e.g., all anti-epileptic agents). In addition, most of these prior reviews have ignored heterogeneity of outcome measures and combined the results of trials utilizing numeric and verbal measures of pain relief, as well as those using composite neuropathy scales that include components not directly linked to pain.

In this chapter, we systematically review data from randomized controlled trials on the efficacy, safety, and tolerability of drugs used to treat painful diabetic neuropathy (DPN), a single type of neuropathic pain that has been the subject of more clinical trials of drugs than any other type of neuropathic pain. While we realize that there is no overwhelming biological rationale for confining our analysis to a single diagnostic entity (since even within this entity, there may be considerable variation between patients in the relative importance of different mechanisms of neuropathic pain), we believe that this variability is less than that which would occur if drug efficacy were examined across multiple neuropathic pain syndromes. We also note that several other reviews (discussed below) have focused on painful DPN. To standardize the assessment of efficacy across studies, we focused on a single primary outcome measure namely, the percentage reduction in pain intensity from baseline to end of study, as measured by a visual analogue scale (VAS) or a numeric rating scale (NRS). In instances where more than one trial is available for a given drug, we have combined results using techniques of meta-analysis. In some respects, we have followed the methodology of two prior meta-analyses that pooled results on the basis of the difference in the mean reduction in VAS pain between the intervention and placebo groups (5, 6).

OUR STUDY

The Medline (1950-2009) and Embase (1974-2009) search engines were used to identify all English-language published original reports of findings from placebo-controlled randomized trials on the efficacy, tolerability, and safety of oral and topical drugs in patients with neuropathic pain. The Medline database was searched with the subject headings (explode mode), "neuralgia" and "diabetic neuropathies", as well as a keyword search on "neuropathic pain". Subject headings that were used to search the Embase database included: 1) "neuralgia"; 2) "neuropathic pain"; 3) "diabetic neuropathy" and 4)"polyneuropathy". We excluded published reports if they concerned: 1) drugs administered in combination with another treatment modality (e.g., acupuncture); 2) drugs administered other than orally or topically; 3) drugs no longer used to treat neuropathic pain (e.g., dextromethorphan) and 4) over-the-counter agents and food supplements. We also excluded reports of clinical trials with treatment duration less than four weeks, and those that involved the treatment of neuropathic pain that was experimentally induced in healthy volunteers.

Searches under subject headings and keywords that did not include the terms "pain" or "neuralgia" (e.g., "diabetic neuropathy") were limited to articles that included the keyword "pain." Searches under subject headings and keywords that might include both nociceptive and neuropathic pain were limited to reports that included the keyword "neuropathic pain." In both the Medline and Embase databases, searches also were conducted under the names of specified drugs, either as subject headings (exploded) or keywords, as appropriate; these drug-oriented searches were limited to those studies that included the keyword "pain." We also searched the most current version of the Cochrane Central Register of Controlled Trials (CENTRAL) as well as all reference lists from identified trial reports and review articles--for reports of RCTs not otherwise identified. From all clinical trials that were identified using these broad criteria, we excluded those that did not focus exclusively on patients with painful DPN or that did not provide results for a subgroup of patients with painful DPN in stratified analyses. A Jadad quality score was calculated for each selected study (7, 8).

A data extraction form was developed for the purpose of recording relevant information from identified qualifying trial reports; data were independently extracted from each report by two reviewers. A unique data extraction form was completed for each RCT identified in the search. Information from completed forms was entered into an Excel database; two independent databases were created (one for each abstractor), and the two databases were compared for discrepancies. When discrepancies were noted between the two abstractors, the information in question was reviewed again by both abstractors as well as the study manager to achieve consensus. Reconciliation was achieved in all cases.

Outcome measures

The principal measure of efficacy from each trial report was the difference between active agent and placebo in the percentage reduction in pain intensity from randomization to end of active treatment, as measured by a NRS, VAS, or other interval-level scale. If the authors of a particular study reported percentage reductions from baseline, these estimates were used. Otherwise, we calculated these values for both active agent and placebo, based on baseline pain intensity and pain intensity at the end of active treatment. If a standard error (or standard deviation) was not reported for the percentage reduction from baseline, we imputed one based on the average coefficient of variation (the standard deviation divided by the effect size) of those studies that did report a standard error (or standard deviation).

We also examined an alternative measure of efficacy—namely, relative risk (RR) of withdrawal due to lack of efficacy (from those trials providing this information)—which we calculated as the percentage of patients in the active treatment arm who withdrew due to lack of efficacy divided by the percentage of patients randomized to placebo who withdrew for this reason. When risk of withdrawal was reported as zero for either active agent or placebo, we substituted the value 0.5 in the numerator of the risk fraction to calculate RR.

We compared tolerability based on RR of withdrawal due to adverse events (again, in those trials providing such information). RR of withdrawal due to adverse events was calculated as the percentage of patients in the active treatment arm who withdrew/ discontinued due to adverse events divided by the percentage of placebo-treated patients who withdrew for this reason.

Serious adverse events are rarely reported in randomized trials of drugs for neuropathic pain. Therefore, we evaluated safety in terms of RR (active agent vs. placebo) of the 10 most frequently reported adverse events among the agents of interest.

Analyses

In analyses of cross-over trials, data from the first treatment period only were considered (if available). For trials using more than one dose of an agent of interest, the highest currently approved dose in the US or Europe was selected. For trials assessing outcomes at different points in time (e.g., weekly, mid-trial), we examined only the change from baseline to the end of active treatment. In those instances in which the measures of interest were reported in more than one trial of a given agent, a pooled estimate of effect was calculated using techniques of meta-analysis. Fixed- or random-effects models were employed based on the results of tests of heterogeneity (χ^2 and I^2 tests). Test for overall effect of each agent versus placebo were based on a Z-score. Analyses were conducted using the computer program, MIX (www.mix-for-meta-analysis.info). Similar analyses were conducted for all measures reported as RRs.

Table 1. Randomized double-blind placebo-controlled clinical trials

Source	Trial Design/Duration	Intervention (No. of Patients)	Dose	Jadad Quality Score	Initial Mean Pain Intensity	Final Mean Pain Intensity
Tandan et al., 1992 (ref. 9)	Parallel/8-wk	Capsaicin (11) Placebo (11)	0.075% cream vehicle cream	4	VAS: NR VAS: NR	VAS: NR* VAS: NR*
Scheffler et al., 1991 (ref. 10)	Parallel/8-wk	Capsaicin (28) Placebo (26)	0.075% cream vehicle cream	3	VAS: 76.80 VAS: 72.80	VAS: NR* VAS: NR*
Wernicke et al., 2006 (ref. 11)	Parallel/12-wk	Duloxetine (114) Placebo (108)	60 mg/d	5	NRS: 6.10 NRS: 5.90	NRS: 3.38 NRS: 4.51
Raskin et al., 2005 (ref. 12)	Parallel/12-wk	Duloxetine (116) Placebo (116)	60 mg/d	4	NRS: 5.50 NRS: 5.50	NRS: 3.00 NRS: 3.90
Goldstein et al., 2005 (ref. 13)	Parallel/12-wk	Duloxetine (115) Placebo (115)	60 mg/d	4	NRS: 6.00 NRS: 5.80	NRS: 3.11 NRS: 3.89
Backonja et al., 1998 (ref. 14)	Parallel/8-wk	Gabapentin (84) Placebo (81)	Titrated from 900-3600 mg/d or max tolerated dosage	4	NRS: 6.40 NRS: 6.50	NRS: 3.90 NRS: 5.10
Simpson, 2001 (ref. 15)	Parallel/8-wk	Gabapentin (27) Placebo (27)	Titrated from 300-3200 mg/d or max tolerated dosage	4	NRS: 6.40 NRS: 6.50	NRS: 4.00 NRS: 6.00
Vinik et al., 2007 (study 1) (ref. 16)	Parallel/12-wk	Lamotrigine (90) Placebo (90)	400 mg/d with 7-wk dose-escalation phase	4	NRS: 6.20 NRS: 6.30	NRS: 3.30 NRS: 4.30
Eisenberg et al., 2001 (ref. 17)	Parallel/6-wk	Lamotrigine (27) Placebo (26)	Titrated from 25-400 mg/d over 4 weeks	3	NRS: 6.40 NRS: 6.60	NRS: 4.20 NRS: 5.30
Vinik et al., 2007 (study 2) (ref. 16)	Parallel/12-wk	Lamotrigine (87) Placebo (86)	400 mg/d with a 7-wk dose escalation phase	4	NRS: 6.50 NRS: 6.10	NRS: 3.80 NRS: 4.50
Beydoun et al., 2006 (ref. 18)	Parallel/16-wk	Oxcarbazepine (87) Placebo (89)	Titrated from 300-1200 mg/d over 4 weeks or max tolerated dose	4	VAS: 75.70 VAS: 70.80	VAS: 46.70 VAS: 51.70

mg/d: milligrams per day
NRS: 11-point Numeric Rating Scale
wk: week
VAS: Visual Analogue Scale
NR: Not reported
* Percentage (%) change from baseline reported

Table 1. (Continued)

Source	Trial Design/Duration	Intervention (No. of Patients)	Dose	Jadad Quality Score	Initial Mean Pain Intensity	Final Mean Pain Intensity
Dogra et al., 2005 (ref. 19)	Parallel/16-wk	Oxcarbazepine (69)	Titrated from 300-1200 mg/d over 4 weeks or max tolerated dose	4	VAS: 71.50	VAS: 47.20
		Placebo (77)			VAS: 74.30	VAS: 59.60
Grosskopf et al., 2006 (ref. 20)	Parallel/16-wk	Oxcarbazepine (71)	Titrated from 300-1200 mg/d over 4 weeks or max tolerated dose	4	VAS: 72.00	VAS: 49.61
		Placebo (70)			VAS: 70.70	VAS: 50.97
Arezzo et al., 2008 (ref. 21)	Parallel/13-wk	Pregabalin (82)	Titrated from 150 mg/d to 600mg/d over the first week	3	NRS: 6.28	NRS: 3.54
		Placebo (85)			NRS: 6.58	NRS: 4.82
Freynhagen et al., 2005 (ref. 22)	Parallel/12-wk	Pregabalin (132)	600mg/d	4	NRS: 6.70	NRS: 3.10
		Placebo (65)			NRS: 6.60	NRS: 4.40
Lesser et al., 2004 (ref. 23)	Parallel/5-wk	Pregabalin (81)	600 mg/d titrated over 6 days	4	NRS: 6.20	NRS: 3.80
		Placbo (97)			NRS: 6.60	NRS: 5.06
Richter et al., 2005 (ref. 24)	Parallel/6-wk	Pregabalin (82)	Titrated from 100 mg/d to 600 mg/d for first 2 weeks and fixed thereafter	3	NRS: 6.70	NRS: 4.30
		Placebo (85)			NRS: 6.90	NRS: 5.80
Rosenstock et al., 2004 (ref. 25)	Parallel/8-wk	Pregabalin (76)	300 mg/d	4	NRS: 6.50	NRS: 4.00
		Placebo (70)			NRS: 6.10	NRS: 5.30
Tölle et al., 2007 (ref. 26)	Parallel/12-wk	Pregabalin (101)	600 mg/d	3	NRS: 6.60	NRS: 3.70
		Placebo (96)			NRS: 6.40	NRS: 4.50
Raskin et al., 2004 (ref. 27)	Parallel/12-wk	Topiramate (208)	Titrated from 25-400 mg/d over 12-week study period	4	VAS: 68.00	VAS: 46.20
		Placebo (109)			VAS: 69.10	VAS: 54.00
Gimbel et al., 2003 (ref. 28)	Parallel/6-wk	CR oxycodone (82)	Titrated from 20-120 mg/d	5	NRS: 6.90	NRS: 4.90
		Placebo (77)			NRS: 6.80	NRS: 5.90
Watson et al., 2003 (ref. 29)	Crossover/8-wk	CR oxycodone (36)	Titrated from 10-80 mg/d	3	VAS: 67.00	VAS: 21.80
		Active Placebo (36)	Benztropine titrated from 0.25-2.0 mg/d		VAS: 67.00	VAS: 48.60

mg/d: milligrams per day
NRS: 11-point Numeric Rating Scale
VAS: Visual Analogue Scale
wk: week
NR: Not reported
* Percentage (%) change from baseline reported

Source	Trial Design/Duration	Intervention (No. of Patients)	Dose	Jadad Quality Score	Initial Mean Pain Intensity	Final Mean Pain Intensity
Atli and Dogra, 2005 (ref. 30)	Parallel/12-wk	Zonisamide (13)	Titrated from 100-600 mg/d over 6 weeks or until max tolerated dose	3	VAS: 58.90	VAS: 41.20
		Placebo (12)			VAS: 63.90	VAS: 57.00
Freeman et al., 2007 (ref. 31)	Parallel/6-wk	Tramadol (160)	37.5 mg/d	3	NRS: 7.13	NRS: 4.43
		Placebo (152)			NRS: 7.12	NRS: 5.29
Agrawal et al., 2009 (study 1) (ref. 32)	Parallel/12-wk	Sodium valproate (20)	20 mg/kg/day	5	NRS: 8.00	NRS: 6.15
		Placebo (21)			NRS: 7.35	NRS: 6.90
Kochar et al., 2004 (ref. 33)	Parallel/12-wk	Sodium valproate (21)	500 mg/d	4	NRS: 6.00	NRS: 3.00
		Placebo (18)			NRS: 5.71	NRS: 6.00
Agrawal et al., 2009 (study 2) (ref. 32)	Parallel/12-wk	Glyceryl trinitrate spray (20)	0.4 mg/day	5	NRS: 7.75	NRS: 4.95
		Placebo (21)			NRS: 7.35	NRS: 6.90
Agrawal et al., 2007 (ref. 34)	Crossover/4-wk	Glyceryl trinitrate spray (22)	0.4 mg/d	4	NRS: 7.18	NRS: 4.68
		Placbo (21)			NRS: 7.57	NRS: 6.90
Kadiroglu et al., 2008 (ref. 35)	Parallel/8-wk	Venlafaxine (30)	75 mg	2	NRS: 7.20	NRS: 3.10
		Placebo (30)			NRS: 7.40	NRS: 5.50
Rowbotham et al., 2004 (ref. 36)	Parallel/6-wk	Venlafaxine (82)	ER150-225	5	VAS: 67.30	VAS: 33.50
		Placebo (81)			VAS: 68.80	VAS: 50.10
Wymer et al., 2009 (ref. 37)	Parallel/18-wk	Lacosamide (91)	400 mg/d	5	NRS: 6.50	NRS: 4.00
		Placebo (93)			NRS: 6.60	NRS: 4.80

mg/d: milligrams per day
NRS: 11-point Numeric Rating Scale
VAS: Visual Analogue Scale
wk: week
NR: Not reported
* Percentage (%) change from baseline reported

John Edelsberg, Claudia Lord and Gerry Oster

FINDINGS

Table 2. Percentage reduction in pain intensity DPN

Source	N	Treatment % Reduction in Pain Intensity, Mean (SE%)	N	Placebo % Reduction in Pain Intensity, Mean (SE%)	Weighted Mean Difference (95% CI)		Weights, %
Capsaicin							
Tandan et al., 1992 (ref. 9)	11	16.00 (5.51)	11	4.10 (1.87)	11.90 (8.46, 15.34)		29.96
Scheffler et al., 1991 (ref. 10)	28	49.10 (2.66)	26	16.50 (5.26)	32.60 (30.35, 34.85)		70.04
Total (95% CI)	39		37		26.40 (24.52, 28.28)		100
Test for Heterogeneity: $\chi^2 = 97.50$ (P<0.0001), $I^2 = 98.97\%$							
Test for Overall Effect: Z= 17.61							
Duloxetine							
Wernicke et al., 2006 (ref. 11)	114	44.59 (3.85)	108	23.56 (4.27)	21.03 (19.96, 22.10)		28.97
Raskin et al., 2005 (ref. 12)	116	45.45 (3.43)	116	29.09 (3.62)	16.36 (15.45, 17.27)		40.38
Goldstein et al., 2005 (ref. 13)	114	48.17 (3.92)	115	32.93 (4.12)	15.24 (14.20, 16.28)		30.65
Total (95% CI)	344		339		17.37 (16.79, 17.95)		100
Test for Heterogeneity: $\chi^2 = 65.65$ (P<0.0001), $I^2 = 96.95\%$							
Test for Overall Effect: Z= 59.03							
Gabapentin							
Backonja et al., 1998 (ref. 14)	84	39.06 (4.86)	81	21.54 (3.61)	17.52 (16.22, 18.82)		85.93
Simpson, 2001 (ref. 15)	27	37.50 (8.24)	27	7.69 (2.23)	29.81 (26.59, 33.03)		14.07
Total (95% CI)	111		108		19.25 (18.04, 20.46)		100
Test for Heterogeneity: $\chi^2 = 48.09$ (P<0.0001), $I^2 = 97.92\%$							
Test for Overall Effect: Z= 31.23							
Lamotrigine							
Vinik et al., 2007 (ref. 16)	90	46.77 (5.63)	90	31.75 (5.05)	15.02 (13.46, 16.58)		21.9
Eisenberg et al., 2001 (ref. 17)	27	34.38 (1.87)	26	19.70 (1.94)	14.68 (13.65, 15.71)		50.74
Vinik et al., 2007 (ref. 16)	87	41.54 (5.08)	86	26.23 (4.27)	15.31 (13.91, 16.71)		27.36
Total (95% CI)	204		202		15.05 (14.58, 15.51)		100
Test for Heterogeneity: $\chi^2 = 0.90$ (P0.64), $I^2 = 0\%$							
Test for Overall Effect: Z= 63.62							
Oxcarbazepine							
Beydoun et al., 2006 (ref. 18)	87	38.20(4.67)	89	27.10 (4.33)	11.10 (9.77, 12.43)		40.32
Droga et al., 2005 (ref. 19)	69	33.99 (4.90)	77	19.78 (4.39)	14.20 (12.70, 15.73)		31.09
Grosskopf et al., 2006 (ref. 20)	71	27.90 (3.78)	70	31.10 (5.61)	-3.20 (-4.78, -1.62)		28.58
Total (95% CI)	227		236		7.98 (7.13, 8.83)		100
Test for Heterogeneity: $\chi^2 = 278.02$ (P<0.0001), $I^2 = 99.28\%$							
Test for Overall Effect: Z= 18.50							
Pregabalin							
Arezzo et al., 2008 (ref.21)	82	43.63 (5.50)	85	26.75 (4.38)	16.88 (15.37, 18.39)		12.49
Freynhagen et al., 2005 (ref. 22)	132	53.73 (5.34)	65	34.33 (6.43)	19.40 (17.59, 21.21)		8.71
Lesser et al., 2004 (ref. 23)	82	41.94 (4.02)	97	23.33 (3.64)	18.61 (17.48, 19.74)		22.25
Richter et al., 2005 (ref. 24)	82	35.82 (4.51)	85	15.94 (2.61)	19.88 (18.76, 21.00)		22.63
Rosenstock et al., 2004 (ref. 25)	76	38.46 (5.04)	70	13.11 (2.37)	25.35 (24.09, 26.61)		17.92
Tölle et al., 2008 (ref. 26)	101	43.94 (4.99)	96	29.69 (4.57)	14.25 (12.92, 15.59)		16.00
Total (95% CI)	555		498		19.26 (18.73, 19.79)		100
Test for Heterogeneity: $\chi^2 = 155.55$ (P<0.0001), $I^2 = 96.79\%$							
Test for Overall Effect: Z= 70.68							
Topiramate							
Raskin et al., 2004 (ref. 27)	214	32.06 (2.50)	109	21.85 (3.16)	10.21 (8.92, 11.49)		100

-10   0   10   20   30   40   50

Weighted Mean Difference, 95% CI

Source	N	Treatment % Reduction in Pain Intensity, Mean (SE%)	N	Placebo % Reduction in Pain Intensity, Mean (SE%)	Weighted Mean Difference (95% CI)		Weights, %
CR Oxycodone							
Gimbel et al., 2003 (ref. 28)	82	28.99 (3.69)	77	13.24 (3.87)	15.75 (14.57, 16.93)		85.88
Watson et al., 2003 (ref. 29)	36	67.46 (5.29)	36	27.46 (7.14)	40.00 (37.10, 42.90)		14.12
Total (95% CI)	118		113		19.17 (18.08, 20.26)		100
Test for Heterogeneity: χ² = 230.25 (P<0.0001), I² = 99.57%							
Test for Overall Effect: Z= 34.46							
Zonisamide							
Atli and Droga, 2005 (ref. 30)	13	30.05 (10.46)	12	10.80 (11.58)	19.25 (11.07, 21.44)		100
Tramadol							
Freeman et al., 2007 (ref. 31)	160	37.87 (3.42)	152	25.70 (3.15)	12.17 (10.30, 12.70)		100
Sodium Valproate							
Agrawal et al., 2009 (ref. 32)	20	23.13 (4.36)	21	6.12 (4.56)	17.01 (14.28, 19.74)		98.96
Kochar et al., 2004 (ref. 33)	21	50.00 (38.89)	18	-5.08 (44.91)	55.08 (28.49, 81.67)		1.04
Total (95% CI)	41		39		17.41 (14.69, 20.12)		100
Test for Heterogeneity: χ² = 7.79 (P=0.005), I² =87.17%							
Test for Overall Effect: Z= 12.56							
Glyceryl trinitrate spray							
Agrawal et al., 2009 (ref. 32)	20	39.06 (2.96)	21	21.54 (3.37)	17.52 (15.58, 19.46)		58.25
Agrawal et al., 2007 (ref. 34)	22	27.82 (4.26)	21	21.91 (3.37)	5.92 (3.62, 8.20)		41.75
Total (95% CI)	42		42		12.67 (11.19, 14.15)		100
Test for Heterogeneity: χ² = 57.49 (P<0.0001), I² =98.26%							
Test for Overall Effect: Z= 16.78							
Venlafaxine							
Kadiroglu et al., 2008 (ref. 35)	30	56.94 (4.42)	30	25.68 (4.12)	31.26 (29.10, 33.42)		37.98
Rowbotham et al., 2004 (ref. 36)	82	50.22 (6.33)	81	27.18 (4.56)	23.04 (21.35, 24.73)		62.02
Total (95% CI)	112		111		26.16 (24.83, 27.50)		100
Test for Heterogeneity: χ² = 34.43 (P<0.0001), I² =97.10%							
Test for Overall Effect: Z= 38.48							
Lacosamide							
Wymer et al., 2009 (ref. 37)	91	38.46 (4.60)	93	27.27 (4.27)	11.19 (10.73, 12.65)		100

-10 0 10 20 30 40 50
Weighted Mean Difference, 95% CI

We identified a total of 31 RCTs of agents used to treat painful DPN (see table 1). Multiple trials were available for most agents: pregabalin (n=6), duloxetine (n=3), oxcarbazepine (n=3),) lamotrigine (n=3), gabapentin (n=2), controlled-release (CR) oxycodone (n=2), venlafaxine (2), lacosamide (2), glyceryl trinitrate (2); sodium valproate (2), and capsaicin (n=2) (a single study only was available for tramadol, topiramate, and zonisamide, respectively). With the exception of three studies, all were published in calendar year 2001 or later. Most clinical trials were relatively small; only the three duloxetine studies, the topiramate study, and the tramadol study included more than 200 patients in the two treatment arms considered in our analysis.

The difference (intervention minus placebo) in the percentage reduction in pain intensity varied from 7.98% (oxcarbazepine) to 26.4% (CR oxycodone) (see table 2). All treatment effects were statistically significant (i.e., 95% confidence interval [CI] did not contain zero). For our secondary measure of efficacy (i.e., withdrawal due to lack of efficacy), RRs varied from 0.11 (CR oxycodone) to 1.15 (oxcarbazepine), among those drugs for which this outcome was reported (see table 3); however, only those for CR oxycodone (0.11) and tramadol (0.33) were statistically significant (i.e., 95% CIs did not contain the value 1.0).

Table 3. Relative risk of withdrawal due to lack of efficacy

Source	Treatment n/N	Placebo n/N	RR (95% CI)		Weights, %
Capsaicin					
Tandan et al., 1992 (ref. 9)	NR	NR			
Scheffler et al., 1991 (ref. 10)	NR	NR			
Duloxetine					
Wernicke et al., 2006 (ref. 11)	1/114	5/108	0.19 (0.02, 1.60)		51.05
Raskin et al., 2005 (ref. 12)	NR	NR			
Goldstein et al., 2005 (ref. 13)	1/115	4/115	0.25 (0.03, 2.20)		48.95
Total (95% CI)	2/229	9/223	0.22 (0.05, 1.00)		100
Test for Heterogeneity: χ^2=0.03 (p=0.86), I^2=0%					
Test for Overall Effect: Z=1.98					
Gabapentin					
Backonja et al., 1992 (ref. 14)	1/84	5/81	0.19 (0.02, 1.62)		62.09
Simpson, 2001 (ref. 15)	1/27	1/27	1.00 (0.07, 1518)		37.91
Total (95% CI)	2/111	6/108	0.36 (0.07, 1.92)		100
Test for Heterogeneity: χ^2=0.87 (p=0.35), I^2=0%					
Test for Overall Effect: Z=1.20					
Lamotrigine					
Vinik et al., 2007 (ref. 16)	NR	NR			
Eisenberg et al., 2001 (ref. 17)	NR	NR			
Vinik et al., 2007 (ref. 16)	NR	NR			
Oxcarbazepine					
Beydoun et al., 2006 (ref. 18)	4/87	2/89	2.05 (0.38, 10.88)		41.09
Dogra et al., 2005 (ref. 19)	0/69	2/77	0.28 (0.01, 6.08)		12.09
Grosskopf et al., 2006 (ref. 20)	3/71	3/70	0.99 (0.21, 4.72)		46.82
Total (95% CI)	7/227	7/236	1.10 (0.40, 3.03)		100
Test for Heterogeneity: χ^2=1.31 (p=0.52), I^2=0%					
Test for Overall Effect: Z=0.24					
Pregabalin					
Arezzo et al., 2008 (ref. 21)	4/82	8/85	0.52 (0.16, 1.66)		12.24
Freynhagen et al., 2005 (ref. 22)	33/132	19/65	0.86 (0.53, 1.38)		71.65
Lesser et al., 2004 (ref. 23)	NR	NR			
Richter et al., 2005 (ref. 24)	1/82	1/85	1.04 (0.07, 16.30)		2.17
Rosenstock et al., 2004 (ref. 25)	1/76	3/70	0.31 (0.03, 2.88)		3.29
Tölle et al., 2007 (ref. 26)	3/101	11/96	0.26 (0.08, 0.90)		10.64
Total (95% CI)	42/473	42/401	0.69 (0.46, 1.030)		100
Test for Heterogeneity: χ^2=3.96 (p=0.41), I^2=0%					
Test for Overall Effect: Z=1.81					
Topiramate					
Raskin et al., 2004 (ref. 27)	31/208	16/109	1.02 (0.58, 1.77)		100
CR Oxycodone					
Gimbel et al., 2003 (ref. 28)	1/82	11/77	0.09 (0.01, 0.65)		50.50
Watson et al., 2003 (ref. 29)	1/36	7/36	0.14 (0.02, 1.10)		49.50
Total (95% CI)	2/118	18/113	0.11 (0.03, 0.45)		100
Test for Heterogeneity: χ^2=0.12 (p=0.73), I^2=0%					
Test for Overall Effect: Z=3.00					
Zonisamide					
Atli and Dogra, 2005 (ref. 30)	NR	NR			
Tramadol					
Freeman et al., 2007 (ref. 31)	8/160	23/152	0.33 (0.15, 0.72)		100
Sodium Valproate					
Agrawal et al., 2009 (ref. 32)	0/20	1/21	0.53 (0.02, 14.80)		64.44
Kochar et al., 2004 (33)	0/21	0/18	0.86 (0.02, 41.05)		35.56
Total (95% CI)	0/41	1/39	0.64 (0.05, 7.92)		100
Test for Heterogeneity: χ^2=0.04 (p=0.85), I^2=0%					
Test for Overall Effect: Z=0.35					

0.01   0.1   1   10   100

Relative Risk, CI%

Source	Treatment n/N	Placebo n/N	RR (95% CI)		Weights, %
Glyceryl trinitrate spray					
Agrawal et al., 2009 (ref. 32)	0/20	0/21	1.05 (0.02, 50.43)		50.03
Agrawal et al., 2007 (ref. 34)	0/22	0/21	0.95 (0.02, 45.95)		49.97
Total (95% CI)	0/42	0/42	1.00 (0.07, 15.47)		100.00
Test for Heterogeneity: χ²=0.00 (p=0.97), I²=0%					
Test for Overall Effect: Z=0.00					
Venlafaxine					
Kadiroglu et al., 2008 (ref. 35)	NR	NR			
Rowbotham et al., 2004 (ref. 36)	3/82	5/81	0.59 (0.15, 2.40)		100.00
Lacosamide					
Wymer et al., 2009 (ref. 37)	1/91	2/93	0.51 (0.05, 5.54)		100.00

```
              0.01   0.1    1    10   100
                   Relative Risk, CI%
```

NR: Not Reported.

RR of withdrawal due to adverse events ranged from 9.6 (zonisamide) to 1.2 (tramadol), and were statistically significant (i.e., 95% CIs did not contain the value 1.0) for six agents: pregabalin (RR=3.6), oxcarbazepine (RR=3.1), topiramate (RR=3.0), lacosamide (RR=2.7), duloxetine (RR=2.1) and lamotrigine (RR=1.8) (Table 4).

Adverse events were erratically and inconsistently reported (appendix available from the authors upon request). Agents and adverse events for which RRs were significantly different than placebo were as follows: 1) duloxetine -- dizziness (RR=2.01, 95% CI: 1.09-3.72), nausea (2.72, 1.32-5.60), somnolence (3.11, 1.30-7.46), diarrhea (6.16, 1.42-26.66), and fatigue (4.42, 1.31-14.96); 2) gabapentin -- dizziness (5.04, 2.03-12.64) and somnolence (3.99, 1.70-9.35); 3) lamotrigine headache (2.28, 1.28-4.08); 4) oxcarbazepine -- dizziness (5.60, 2.18-14.39) and nausea (2.86, 1.20-6.79); 5) pregabalin -- dizziness (5,54, 3.71-8.29), somnolence (5.07, 2.97-8.67), dry mouth (3.08, 1.24-7.70), and asthenia (3.83, 1.71-8.56); 6) topiramate -- dizziness (3.11, 1.51-6.38) and diarrhea (3.14, 1.11-8.83); 7) CR oxycodone -- dizziness (2.87, 1.52-5.39), nausea (2.98, 1.29-6.91), vomiting (4.69, 1.51-14.56), constipation (3.06, 1.81-5.15), and dry mouth (4.72, 1.90-11.82); 8) tramadol -- dizziness (4.75, 1.06-21.33), nausea (3.61, 1.38-9.43), and somnolence (4.75, 1.06-21.33); and 9) venlafaxine -- somnolence (14.82, 2.00-109.58). We note that absence of a significant finding for a particular drug and adverse event simply may reflect failure to report such information. For example, the highest risk of withdrawal due to adverse events was reported in the zonisamide study, but individual adverse events were not reported. Lack of statistical significance also may reflect small numbers of patients and inadequate statistical power; RR of constipation with tramadol, for instance, was nominally high (RR=3.80) but not significantly different than placebo (95%CI: 0.82, 17.61).

DISCUSSION

We undertook a systematic review of data from reports of placebo-controlled, randomized trials of oral and topical agents used to treat painful DPN that were published between 1950 and 2009. Only two agents were found to have a 20% or greater reduction in pain intensity versus placebo--capsaicin (28.9%) and venlafaxine (26.16%). Reductions in pain intensity for the other agents ranged from 8% to 19%; all were significantly better than placebo. In terms of our secondary measure of efficacy, RR of withdrawal due to lack of efficacy, only the two opioids were found to be statistically superior to placebo: CR oxycodone (RR=0.11, 95% CI .03-.47) and tramadol (0.33, 0.15-0.72); the result for duloxetine was of borderline significance (0.22, 0.05-1.00).

Our examination of findings with respect to safety is less complete than that of efficacy due to highly variable reporting of adverse events in individual studies. The highest significant RRs of withdrawal due to adverse events were reported for oxcarbazepine, pregabalin, and topiramate, while the drugs with the greatest number of adverse events significantly different from placebo were CR oxycodone (n=5) and duloxetine (n=5).

One major limitation of our study is the assumption that all studies were of sufficiently similar design to permit meta-analysis of the data. In fact, differences among the study populations may explain some of the differences in results across trials of different drugs and among studies of the same drug. Mean pain intensity at baseline, for example, varied from 5.7 (NRS) to 8.0 (NRS) (see table 1). We note, however, that such differences are adjusted for, to a large extent, by the technique of random effects meta-analysis. Another major limitation is the paucity of published trials and the relatively small numbers of patients in most of them.

While we have identified drugs that have demonstrated efficacy in patients with painful DPN and have examined the strength of supportive data for each, we believe that our study provides only limited practical guidance as to which drugs are best to treat this condition. One reason for this is that a whole class of drugs commonly used to treat painful DPN—tricyclic antidepressants (TCAs)—was not included in our analysis because no trials met our inclusion criteria. TCAs, however, have been the subject of several active-controlled RCTs among patients with painful DPN, and these trials generally have shown TCAs to be equivalent in efficacy to some of the agents we examined (38-43). Second, some of the highest estimates of efficacy are based on quite small numbers of patients. For example, the efficacy estimate for capsaicin—a 26.4% reduction in pain intensity—is based on data for 76 patients, and the 19.3% reduction for zonisamide is based on only 25 patients. Although these drugs might be good choices for the treatment of painful DPN, one hesitates to recommend them on the basis of such scanty data. Finally, choice of therapy for any given patient depends not only on efficacy but also on cost, patient preferences (e.g., some patients may be wary of opioids), patient susceptibility to an agent's adverse effects (e.g., elderly patients with coronary heart disease probably should not receive TCAs), and anticipated tolerability. In this regard, the drug with the lowest risk of withdrawal due to lack of efficacy CR oxycodone appears to have a less favorable safety profile than several other drugs with lower efficacy. We suspect that most physicians would not view oxycodone as the drug of choice for the treatment of painful DPN due to the relatively unfavorable adverse event profile of opioids. In fact, the American Diabetes Association's Standards of Medical Care in Diabetes - 2009 does not even include opioids among the drugs recommended for the treatment of DPN (44).

Table 4. Relative risk of withdrawal due to adverse events

Source	Treatment n/N	Placebo n/N	RR (95% CI)		Weights, %
Capsaicin					
Tandan et al., 1992 (ref. 9)	NR	NR			
Scheffler et al., 1991 (ref. 10)	5/28	0/26	9.46 (0.54, 164.97)		100
Duloxetine					
Wernicke et al., 2006 (ref. 11)	17/114	8/108	2.01 (0.91, 4.47)		47.87
Raskin et al., 2005 (ref. 12)	5/113	3/116	1.71 (0.42, 6.99)		15.38
Goldstein et al., 2005 (ref. 13)	15/115	6/115	2.50 (1.01, 6.22)		36.75
Total (95% CI)	37/342	17/339	2.13 (1.23, 3.70)		100
Test for Heterogeneity: χ^2=0.23 (p=0.89), I^2=0%					
Test for Overall Effect: Z=2.69					
Gabapentin					
Backonja et al., 1992 (ref. 14)	7/84	5/81	1.35 (0.45, 4.08)		74.40
Simpson, 2001 (ref. 15)	2/27	2/27	1.00 (0.15, 6.59)		25.60
Total (95% CI)	9/111	7/108	1.25 (0.48, 3.25)		100
Test for Heterogeneity: χ^2=0.92 (p=0.63), I^2=0%					
Test for Overall Effect: Z=0.92					
Lamotrigine					
Vinik et al., 2007 (ref. 16)	19/90	9/90	2.11 (1.01, 4.41)		39.21
Eisenberg et al., 2001 (ref. 17)	4/27	4/26	0.96 (0.27, 3.45)		13.07
Vinik et al., 2007 (ref. 16)	21/90	11/90	1.91 (0.98, 3.72)		47.71
Total (95% CI)	44/207	24/206	1.83 (1.15, 2.89)		100
Test for Heterogeneity: χ^2=1.13 (p=0.57), I^2=0%					
Test for Overall Effect: Z=2.53					
Oxcarbazepine					
Beydoun et al., 2006 (ref. 18)	20/87	9/89	2.27 (1.10, 4.71)		45.03
Dogra et al., 2005 (ref. 19)	19/69	6/77	3.53 (1.50, 8.34)		32.49
Grosskopf et al., 2006 (ref. 20)	18/71	4/70	4.44 (1.58, 12.45)		22.48
Total (95% CI)	57/227	19/236	3.13 (1.92, 5.09)		100
Test for Heterogeneity: χ^2=1.24 (p=0.54), I^2=0%					
Test for Overall Effect: Z=4.47					
Pregabalin					
Arezzo et al., 2008 (ref. 21)	14/82	10/85	1.45 (0.68, 3.08)		34.08
Freynhagen et al., 2005 (ref. 22)	11/132	5/65	1.08 (0.39, 2.99)		18.76
Lesser et al., 2004 (ref. 23)	10/82	3/97	3.94 (1.12, 13.85)		12.23
Richter et al., 2005 (ref. 24)	7/82	4/85	1.81 (0.55, 5.97)		13.62
Rosenstock et al., 2004 (ref. 25)	8/76	2/70	3.68 (0.81, 16.76)		8.41
Tölle et al., 2007 (ref. 26)	13/101	3/96	3.56 (1.02, 12.35)		12.89
Total (95% CI)	63/555	27/498	3.61 (1.38, 9.44)		100
Test for Heterogeneity: χ^2=0.00 (p=0.97), I^2=0%					
Test for Overall Effect: Z=2.61					
Topiramate					
Raskin et al., 2004 (ref. 27)	52/208	9/109	3.03 (1.55, 5.91)		100
CR Oxycodone					
Gimbel et al., 2003 (ref. 28)	7/82	4/77	1.64 (0.50, 5.39)		74.73
Watson et al., 2003 (ref. 29)	7/36	1/36	7.00 (0.91, 54.04)		25.27
Total (95% CI)	14/118	5/113	2.65 (0.70, 10.13)		100
Test for Heterogeneity: χ^2=1.44 (p=0.23), I^2=30.72%					
Test for Overall Effect: Z=1.65					
Zonisamide					
Atli and Dogra, 2005 (ref. 30)	NR	NR			
Tramadol					
Freeman et al., 2007 (ref. 31)	13/160	10/152	1.24 (0.56, 2.73)		100
Sodium Valproate					
Agrawal et al., 2009 (ref. 32)	0/20	0/21	1.05 (0.02, 50.43)		42.53
Kochar, 2004 (33)	1/21	0/18	1.71 (0.06, 48.18)		52.47
Total (95% CI)	1/41	0/39	1.40 (0.11, 17.20)		100
Test for Heterogeneity: χ^2=0.04 (p=0.85), I^2=0%					
Test for Overall Effect: Z=0.26					

Relative Risk, CI%
0.01   0.1   1   10   100

NR: Not Reported.

Table 4. (Continued)

Source	Treatment n/N	Placebo n/N	RR (95% CI)		Weights, %
Glyceryl trinitrate spray					
Agrawal et al., 2009 (ref. 32)	0/20	0/21	1.05 (0.02, 50.43)		42.69
Agrawal et al., 2007 (ref. 34)	1/22	0/21	1.91 (0.07, 53.96)		57.31
Total (95% CI)			1.48 (0.12, 18.56)		100
Test for Heterogeneity: χ^2=0.05 (p=0.82), I^2=0%					
Test for Overall Effect: Z=0.30					
Venlafaxine					
Kadiroglu et al., 2008 (ref. 35)	NR	NR			
Rowbotham et al., 2004 (ref. 36)	8/82	3/81	2.63 (0.72, 9.58)		100
Lacosamide					
Wymer et al., 2009 (ref. 37)	21/91	8/93	2.68 (1.25, 5.74)		100

Relative Risk, CI%

NR: Not Reported.

There have been several reviews of pharmacotherapy for painful DPN in the past few years. Of these, only one has been rigorously systematic, with clear definitions and descriptions of methods. Quilici and colleagues performed a meta-analysis of duloxetine, pregabalin, and gabapentin in the treatment of painful DPN using methods similar to ours (45). They concluded that the three drugs show "comparable efficacy and tolerability." Gutierrez-Alvarez and colleagues reviewed antiepileptic drugs for painful DPN (46). Their primary focus was on studies that presented data concerning the proportion of patients with a ≥50% reduction in pain from baseline, but the scales used to evaluate this measure were not described, and results were reported in terms of numbers needed to treat (NNT). Of the three drugs included in their analysis--pregabalin, oxcarbazepine, and topiramate--pregabalin was found to have the lowest NNT, but the authors did not recommend this drug over the others, concluding "there are few differences between the studied drugs." Chong and Hester reviewed pharmacotherapy for painful DPN and present a table of NNTs for a group of randomized studies with at least 50 subjects and "positive results" (47). The measures used to calculate NNTs were not described, and data were not meta-analyzed. The authors concluded that "it is not possible to nominate a single drug as the first-line treatment for DPN." Finally, Adriaensen and colleagues reviewed oral drugs for painful DPN with a focus on reduction in pain intensity as the efficacy measure of principal interest, but they did not undertake a meta-analysis of data from multiple studies of the same drug (48). They concluded that gabapentin "may be a first choice treatment in painful diabetic neuropathy, especially in the elderly." Our analysis is more comprehensive than that of Quilici and colleagues, and more systematic and up-to-date than that presented in the other reviews.

In its table of drugs to treat painful DPN, the American Diabetes Association's Standards of Medical Care in Diabetes—2009 recommends three TCAs, gabapentin, carbamazepine, pregabalin, duloxetine, and capsaicin, but does not discuss the reasons for these choices (44). (Carbamazepine was not included in our analysis because the single randomized trial, although otherwise fulfilling our criteria for inclusion, was a crossover study with a total duration of only two weeks (49)). More recently, the National Institute for Health and Clinical Excellence (NICE) in the UK issued guidance for the pharmacological management of neuropathic pain in adults in non-specialist settings (50). Recommendations for the treatment of painful DPN are separate from those for other neuropathic pain conditions. For painful DPN, duloxetine is recommended as a first-line treatment, and amitriptyline is recommended for first-line use if duloxetine is contraindicated. Pregabalin is recommended for second-line treatment, either alone or in combination with first-line agents. For other neuropathic pain, amitriptyline or pregabalin are recommended as first-line treatment (randomized controlled trials of duloxetine have not been conducted in neuropathic pain conditions other than DPN). For additional guidance as to the treatment of neuropathic pain in general (not specific to DPN), algorithms and recommendations based on reviews of existing literature are available from professional organizations and independent reviewers (51-53).

ACKNOWLEDGMENTS

The analyses were conducted by John Edelsberg, Claudia Lord, and Gerry Oster, all of whom are employees of Policy Analysis Inc (PAI). PAI received financial support from Pfizer, Inc. for the conduct of this analysis and development of this manuscript.

REFERENCES

[1]   Woolf CJ. Pain: Moving from symptom control toward mechanism-specific pharmacologic management. Ann Intern Med 2004;140:441-51.

[2]   Hansson PT, Dickenson AH. Pharmacological treatment of peripheral neuropathic pain conditions based on shared commonalities despite multiple etiologies. Pain 2005;113:215-54.

[3]   Gallagher RM. Management of neuropathic pain: Translating mechanistic advances and evidence-based research into clinical practice. Clin J Pain 2006;22(suppl 1):S2-8.

[4]   Edelsberg J, Oster G. Summary measures of number needed to treat: How much clinical guidance do they provide in neuropathic pain? Eur J Pain 2009;13:11-6.

[5]   Eisenberg E, McNicol ED, Carr DB. Efficacy and safety of opioid agonists in the treatment of neuropathic pain of nonmalignant origin: Systematic review and meta-analysis of randomized controlled trials. JAMA 2005;293:3043-52.

[6]   Tremont-Lukats IW, Challapalli V, McNicol ED, Lau J, Carr DB. Systemic administration of local anesthetics to relieve neuropathic pain: A systematic review of meta-analysis. Anesth Analg 2005; 101:1738-49.

[7]   Jadad AR, Moore RA, Carroll D, Jenkinson C, Reynolds DJ, Gavaghan DJ, McQuay HJ. Assessing the quality of reports of randomized clinical trials. Is blinding necessary? Control Clin Trials 1996;17:1-12.

[8]   Explanation of Columns in Natural Standard Evidence Table. Accessed 2013 Jul 8. URL: http://www.naturalstandard.com/ explanation_columns.html

[9]   Tandan R, Lewis GA, Krusinski PB, Badger GB, Fries TJ. Topical capsaicin in painful diabetic neuropathy: Controlled study with long-term follow-up. Diabetes Care 1992;15:8-14.

[10]   Scheffler N, Sheitel P, Lipton M. Treatment of painful diabetic neuropathy with capsaicin 0.075%. J Am Podiatr Med Assoc 1991; 81:288-93.

[11]   Wernicke JF, Pritchett YL, D'Souza DN, Waninger A, Tran P, Iyengar S, Raskin J. A randomized controlled trial of duloxetine in diabetic peripheral neuropathic pain. Neurology 2006;67:1411-20.

[12]   Raskin J, Pritchett Y, Wang F, D'Souza DN, Waninger AL, Iyengar S, Wernicke JF. A double-blind, randomized multicenter trial comparing duloxetine with placebo in the management of diabetic peripheral neuropathic pain. Pain Med 2005;6:346-56.

[13] Goldstein D, Lu Y, Detke M, Lee T, Iyengar S. Duloxetine vs. Placebo in patients with painful diabetic neuropathy. Pain 2005; 116:109-118.

[14] Backonja M, Beydoun A, Edwards KR, Schwartz SL, Fonseca V, Hes M, LaMoreaux L, Garofalo E. Gabapentin for the symptomatic treatment of painful neuropathy in patients with diabetes mellitus. JAMA 1998;280:1831-6.

[15] Simpson DA. Gabapentin and venlafaxine for the treatment of painful diabetic neuropathy. J Clin Nueromuscular Dis 2001;3:53-62.

[16] Vinik AI, Tuchman M, Safirstein B, Corder C, Kirby L, Wilks K, Quessy S, Blum D, Grainger J, White J, Silver M. Lamotrigine for treatment of pain associated with diabetic neuropathy: Results of two randomized, double-blind, placebo-controlled studies. Pain 2007; 128:169-79.

[17] Eisenberg E, Lurie Y, Braker C, Daoud D, Ishay A. Lamotrigine reduces painful diabetic neuropathy: A randomized, controlled study. Neurology 2001;57:505-9.

[18] Beydoun A, Shaibani A, Hopwood M, Wan Y. Oxcarbazepine in painful diabetic neuropathy: Results of a dose-ranging study. Acta Neurol Scand 2006;113:395-404.

[19] Dogra S, Beydoun S, Mazzola J, Hopwood M, Wan Y. Oxcarbazepine in painful diabetic neuropathy: A randomized, placebo-controlled study. Eur J Pain 2005;9:543-54.

[20] Grosskopf J, Mazzola J, Wan Y, Hopwood M. A randomized, placebo-controlled study of oxcarbazepine in painful diabetic neuropathy. Acta Neurol Scand 2006;114:177-80.

[21] Arezzo JC, Rosenstock J, LaMoreaux L, Pauer L. Efficacy and safety of pregabalin 600 mg/d for treating painful diabetic peripheral neuropathy: A double-blind placebo-controlled trial. BMC Neurology 2008;8:33

[22] Freynhagen R, Strokek K, Griesing T, Whalen E, Balkenohl M. Efficacy pregabalin in neuropathic pain evaluated in a 12-week, randomized, double-blind, multicentre, placebo-controlled trial of flexible- and fixed-dose regimens. Pain 2005;115:254-63.

[23] Lesser H, Sharma U, LaMoreaux L, Poole. Pregabalin relieves symptoms of painful diabetic neuropathy: A randomized controlled trial. Neurology 2004;63:2104-10.

[24] Richter RW, Portenoy R, Sharma U, Lamoreaux L, Bockbrader H, Knapp LE. Relief of painful diabetic peripheral neuropathy with pregabalin: A randomized, placebo-controlled trial. J Pain 2005; 6:253-60.

[25] Rosenstock J, Tuchman M, LaMoreaux L, Sharma U. Pregabalin for the treatment of painful diabetic peripheral neuropathy: A double-blind, placebo-controlled trial. Pain 2004;110:628-38.

[26] Tölle T, Freynhagen R, Versavel M, Trostmann U, Young Jr. JP. Pregabalin for relief of neuropathic pain associated with diabetic neuropathy: A randomized, double-blind study. Eur J Pain 2008; 12:203-13.

[27] Raskin P, Donofrio PD, Rosenthal NR, Hewitt DJ, Jordan DM, Xiang J, Vinik AI. Topiramate vs. placebo in painful diabetic neuropathy: Analgesic and metabolic effects. Neurology 2004;63:865-73.

[28] Gimbel J, Richards P, Portenoy K. Controlled-release oxycodone for pain in diabetic neuropathy: A randomized controlled trial. Neurology 2003;60:927-34.

[29] Watson C, Moulin D, Watt-Watson J, Gordon A, Eisenhoffer J. Controlled-release oxycodone relieves neuropathic pain: A randomized controlled trial in painful diabetic neuropathy. Pain 2003; 105:71-8.

[30] Atli A, Dogra S. Zonisamide in the treatment of painful diabetic neuropathy: A randomized, double-blind, placebo-controlled pilot study. Pain Med 2005;6:225-34.

[31] Freeman R, Raskin P, Hewitt DJ, Vorsanger GJ, Jordan DM, Xiang J, Rosenthal NR. Randomized study of tramadol/acetaminophen versus placebo in painful diabetic peripheral neuropathy. Curr Med Res Opin 2007;23:147-61.

[32] Argawal RP, Goswami J, Jain S, Kochar DK. Management of diabetic neuropathy by sodium valproate and glyceryl trinitrate spray: A prospective double-blind randomized placebo=controlled study. Diabetes Res Clin Practice 2009;83:371-378.

[33] Kochar DK, Rawat N, Agrawal RP, Vyas A, Beniwal R, Kochar SK, Garg P. Sodium valporate for painful diabetic neuropathy: A randomized double-blind placebo-controlled study. Q J Med 2004; 33-38.

[34] Agrawal RP, Choudhary R, Sharma P, Sharma S, Beniwal R, Kaswan K, Kochar DK. Glyceryl trinitrate spray in the management of painful diabetic neuropathy: A randomized double blind placebo controlled cross-over study. Diabetes Res Clin Practice 2007;77:161-7.

[35] Kadiroglu AK, Sit D, Kayabasi H, Tuzcu AK, Tasdemir N, Yilmaz ME. The effect of velafaxine HCI on painful peripheral diabetic neuropathy in patients with type 2 diabetes mellitus. J Diabet Complications 2008;22:241-5.

[36] Rowbotham MC, Goli V, Kunz NR, Lei D. Venlafaxine extended release in the treatment of painful diabetic neuropathy: A double-blind, placebo-controlled study. Pain 2004;110:697-706.

[37] Wymer JP, Simpson J, Sen D, Bongardt S. Efficacy and safety of lacosamide in diabetic neuropathic pain. An 18 week double-blind placebo-controlled trial of fixed-dose regimens. Clin J Pain 2009; 25:376-85.

[38] Biesbroeck R, Bril V, Hollander P, Kabadi U, Schwartz S, Singh SP, et al. A double-blind comparison of topical capsaicin and oral amitriptyline in painful diabetic neuropathy. Adv Ther 1995; 12:111-120.

[39] Dallocchio C, Buffa C, Mazzarello P, Chiroli S. Gabapentin vs. amitriptyline in painful diabetic neuropathy: An open-label pilot study. J Pain Symptom Manage 2000;20:280-5.

[40] Gómez-Pérez FJ, Choza R, Ríos JM, Reza A, Huerta E, Aguilar CA, Rull JA. Nortriptyline-fluphenazine vs. carbamazepine in symptomatic treatment of diabetic neuropathy. Arch Med Res 1996; 27:525-9.

[41] Jose VM, Bhansali A, Hota D, Pandhi P. Randomized double-blind study comparing the efficacy and safety of lamotrigine and amitriptyline in painful diabetic neuropathy. Diabet Med 2007; 24:377-83.

[42] Max MB, Lynch SA, Muir J, Shoaf SE, Smoller B, Dubner R. Effects of desipramine, amitriptyline, and fluoxetine on pain in diabetic neuropathy. N Engl J Med 326:1250-6.

[43] Morello CM, Leckband SG, Stoner CP, Moorhouse DF, Sahagian GA. Randomized double-blind study comparing the efficacy of gabapentin with amitriptyline on diabetic peripheral neuropathy pain. Arch Intern Med 1999;159:1931-7.

[44] American Diabetes Association. Standards of Medical Care in Diabetes – 2009. Diabetes Care 2009;32:S13-S61.

[45] Quillici S, Chancellor J, Löthgren M, Simon D, Said G, Le TK, Garcia-Cebrian A, Monz B. Meta-analysis of duloxetine vs. pregabalin and gabapentin in the treatment of diabetic peripheral neuropathic pain. BMC Neurology 2009;9:1471-7.

[46] Gutierrez-Alvarez AM, Beltran-Rodriguez J, Moreno CB. Antiepileptic drugs in treatment of pain caused by diabetic neuropathy. J Pain Symptom Manag 2007;34:201-8.

[47] Chong SM, Hester J. Diabetic painful neuropathy. Current and future treatment options. Drugs 2007;67:569-85.

[48] Adriaensen H, Plaghki L, Joffroy A, Vissers K. Critical review of oral drug treatments for diabetic neuropathic pain –Clinical outcomes based on efficacy and safety data from placebo-controlled and direct comparative studies. Diabetes Metab Res Rev 2005;1:231-40.

[49] Wilton TD. Tegretol in the treatment of diabetic neuropathy. S Afr Med J 1974;48:18.

[50] National Institute for Health and Clinical Excellence (NICE). Neuropathic pain: The pharmacological management of neuropathic pain in adults in non-specialist settings. London: NICE 2010. Accessed 2013 May 20.URL: http://www.nice.org.uk/ nicemedia/live/12948/47936/ 47936.pdf.

[51] Gilron I, Watson CP, Cahill CM, Moulin DE. Neuropathic pain: A practical guide from the clinician. CMAJ 2006;175:265-75.

[52] Mendell J, Sahenk Z. Painful sensory neuropathy. N Engl J Med 2003;348:1243-55.

[53] Attal N, Cruccu G, Haanpää M, Hansson P, Jensen TS, Nurmikko T, eta l. EFNS guidelines on pharmacological treatment of neuropathic pain. Eur J Neurology 2006;13:1153-69.

In: Food, Nutrition and Eating Behavior
Editors: Joav Merrick and Sigal Israeli

ISBN: 978-1-62948-233-0
© 2014 Nova Science Publishers, Inc.

Chapter 10

LOW W-6/W-3 RATIO DIETARY PATTERN AND RISK OF CARDIOVASCULAR DISEASE AND DIABETES MELLITUS

Ram B Singh, MD[*1], *Mahmood Moshiri, MD*[1],
Fabien DeMeester, PhD[1], *Lekh Juneja, PhD*[2],
Veerappan Muthusami, DM[3]
and Shanmugam Manoharan, PhD[4]

[1]The Tsim Tsoum Institute, Krakow, Poland
[2]Taiyo Kagaku Limited, Yokkaichi, Japan
[3]Department of Cardiology, Sugapriya Hospital, Madurai and [4]Department of Biochemistry, Annamalai University, Annamalai Nagar, India

Diet and physical inactivity appear to be important in the pathogenesis of cardiovascular disease (CVD) and type 2 diabetes. However, the exact nutrients and their pathogenesis are difficult to define. The evolutionary aspects of diet and lifestyle appear to be important. Methods: Review of literature from the internet and discussion with colleagues. Results: Cereal grains (refined), and vegetable oils that are rich in w-6 fatty acids and trans fats are relatively recent addition to the human dietary patterns that represent dramatic departure from natural foods and nutrients to which we are adapted. Excess of trans, saturated and total fat as well as refined starches and sugar in presence of high w-6/w-3 ratio of the diet, are proinflammatory. These foods, can enhance sympathetic activity and oxidative stress that appear to be underlying mechanisms of inflammation, obesity and metabolic syndrome. Excess secretion of these neurotransmitters in conjunction of underlying w-3 fatty acid deficiency, may damage the neurons via proinflammatory cytokines, resulting into their dysfunction. Since, 30–50% of the fatty acids in the brain are omega-3 fatty acids, incorporated in the cell membrane phospholipids, it is possible that their supplementation may be protective. Conclusions. High w-6/w-3 ratio Western diet appear to be risk factor of CVD and type 2 diabetes mellitus. However, Mediterranean diet characterised with low w-6/w-3 ratio of 1:1, in

* Correspondence: Professor Ram B Singh, MD, Halberg Hospital and Research Institute, Civil Lines, Moradabad-10(UP), 244001 India. E-mail: rbs@tsimtsoum.net or drkk@dataone.in.

conjunction with other nutrients; essential amino acids, soluble fibre, vitamins, minerals and antioxidants may be protective.

INTRODUCTION

Hypertension and stroke as well as coronary artery disease (CAD), diabetes and cancers have become a major cause of morbidity and mortality in Asia (1-13). The epidemic of these problems, in the western world and in middle income countries, indicates major increases in the incidence of generalized atherosclerosis and the total burden of cardiovascular diseases (CVD) due to changes in the lifestyle factors (3-6). Maladaptation, genetic predisposition, environmental; dietary and lifestyle factors, in relation to mind-body interactions predispose CVD and type two diabetes mellitus (1-5). Lifestyle factors such as physical inactivity and unhealthy and unbalanced nutritional consumption of excess calories, simple refined carbohydrates with a high glycemic index and load of high saturated fat (SF), high trans fatty acids (TFA), high n-6 fatty acids and lack of monounsaturated fatty acids(MUFA) and n-3 fatty acids in the diet and reduced exercise, can damage the genes and gut-liver- brain axis, contributing to the escalating rates of obesity and mortality due to CVD (3-9). The obesity and CVD are contributing to major economic and public health concerns and problems that mandate aggressive, urgent and dedicated identification, prevention, treatment and education of public. private (4-7).

Indians from the ancient times, were aware with adverse role of diet, which is evident from the following verse from an ancient scripture Bhagwatgeeta: "Foods which are bitter, acid, salted, burnet, fried and pungent, give rise to pain, mental stress and diseases" (3100 BCE). Charaka (600 BCE), a great physician of India, knew about the role of diet and lifestyle in the pathogenesis of heart attack, which would be clear from the following verse: "Heart attack is born by the intake of fatty meals, overeating, excess of sleep, lack of exercise and anxiety" (Charaka Sutra, 600 BCE). In Ayurveda, three types of diets have been proposed (see table 1).

Table 1. Dietary advice in ancient Ayurveda (Maha-anaarany Upanishad, 5000 BCE)

1. Satvic diet. Advised to saints. Contains fruits, vegetables, sprouted grains, roots, nuts, cow milk, curd, honey. It would cause, longevity, health and happiness in mind and enhances spirituality and possible survival may be 100-150 years. Good for mental, social and spiritual health.
2. Rajsic diet. Advised to kings and fighters. Contains fruits, vegetables, nuts, meats from hunted animals, clarified butter, butter, curd, honey, spices, wines. It may cause excitement and increase intelligence with life expectancy of about 100 years. Good for physical, mental and social health.
3. Tamsic diet. Not advised. Contains high fat fried foods, rich in salt, sugar, spices, chilies, meats from big tamed animals, butter and liquor. This diet makes dull, enhances anger and criminal tendency and impedes spiritual progress. Life expectancy was much lower. Bad for health.

While Charak was supposed to live in Taxila University in the north of India and a Brahman physician, Sushruta was a surgeon from the Vishwamitra family from Varanasi. In

Mahabharata, he is represented as a son of that royal sage. The garuda puranam places Divodasa as 4th in descent from Dhanavantari, the first propounder of the medical sciences upon earth, whereas the sushruta samhita describes both as the same person. Sushruta who was a surgeon, gave a more clear description of atherosclerosis or madroga: "Excess intake of fatty foods and lack of exercise causes obesity and narrowing of the channels taking blood to the heart. It is useful to use guggul, triphala and silajit in the treatment." These herbs are known to have high content of antioxidant flavonoids, vitamins and minerals as well as fibres.

A Chinese physician proposed that "increased consumption of salt may cause hardening of the pulse (7th century BCE). About 2000 years ago, Confucius, the Chinese philosopher taught his students that "the higher the quality of foods, the better and never rely upon the delicacy of cooking." Thus a dietary guideline based on experience, observation and thinking was given as "cereals, the basic, fruits the subsidiary, meat the beneficial and vegetable the supplementary." Therefore, according to WHO experts in 1990, the concept of eating a diet high in animal foods and preference for meat and greasy foods was shaped in China. However, possibly the meat had a low w-6/w-3 ratio and the total fat intake remained within desirable limits and did not exceed as in the west. These dietary patterns were associated with enormous physical activity and sports, such as hunting and also possibly meditation due to introduction of Buddhism, causing possibly, a beneficial effect on mind-body connection showing no significant problem of noncommunicable diseases during that period. Moreover, the meat may have been from the running animals which has useful fatty acid composition.

CAUSES OF DEATH

CVD is the number one cause of death globally and projected to remain the leading cause of death. According to WHO estimates, 17.5 million people died from CVD in 2008, representing 30% of all global deaths. Coronary artery disease was the cause of death, among 7.6 million and 5.7 million deaths were due to stroke (3-7). The majority of these deaths (80%) occurred in low and middle income countries. *The PURE Investigators reported prevalence of a healthy lifestyle among individuals with cardiovascular disease in high-, middle- and low-income countries, showing greater rates in developed countries (5).*

In the year 1994 to 1998, trends indicated that there had been a significant decline of proportionate deaths from infectious diseases from 22% to 16%, according to Registrar General of India. However, mortality from cardiovascular disease(CVD) increased from 21% to 25%, which is lower than death rate of 29.1 reported by Singh et al. in 2005 (7). Mohan et al. (9) studied the mortality rates due to diabetes in selected urban population from south India among 1,399 subjects (respondents 1,262). During a median follow up of six years, deaths were significantly greater among diabetics compared to nondiabetics (18.9 vs 5.3 per 1,000 person years, P=0.004). Mortality due to CVD were 52.9% among diabetics and 24.2 among nondiabetics. It is clear that the burden of CVD and diabetes appears to be quite significant in India indicating urgency for prevention program (4-11). The higher risk of CAD mortality is not explained by conventional risk factors common among Indian immigrants to industrialized countries (12, 13). Indian Society of Hypertension and International College of Nutrition and other experts have proposed guidelines for prevention of CVD and diabetes in Indians and Asians, which are being used for public education by the health workers. Social class is also a determinant of mortality including cardiovascular mortality (4,7). It thus seems logical to examine whether differences in nutritional intake exist between the social classes, which could explain part of the existing differences in mortality due to CVD, diabetes and cancers (4-13). About one fifth of the adult population in developing countries and one forth in industrialized countries, may have CVD and diabetes (3-6). The prevalence of diabetes and prediabetes were about 6% each in the year 2007 in South East Asia, indicating that 46.5 million subjects above 20 years had this problem which would be doubled by the year 2025. Similar targets have been calculated for CAD.

The burden of hypertension would be four fold greater compared to diabetes. In various studies, the prevalence of hypertension (>140/90 mmHg) has been reported to be 22-30% in India among urban subjects above 20 years of age. The prevalence of CAD varies between 8% to 14% in various cities of India. In rural population, the prevalence of diabetes, hypertension and CAD is 2-3 fold lower compared to urban subjects. Dietary intake of total fat amounts to 25-45% in developed countries and 15%-35% of total energy in developing countries (7). Most of the dietary fatty acids are derived from meats, vegetable oils and dairy products, resulting in to marked increase in saturated and w-6 fatty acids but relatively modest of monounsaturated fatty acids (MUFA) and long chain polyunsaturated fatty acids (PUFA) (10) particularly w-3 fatty acids. Refining of vegetable oils has been a major cause for increased consumption of w-6 fatty acids and hydrogenation of these oils caused greater intake of TFA, that may be the cause of mitochondrial damage in the related organs; endothelial cells, cardiomyocytes, smooth muscle cells, neurons, beta cells, and liver, causing mitochondrial damage, leading to increased prevalence of CVD, diabetes and cancers, and neurodegenerative diseases, in most countries of the world (1-9). The increase in CVD morbidity and mortality may be related to changes in diet and w-3 fatty acid consumption (see tables 1-5). While Japan, Eskimos in Greenland and Mediterranean countries consuming high w-3 fatty acid have lower CVD mortality, death rates are much higher in the northern Europe, USA and South Asia consuming high w-6/3-3 ratio of 20-50 in the diets due to increased consumption of vegetable oils rich in w-6 fatty acids (see tables 4,5).

Table 2. Food and nutrient intake among hunter-gatherer and western population.
Modified from Simopoulos (57)

Food and nutrient	Hunter gatherer	Western population
Energy density	Low	High
Protein	High	Low-moderate
Animal	High	Low –moderate
Vegetable	Very low	Low –moderate
Carbohydrate	Low-moderate(slowly absorbed)	Moderate-rapidly absorbed
Fiber	High	Low
Fat	Low	High
Animal	Low	High
Vegatable	Very low	High
Total w-3	High(2.3g/day)	Low (0.2g/day)
Ratio w-6:w-3	Low 2.4	High 15-20
Vitamins and minerals	high	low

EVOLUTION AND HEALTH PROMOTION

A fundamental view of evolution in relation to health promotion has been that the genetic makeup of contemporary humans shows minor difference from that of the modern humans who appeared in Africa between 100,000 and 50,000 years ago. The human evolution has been comparatively rapid during the past 50,000 years, as revealed by the molecular geneticists. There have been marked changes in the food supply with the development of agriculture about 10,000 years ago. However, only insignificant changes in our genes have occurred during the past 10 centuries, due to the presence of w-3 fatty acids, amino acids, vitamins and minerals in the diet. There have been some structural modifications in individual DNA sequence and altered gene regulation has been the dominant mechanism involved. Increased evolutionary rapidity in humans compared with rates for other primates, has resulted from unprecedented demographic expansion, which has provided a far larger pool of mutations, upon which natural selection can operate. The human diaspora which has exposed humans environmental changes appears to be quite different from those of their ancestral land in Africa.

Table 3. Estimated fatty acid consumption in the late Paleolithic period. Modified from Simopoulos (57)

Sources	Fatty acids(g/day) en 35.65/day
Plants	
Linoleic acid	4.28
Alpha-linoleic acid	11.40
Animal	
Linoleic acids	4.56
Alpha-linolenic acid	1.21
Total	
Linoleic acid	8.84
Alpha linolenic acid	12.60
Animal	
Arachidonic acid(w-6) (AA)	1.81
Eicosapentaenoic acid(w-3)(EPA)	0.39
Docosatetraenoic acid(w-6) (DTA)	0.12
Docosapentaenoic acid(w-3)(DPA)	0.42
Docosahexaenoic acid(w-3)(DHA)	0.27
Ratios of w-6/w-3	
Linoleic acid/alpha linolenic acid	0.70
AA+DTA/EPA+DPA+DHA	1.79
Total w-6/w-3	0.79

The spontaneous mutation rate for nuclear DNA is estimated at 0.5% per million years. Hence, over the past 10,000 years there has been time for very little change in our genes, possibly 0.005%. Our genes appear to be similar to the genes of our ancestors during the Paleolithic period 40,000 years ago, the time when our genetic profile was established. Man appears to live in an nutritional environment which completely differs from that for which our genetic constitution was selected. However, it was only during the last 100-160 years that dietary intakes have changed significantly, causing increased intake of saturated fatty acids

(SFA) and linoleic acid, and decrease in w-3 fatty acids, from grain fed cattle, tamed at farm houses, rather than meat from running animals. There is marked decrease in the intake of vitamins and antioxidants. The food and nutrient intake among hunter-gatherers and during Paleolithic period are given in tables 2-4. There is marked reduction in consumption of w-3 fatty acids, vitamins and minerals and proteins and significant increase in the intakes of carbohydrates, (mainly refined,), fat (saturated, trans fat, linoleic acid) and salt compared to Paleolithic period (see tables 2-7, Figure 1).

Table 4. Nutrient composition in the late Paleolithic and current recommendations. Modified from Simopoulos (57)

Nutrient	Late Paleolithic	Current recommendation
Total dietary energy%		
Protein	33	12
Carbohydrate	46	58
Fat	21	30
Alcohol	-0	moderate alcohol
P/S ratio	1.41	1.00
Cholesterol, mg	520	300
Fiber,g	100-150	30-60
Sodium,mg	690	1100-3300
Calcium,mg	1500-2000	800-1600
Ascorbic acid, mg	440	60
W-6/W-3 ratio	1:1	1:1

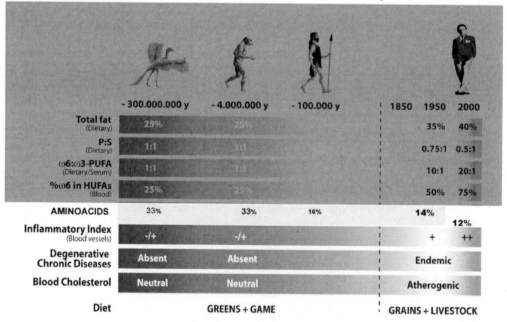

Figure 1. Nutrient intake among Paleolithic societies; *Homo sapiens and Homo economicus.*

The Columbus concept of diet means that humans evolved on a diet that was low in saturated fat and the amount of w-3 and w-6 fatty acids was quite equal (14). Nature recommends to ingest fatty acids in a balanced ratio (polyunsaturated:saturated=w-6:w-3=1:1) as part of dietary lipid pattern in monounsaturated fatty acids (P:M:S=1:6:1).These ratios represent the overall distribution of fats in a natural untamed environment. (www.columbus-concept.com). The Columbus foods include egg, milk, meat, oil , and bread, all rich in w-3 fatty acids, similar to wild foods, consumed about 160 years ago from now. Blood lipid composition does reflect one's health status: (a) circulating serum lipoproteins and their ratio provide information on their atherogenicity to blood vessels and (b) circulating plasma fatty acids, such as w-6/w-3 fatty acid ratio, give indication on proinflammatory status of blood vessels; (a) and (b) are phenotype-related and depend on genetic, environmental and developmental factors. As such, they appear as universal markers for holistic health. Blood cholesterol is central to this approach. Its 3D-representation shows how circulating lipoproteins affect blood vessels integrity upon their circulating throughout the body. Of major importance appear the essential dietary nutrients (essential amino acids, fatty acids, antioxidant vitamins and minerals) and the functional component of the regimen (diet, sport, spiritualism, etc.). An example is given of an essential dietary nutrient and of a functional component of man's regimen that affect health in a predictive way derived from the 3Drepresentation of blood cholesterol. Caption The Columbus Concept and its 3D representation of blood lipoprotein behaviors. "Bad" LDL-C, "good" HDLC, and "healthy" LDL-CC:HDL-CC ratios. CC= Columbus Concept. The Tsim Tsoum Concept is an extension of the Columbus concept which includes the simultaneous approach of controlling of brain-body connection. Sachs and group (15-17) used Dietary Approaches to Stop Hypertension (DASH) for decreasing blood pressures, blood lipoproteins and coronary risk. Similar dietary (18-23) interventions have been used by other workers for the last three decades, to modulate blood pressure, obesity, diabetes and dyslipidemia and coronary risk, in patients with high risk of CAD. These strategies appear to be similar to Columbus diet and lifestyle which may be protective, due to a favourable fatty acid ratio, antioxidants and slowly absorbed nutrients, in the diet.

DEVELOPMENT OF CARDIOVASCULAR DISEASE AND DIABETES

Overweight and central obesity, may cause clustering of risk factors which may be characterized with impaired glucose tolerance, with an adverse lipid profile and oxidative stress leading to hypertension and may be seen as early as in childhood and adolescence. These risk factors which are indicator of metabolic syndrome and CVD, tend to be clustered more rapidly in children and adolescents with unhealthy lifestyles and diets such as those with excessive intakes of saturated fats, cholesterol, refined carbohydrates and salt and inadequate consumption of dietary fibre, antioxidants, vitamins, minerals, coenzyme Q10 and w-3 fatty acids. Low power mitochondria, due to coenzyme Q deficiency, may be associated with reduced aerobic capacity and predispose the metabolic syndrome and CVD (31-36). Lack of physical activity and increased television viewing are other factors which further increase the risk by decreasing BMR (1-3). In older children and adolescents, habitual alcohol and tobacco use also contribute to high blood pressure and to the development of other risk factors in early adulthood which continue to act in later life course. Such clustering of risk factors which is characteristic of metabolic syndrome and CVD, represents an opportunity to address more than one risk factor at a time and may be due to clustering of health related behaviours (36). Of the several characteristics of metabolic syndrome, at least three should be present for its diagnosis.

Obesity in conjunction with type 2 diabetes, hypertension, coronary artery disease (CAD), and dyslipidemia are important features of the metabolic syndrome which is usually associated with hyperinsulinemia and insulin resistance (30-32). There is coexistence of nutritional deficiencies and appreciable overnutrition in the form of central obesity and overweight in both developed and developing countries (11-36). Cohort studies clearly showed that the gratifying gains in cardiovascular health occurred in developed countries, in association with an epidemic of CVD in the developing world (30-33). We have been in a position to learn, the mechanism of transition from poverty to economic development and emergence of cardiovascular disease (CVD) (11, 24). It seems that metabolic syndrome is an important pathway for development of CVD and type 2 diabetes (see figure 1). We proposed that "overweight comes first in conjunction with hyperinsulinemia, increased angiotensin activity, increased proinflammatory cytokines and central obesity followed by glucose intolerance, type 2 diabetes, hypertension, low high density lipoprotein cholesterol (HDL) and hypertriglyceridemia (Metabolic syndrome) (31-33). This sequence is followed by CAD, gall stones and cancers and finally dental caries, gastrointestinal diseases and bone and joint diseases, during transition from poverty to affluence". As people become rich, they begin to increase their dietary fat, salt and sugar (proinflammatory foods) intake in the form of ready prepared foods, syrups, dairy products and flesh foods in place of grain based diet (33). There is a greater use of automobiles, television viewing and decrease in sports, walking and dancing as recreation. These changes in the diet and lifestyle in conjunction with increased tobacco and alcohol intake, appear to be basic factors in the pathogenesis of noncommunicable diseases, including CVD (3, 30). The last few decades of the 20th century offered us an opportunity to initiate action to counter growing epidemics of CVD and type 2 diabetes, on both sides of the Atlantic (31-37). When people learned the methods of prevention, there was a decrease in CVD in the western world but obesity continued to increase, resulting into an increase in the metabolic syndrome in both developed and developing economies (30-32). It is possible that these adverse diet and lifestyle factors damage the mitochondria of the cardiovascular system and ventromedial hypothalamus, leading to CVD and diabetes.

There has been an enormous increase in w-6 fatty acid (about 30 g/day) in the diet due to the production of oils from vegetable seeds such as corn, sunflower, safflower, soybean and cotton. Increased intake of meat has resulted into greater intake of arachidonic acid (0.2-1.0mg/day), whereas the consumption of alpha-linolenic acid (ALA) has decreased (about 0.55 g/day) and the amounts of eicosapentaenoic acid (EPA) and docosahexaenoic acid (DHA) are 48 and 72mg/day respectively (29-35). A relative and absolute decrease in w-3 fatty acids has led to an imbalance and increase in the ratio of w-6/w-3 fatty acids to up to 50 in India and other developing countries, consuming vegetable seed oils (corn, soyabean, sunflower, cotton) (33-39). Saturated fatty acids (SFA) and trans fatty acids (TFA) elevate, PUFA decrease and MUFA have beneficial effects on total and low density lipoprotein cholesterol (LDL)as well as on HDL cholesterol. Omega-6 PUFA and TFA also decrease HDL cholesterol, and increase insulin resistance, free radical stress and inflammation, which may enhance atherosclerosis (33-35). Increased intake of total fat, TFA, SFA and w-6 fatty acids and refined carbohydrates, may cause insulin resistance resulting into metabolic syndrome(22-30).Decreased intake of MUFA,w-3 fatty acids, fiber and phytochemicals, may enhance the metabolic syndrome (14-36).

CARDIOVASCULAR DISEASE IN THE DEVELOPING WORLD

Coronary risk factors in the developing world, include low concentration of HDL cholesterol, hypertriglyceridemia, abdominal obesity, high prevalence of type 2 diabetes and CAD, hypertension, indicating presence of metabolic syndrome and CVD (37-40). Sedentary lifestyle, increase in dietary fat and refined carbohydrate and alcohol consumption are common behaviour patterns, underlying above risk factors. Insulin resistance is nearly universal in all these conditions and South Asians are at the greatest risk of developing CAD and diabetes (36-39). These behaviour patterns, result into hyperinsulinemia but insulin resistance may differ and may not occur in all tissues of the body. Adipose tissue is not resistant to insulin in the early stages of whole-body insulin resistance, but muscle is resistant very early in the progression of metabolic syndrome X. Therefore, physical activity and yogasans, appear to be important in the prevention and treatment of insulin resistance. There is no scientific evidence to demonstrate that metabolic syndrome among South Asians is genetic in origin. It is possible that populations in developing countries, under scarcity, may have adapted to survive at low fat intake and physically demanding occupations, which made them more susceptible to dietary energy, sedentary behaviour and to established risk factor (47-55). Abdominal obesity (central deposition of fat) in South Asians, appears to be universal in all the countries, wherever they are living, but whether the development of this type of obesity is genetic, dietary, caused by low physical activity, or a combination of these factor has not been established. Central obesity appears to be more prominent in the South Asian population than in the other Asian and Western populations. It is possible that transgenic mice overexpressing 11β hydroxysteroid dehydrogenase type 1 (11βHSD-1) selectively in adipose tissue can develop abdominal obesity and exhibit insulin-resistant diabetes, hyperlipidemia and hyperphagia despite hyperleptinemia (55). It is not known whether adipose tissue from the abdomens of South Asians show increased 11βHSD-1 activity. If this is true, peroxisome proliferator-activated receptor-γ ligands, which markedly reduce adipocyte 11βHSD-1 activity in vitro and in vivo preferentially reduce abdominal fat, may be the drugs of choice in South Asians to reduce insulin resistance and obesity (48, 55). South Asians may be genetically programmed or due to maladaptation may overexpress 11βHSD-1 in their adipose tissue, which may account for their higher risk of metabolic syndrome. It is possible, that treatment of central obesity with these agents, may be protective against metabolic syndrome, in South Asians (48, 55).

Singh et al. (48) in one cross sectional survey among 255 rural and 311 urban elderly subjects showed, that mean blood pressures, body mass index and insulin levels and the prevalence of hypertension were significantly greater among urban compared to rural population. Total fat intake was significantly greater among urban and hypertensive subjects compared to rural normotensive and hypertensive subjects, respectively. A recent study (51) among 54 patients of acute myocardial infarction (AMI) showed that the intake of large meals and large breakfast >1000 cal especially rich in TFA was significantly associated with AMI compared to control subjects. Those consuming large meals, showed significantly greater levels of tumour necrosis factor-alpha (TNF-α) and interleukin-6 (IL-6)) compared to subjects taking small breakfast. In another study (26) among 202 patients, large meals was a trigger for development of AMI among half of the patients. TNF-α and IL-6, incidence of known hypertension and type-2 diabetes were significantly greater among AMI patients compared to healthy subjects. These proinflammatory markers are risk factors of AMI and metabolic syndrome (47). In one cross-sectional survey (52),among 3,257 women, aged 25-64 years, social class 1-3 were consuming significantly greater amount of total visible fat, including TFA and clarified butter (Indian ghee) and vegetable oils, compared to lower social classes 4 and 5. Mean body mass index (BMI), over weight (BMI>25Kg/M2) and central obesity (Waist-hip ratio >85) were significantly greater among higher social classes than lower social classes. Higher social classes 1-3 are known to have greater prevalence of CAD, type 2 diabetes and hypertension, indicating metabolic syndrome in Indians. It is possible that lower intake of w-3 fatty acids and MUFA, as well as increased consumption of w-6 fatty acids, SFA and TFA may be responsible for central obesity and metabolic syndrome among these patients (39, 52-54). In another study (55), among 850men, aged 25-64 years, subjects were divided into high fat, over-fat, normal-fat and under fat based on criteria of body fat analysis by bioelectrical impedance. The prevalence of CAD, type 2 diabetes, and hypertension, as well as low HDL cholesterol, BMI and WHR were significantly associated with high body fat percent.

NUTRITIONAL MODULATION OF GENETIC EXPRESSION

Dietary factors and physical activity, mental stress and environmental toxicants can influence gene expression and have shaped the genome over several million years of human evolution (49, 54, 57), which has given an opportunity for health, as well as susceptibility to diseases, through genes, while environmental factors determine which susceptible individuals will develop metabolic syndrome. Rapid changes in diet and lifestyle due to socioeconomic changes provide added stress causing exposure of underlying genetic predisposition to chronic diseases such as type 2 diabetes, obesity, hypertension, CAD and atherosclerosis. Several studies are continuing on the role of nutrients in gene expression (54). It is not clear how n-3 fatty acids suppress or decrease the mRNA of interleukin, which is elevated in atherosclerosis, arthritis and other autoimmune diseases, whereas n-6 fatty acids have no such effects (54). Metabolic syndrome appears to be polygenic in nature and rapidly escalating rates suggest the importance of environmental change, rather than changes in genetic susceptibility

It has been proposed (47-55) that genetic and other factors, including oxidative stress; superoxide anion (O2) and hydrogen peroxide (H2O2), endothelial nitric oxide (eNO), lipid peroxides, anti-oxidants, endothelin, angiotensin converting enzyme (ACE) activity, angiotensin-II, transforming growth factor-β (TGF-β), insulin, homocysteine, asymmetrical dimethyl arginine, pro-inflammatory cytokines: interleukin-6 (IL-6), tumor necrosis factor-α (TNF-α), C-reactive protein (hs-CRP), and long-chain polyunsaturated fatty acids (LCPUFAs) and activity of NAD(P)H oxidase have a role in human essential hypertension.

There is a close interaction between endogenous molecules like e NO, endothelin, cytokines and nutrients with folic acid, coenzyme Q10, L-carnitine, L-arginine, tetrahydrobiopterin (H4B), vitamin B6, vitamin B12, vitamin C and LCPUFAs. Statins can mediate some of their actions through (LCPUFAs), whereas these fatty acids (especially ω-3 fatty acids) suppress cyclo-oxygenase activity and the synthesis of pro-inflammatory cytokines, and activate parasympathetic nervous system. This activity can reduce the risk of major vascular events. LCPUFAs such as EPA, DHA from precursors to lipoxins and resolvins may have anti-inflammatory actions. Low-grade systemic inflammation seen in hypertension seems to have its origins in the perinatal period and availability of adequate amounts of LCPUFAs during the critical periods of brain growth prevents the development of hypertension (57). This indicates that preventive strategies aimed at decreasing the incidence of hypertension and its associated conditions such as atherosclerosis, type 2 diabetes, CAD and cardiac failure in adulthood need to be prevented during the perinatal period for primordial prevention of metabolic syndrome.

DIETARY FACTORS AND CARDIOVASCULAR DISEASE

Experimental studies indicate that type and amount of dietary fatty acids may cause insulin resistance and metabolic syndrome (58). MUFA or w-3 fatty acids appear to have beneficial effects on insulin action, whereas w-6 fatty acids, saturated fats and diets with high total-fat content, appear to decrease insulin sensitivity in animal studies (36-38). It is hypothesized that dietary fats affect the phospholipid composition of cell membranes in skeletal muscle and other tissues. Several clinical studies showed a decrease in insulin sensitivity with high fat diets (61, 62). A few studies diminish the strength of their conclusions, including large difference in diets, the nonrandomized assignment of diets and lack of standardized methods to measure insulin sensitivity. A few studies using more standard measures reported a relationship between fat content and insulin sensitivity (63). One reason may be the relatively short duration of intervention in many of these studies. A recent multicenter, 3-month investigation found that a diet high in saturated fat (18% of energy) decreased insulin sensitivity more than a diet high in monounsaturated fat (21% of energy) among 162 healthy men and women (64). Many cross-sectional epidemiologic studies also demonstrated positive association between intake of saturated fat and hyperinsulinemia, after adjustment for measure of body fat (43, 44), but, at least one large, well-designed study showed no association (67).

Prospective studies including the Nurses' Health Study (68) suggest the role of specific types of fat in the development of type 2 diabetes mellitus. In the Nurses' Health Study, investigators reported an inverse association between development of diabetes and intake of vegetable fat and polyunsaturated fat, a positive association for trans-fatty acids, but no association for total fat in the diet. In a more recent study (69) among 15 obese, hyperinsulinemic subjects, a hypoenergetic, MUFA rich diet containing 35% carbohydrate, 45% fat and 20% protein was compared with a diet containing 60% carbohydrate, 20% fat and 20% protein. After four weeks, fasting insulin levels, insulin to glucose ratio and homeostatic model and assessment index decreased to normal ranges and were significantly lower in high MUFA group as compared with the control group. However, insulin sensitivity score increased significantly more, waist circumference showed significant decline, in the high MUFA group compared to high carbohydrate group, indicating improved insulin sensitivity and decreased central obesity respectively with MUFA rich diet. In a cross-sectional population study Folsom et al. (70) reported among 4,000 healthy subjects that fasting insulin levels were positively associated with the percentage of saturated fat in plasma and inversely associated with present age of MUFA. Lovejoy et al. (71) observed that certain class of fatty acids such as w-6, saturated and TFA have more deleterious effects on insulin action than others, and increase the risk of type 2 diabetes mellitus and therefore metabolic syndrome. Low and coworkers (72) found that a high MUFA diet induced improvement in the control of type 2 diabetes as compared to high carbohydrate diet. Similar results were noted by other workers (69, 73). In one study, MUFA rich diet also reduced the total cholesterol to HDL-cholesterol ratio, compared to high carbohydrate diet (74).

A greater reduction in triglyceride levels was observed in the high MUFA group than in the high carbohydrate group (74, 75). These results were observed in earlier studies (56) showing that dietary fatty acid composition affects the fatty acid composition of VLDL-triglyceride and alterations in composition of VLDL and in the enzymes involved in its catabolism, are two mechanisms observed in the hypotriglyceridemic effect of high MUFA diets (76). Oleic acid has also been found to cause a reduction in triglyceride levels, possibly through increasing the removal of triacylglycerol (77). Moreover, olive oil has been found to promote gastrointestinal secretions and stimulate stomach emptying thereby increasing the rate of supply of fatty acids to the enterocytes (78), thus accelerating the rate of digestion and absorption and faster rate of entry of chylomicrons into the circulation. This implies that the long-term use of olive oil may cause up-regulation of the enterocytes' ability to process dietary triacylglycerol and synthesize chylomicrons (79). However, high carbohydrate diets are known for their hypertriglyceridemic effects and glucose intolerance (80), which appear to be due to down-regulation of muscle lipoprotein lipase (LPL) activity (81).These adverse effects of such diets can enhance diabetes and cardiovascular disease or metabolic syndrome (82-86). The Columbus concept of diet; including fruits, vegetables, whole grains, nuts, w-3 fatty acid rich egg and meats and Columbus oil (olive oil+linseed oil) in conjunction with physical activity addresses both diet and lifestyle, and may be useful in the prevention of metabolic syndrome as well as its components (57, 87-89).

ENDOTHELIAL DYSFUNCTION

Vascular indexes should be independently considered as risk factors of atherothrombosis, because of anti-inflammatory effects of statins, hormone replacement therapy (HRT) and post-prandial endothelial dysfunction, in relation to inflammation (33-35) impaired vascular biology, physiology and biochemistry resulting into inflammation and endothelial dysfunction may be independently atherothrombotic (33, 90). There is evidence that abnormalities of the post-prandial state are important contributing factors to the development of atherosclerosis (50, 51, 90). Recent studies indicate that changes in LDL cholesterol and C-reactive protein independently correlated with coronary atherosclerosis progression and coronary events (91, 92). However, on treatment, C-reactive protein was as predictive of subsequent coronary events as was LDL cholesterol. HRT increases HDL cholesterol, and endothelial function, as well as inflammation and coagulation which are atherogenic, hence HRD has been discarded.

Clinical data indicate that post-prandial hypertriglyceridaemia is a risk factor for cardiovascular disease in non-diabetic subjects and may be a predictor of carotid intima-media thickness in type 2 diabetic patients (93). Meal absorption is a complex phenomenon, and post-prandial hyperlipidaemia and hyperglycaemia are simultaneously present in the post-absorptive phase, particularly in diabetic patients or in subjects with impaired glucose tolerance (9, 90, 93, 94). Both post-prandial hyperglycaemia and hypertriglyceridaemia may cause endothelial dyfunction, which is considered an early marker of atherosclerosis (33). Effect of different isocaloric meals on endothelial function in both normal subjects and type 2 diabetic patients, may be that the level of triglycerides after a high-fat (saturated) meal may be associated with endothelial dysfunction, with maximal impairment occurring at the time of the simultaneous presence of post-prandial hyperglycaemia and hypertriglyceridaemia (33). The effect of liquid meals rich in carbohydrates or saturated fats may be similar. It is possible that endothelial dysfunction induced by a high-fat meal in type 2 diabetic patients or associated with fasting hypertriglyceridaemia in young men could be associated with increased plasma concentrations of asymmetric dimethylarginine, an endogenous nitric oxide synthase inhibitor, suggested as a novel cardiovascular risk factor (95).

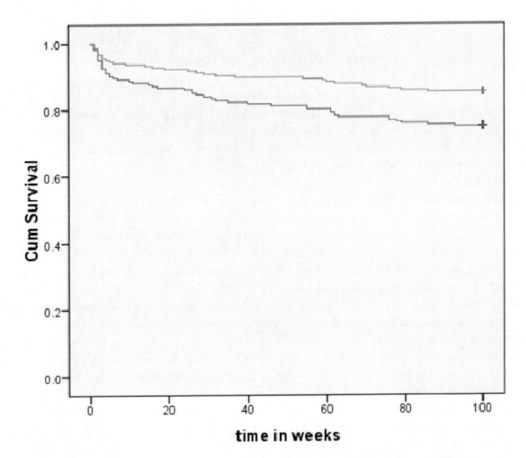

Figure 2. Kaplan Meier survival curve: proportions of deaths after 2 years. Singh et al. (137).

A mild prooxidative state accompanies meal ingestion, which results in raised circulating biomarkers of inflammation, adhesion and endothelial dysfunction, all of which are factors in the development of cardiovascular disease (96). The effect of hyperglicaemia, hypertriglyceridaemia and raised free fatty acids (FFA) levels both fasting and post-prandial, on endothelial function may be mediated through the generation of an oxidative stress (33, 96) (see figure 1, 2). The process is supposed to involve increased superoxide generation, which in turn inactivates nitric oxide. Superoxide and nitric oxide combine to produce peroxynitrite, a potent and long-lived oxidant that is cytotoxic, initiates lipid peroxidation and nitrates amino acids such as tyrosine which affects many signal transduction pathways. The production of the peroxynitrite anion can be indirectly inferred by the presence of nitrotyrosine (NT). An increase in plasma NT levels has been reported in association with post-prandial hyperglycaemia or hypertrigly- cidaemia, with a cumulative effect occurring in the presence of both conditions (33-35). It seems therefore that oxidative stress is a mediator of the effect of raised substrate concentration in the post-prandial phase (97, 98). It is clear that what happens during the absorption phase may be of considerable importance, because it occurs several times every day and human beings now spend an increasingly greater part of their lives in the post-prandial phase without periods of fasting. These biological markers after a high fat meal, also rich in refined carbohydrates, appear to be basic underlying mechanism for insulin resistance and metabolic syndrome leading to CVD (99).

PROINFLAMMATORY NUTRIENTS

Proinflammatory macronutrients such as w-6 fatty acids, TFA and SFA as well as refined carbohydrates intake may produce oxidative stress and proinflammatory substances (33) (see figure 1, 2). Glucose ingestion in normal subjects is associated with increased superoxide generation in leukocytes and mononuclear cells, as well as with raised amount and activity of nuclear factor-κB (NF-κB), a transcriptional factor regulating the activity of at least 125 genes, most of which are pro-inflammatory (99). Increased consumption of refined carbohydrates also causes an increase in two other pro-inflammatory transcription factor, activating protein-1(AP-1) and Egr-1, the first regulating the transcription of matrix metallo-proteinases and the second modulating the transcription of tissue factor and plasminogen activator inhibitor-1 (33, 99). A mixed meal from a fast-food chain has also been shown to induce activation of NF-κB associated with the generation of reactive oxygen species (ROS) by mononuclear cells. Superoxide anion appears to be an activator of at least two major pro-inflammatory transcription factor, NF-κB and AP-1. These observations are consistent with previous findings, demonstrating that after oral or intravenous glucose challenges, in both normal subjects and patients with type 2 diabetes mellitus, there is an increased generation of ROS and raised circulating levels of proinflammatory cytokines, such as TNF-α, IL-6 and IL-18 (33, 100-102). In apparently healthy subjects, a single high-fat meal produces endothelial activation, as evidenced by increased concentrations of the adhesion molecules VCAM-1 (vascular cell adhesion molecule-1) and ICAM-1 (intercellular adhesion molecule-1), in association with raised plasma concentrations of IL-6 and TNF-α (33). A high-fat meal (102) may increase the circulating levels of IL-18, a pro-inflammatory cytokine supposed to be involved in plaque destabilization associated with the simultaneous decrease of circulating adiponectin, an adipocyte-derived protein with insulin sensitizing, anti-inflammatory, and antiatherogenic properties (103).

NUTRITION AND INSULIN RESISTANCE

Biological dysfunctions, found in diabetes, obesity and the metabolic syndrome include, among others, increases in the circulating levels of metabolites, such as FFA and triglycerides and cytokines such as TNF-α and IL-6.Administration of a macronutrient, causes a shift towards oxidative stress and inflammation, which in turn may reduce insulin sensitivity. FFA as well as proinflammatory markers have been shown to predict type 2 diabetes independent of known risk factor (104,105). Both FFA and TNF-α have also been shown to activate inhibitor K kinase β (IKK-β) in adipocytes and hepatocytes, which can then increase the serine phosphorylation of insulin receptor substrate1(IRS-1) with subsequent reduction in insulin- dependent tyrosine phosphorylation of IRS-1, and ultimately glucose transport (106). IKKβ is a serine kinase that controls the activation of NK-κB, a transcription factor associated with inflammation. IRS-1 may be directly phosphorylated by IKK-β at serine residues, representing a novel class of substrates for IKKβ (107). In one recent study (108) in which hepatic expression of the lkappa Balpha super-repressor, which reduces IKKβ activity, reversed the phenotype of wild-type mice fed diet. It is possible that lipid accumulation in the liver leads to subacute hepatic 'inflammation' through NK-κB activation and downstream cytokine production resulting into insulin resistance both locally in liver as well as systemically. Circulation of IL-6 in plasma is at high concentrations and is associated with insulin resistance in men and in obese or hyperandrogenic women (33). Circulating IL-6 levels and insulin sensitivity relationships seem to occur in parallel to increases in plasma FFA. In contrast to IL-6 and TNF-α, adiponectin mRNA is reduced in adipose tissue from patients with type 2 diabetes (103).

It seems that low adiponectin production contributes to insulin resistance and there is evidence that adiponectin decreases circulating FFA levels by increasing fatty acid oxidation by skeletal muscle (109). The endogenous proinflammatory potential may be greater, in the post-prandial phase, due to imbalance in pro and anti-inflammatory cytokines, particularly following the ingestion of rapidly absorbed foods. Modification of circulating FFA levels may mediate a part of this effect and blunting of antiinflammatory actions of insulin might also play a role. Insulin causes a suppression of NK-κB, at physiologically relevant concentrations, thus reducing the production of some of its transcripts, namely IL-6 and TNF-α (33). This benefit of insulin, has been related to its ability to induce the release of nitric oxide and to enhance the expression of constitutive nitric oxide synthase.

NUTRITIONAL APPROACHES TO STOP ENDOTHELIAL DYSFUNCTION

The vascular effects of high sugar and high fat meals have greatly increased our understanding about the role of diet on atherothrombosis (34). There is increased flux of nutrients in the post-prandial state which is associated with an increase in circulating levels of pro-inflammatory cytokines, recruitment of netrophils and oxidative stress. The generation of reactive oxygen species (ROS) may be a common ground for all these findings and may help understanding current dietetic recommendations of the International College of Cardiology, emphasizing increased consumption of fruits, vegetables (400g/day), nuts (50g/day) and grains (400g/day), spices and MUFA+w-3 fatty acids rich oils (30-50g/day). Fruits, vegetables, nuts and spices are rich in natural antioxidants, phytochemicals and fibre that help fighting the oxidant wave of meals. Decreasing the intake of w-6, trans-and saturated fatty acids and increasing the consumption of omega-3 fatty acids (lin, mustered, canola oil) and MUFA (olive oil) are also considered important strategies to reduce CAD and metabolic syndrome (30-32). There is evidence that these two strategies are also associated with a reduced inflammatory status. In the Nurses Health Study, levels of C-reactive protein and markers of endothelial dysfunction were 73% higher in the highest quintile of trans-fatty acids intake, compared with the lowest quintile (110) and low-cholesterol/low-saturated fat diets are associated with mitigation of low-grade systemic inflammation, which correlated with reduction of plasma C-reactive protein levels (111). Cross-sectional study from the Nurses Health Study I cohort demonstrated lower concentrations of many markers of inflammation and endothelial activation, including C-reactive protein, IL-6 and E-selectin, among those in the highest quintile of omega-3 fatty acids, when compared with the lowest quintile (112). Since a high intake of omega-6 fatty acids may reduce the known beneficial effects of omega-3 fatty acids on CAD risk (54); a combination of both types of fatty acids in a ratio of 1:1 as advised by Columbus Concept Institute, which may be associated with the lowest level of inflammation (113).

However, it seems that w-6/w-3 ratio in the diet should be <5.0 to have optimal benefit of these fatty acids in the prevention of CVD, type 2 diabetes and metabolic syndrome.

Since free radical stress is supposed to play a key role in the development of atherosclerosis, antioxidant-vitamin supplementation has been suggested for the treatment and prevention of chronic diseases, including CAD (49). The encouraging results of short-term trials in participants with coronary atherosclerosis were not confirmed in large-size intervention trials. It seems that it is wrong to focus on a single element of the diet; guideline from some professional or governmental panels recommend to consume vitamins and minerals from food sources, rather than from supplements (49, 113). A shift towards energy dense, refined, ready prepared foods with high glycemic index (refined starches and sugar) and unhealthy lipids (TFA,SF,w-6 rich oils) poor in phytochemicals and fibre have been adopted by increased number of people and populations in the western world and in the urban populations of middle income countries in the last few decades (32,47-53). These changes in diet can cause an inactivation of innate immune system, by excessive production of proinflammatory cytokines and reduced production of anti-inflammatory cytokines, which may result into generation of inflammatory milieu, causing insulin resistance and endothelial dysfunction. These changes in diet in conjunction with inadequate physical activity appear to be responsible for the development of positive energy balance, weight gain and central obesity, which is widely acknowledged as an endocrine organ, secreting an increasing number of mediators, including proinflammatory cytokines (114). Central obesity is a key promoter of low grade systemic inflammatory state (93, 94) and is characterized by the most severe metabolic abnormalities (34).It seems that subjects with abdominal adiposity are particularly prone to the pro-inflammatory effects of unhealthy diets. The changes in dietary patterns that occurred in recent years are characterised with the intake of large amount of foods that seem faster in preparations and producing health damage. One prospective CARDIA (Coronary artery risk development in young adults) study indicated that frequent fast food intake causes weight gain and risk of insulin resistance, over 15 years (117).

The Quebec Family Study has shown that a decrease in the consumption of fat-foods or an increase in consumption of whole grains and fruits predicted a lower increase in body weight and adiposity indicators, over a 6-year follow-up (118). However, no specific dietary recommendations have been advocated by health agencies for the treatment of insulin resistance or the metabolic syndrome (49, 88, 89). Given that the metabolic syndrome is an identifiable and potentially modifiable risk state for both type 2 diabetes and cardiovascular disease, adopting a dietary pattern as that used by other workers may reduce the potential risk of these diseases (49, 122-126). In one study, Knoops et al. (119) colleagues from the Netherlands, France, Spain and Italy demonstrated that in European men and women aged 70-90 years, adherence to a Mediterranean-style diet, which represents a solid example of a healthy dietary pattern, moderate alcohol consumption, non-smoking status and physical activity was associated with a lower rate of all-cause mortality. This combination of healthy diet and lifestyle, was associated with a mortality rate of about one-third that of those with none or only one of these protective factors. In another larger study, involving about 22,000 adults, showed an inverse correlation between a greater adherence to a Mediterranean-style diet and death (120). Approximately a 2/9 increment in the Mediterranean diet score, was associated with a 25% reduction in total mortality and a 33% reduction in CAD mortality. Intervention trials, using the whole diet approach so far produced are also in line with this epidemiological evidence.

THE LYON DIET HEART STUDY

The Lyon Diet Heart Study hypothesis was that the lowest rates of cardiovascular diseases in the world were observed in populations either following a Mediterranean diet or a diet low in omega-6 fatty acids, but rich in omega-3 fatty acids (121). Therefore, the main strategy to reduce the rate of complications in patients with established CHD should be to adopt an omega-3 fatty acid-rich Mediterranean diet, which is characterised with fruits, vegetables, nuts, poultry and olive oil. This study is a secondary prevention trial designed to test the hypothesis that a Mediterranean ALA-rich diet may improve the prognosis of patients having survived a first acute myocardial infarction (AMI). In this study, 605 patients who had a myocardial infarction were randomly assigned to a 'Mediterranean-style' diet or a control diet resembling the American Heart Association Step I diet. The Mediterranean diet model supplied 30% of energy from fats and < 10% of energy from saturated fatty acids, whereas the intake of 18:3 (n-3) (α-linolenic acid) provided >0.6% of energy. After a mean follow-up of 27 months, the risk of new acute myocardial infarction and episodes of unstable angina was reduced by about 70% by the Mediterranean diet and total mortality was also reduced by 70%.

A striking protective effect of the Mediterranean diet was reported with a 50-70 % reduction of the recurrence also after four years of follow-up. Briefly, as regards lipids the experimental Mediterranean diet tested in the trial supplied less than 30% of energy from fats and less than 8% of energy from saturated fats. Regarding essential fatty acids, the intake of linoleic acid was restricted to 4% of energy and the intake of ALA made up more than 0.6% of energy. In practical terms, the dietary instructions were detailed and customized to each patient and can be summarized as: more bread, more cereals, more legumes and beans, more fresh vegetable, nuts and fruits, more fish, less meat (beef, lamb, pork) and delicatessen, which were to be replaced by poultry; no more butter and cream to be replaced by an experimental canola oil-based margarine. This margarine was chemically comparable with olive oil but slightly enriched in linoleic acid and mostly in ALA, the two essential fatty acids. Finally, the oils recommended for salad and food preparation were exclusively olive and canola oils. Two other major components of the traditional Mediterranean diet, in addition to a low omega-6/omega-3 fatty acids ratio, are low saturated fat intake and high oleic acid intake. Patients also had to meet these two major criteria of a healthy diet. Thus, to meet the criteria of a Mediterranean diet, patients had to drastically reduce the consumption of foods rich in saturated (essentially animal) fat. Among vegetable oils, only olive oil (despite its lack of ALA) and canola oil (despite its very high amounts of linoleic acid) have a fatty acid composition in line with our strategy. Thus, the patients were advised to use both oils. Because of their high content in linoleic acid; soybean, sunflower and safflower oils should not be used daily for food preparation and salad dressing. Peanut oil is too rich in saturated fatty acids and linoleic acid, and linseed (flaxseed) oil is too rich in polyunsaturated fatty acids. In theory, the best option should be to vary the use of several oils. To simplify, all subjects were advised and to the exclusive use of olive and canola oils. This exclusive use of olive and canola oils (and of canola-oil based margarine instead of butter to spread on the bread) to prepare meals and salad was a major issue in that trial as it resulted in significant differences in the fatty acid composition of both circulating plasma (essentially lipoproteins) and cell membrane phospholipids. The main differences between groups in platelet phospholipid fatty acids were not seen at the level of individual fatty acids (ALA is almost undetectable in cell membranes), but for the entire family of each group.

Significant differences were also seen for the ratio of omega-6 to omega-3 fatty acids. When comparing the dietary fatty acids in the two groups, control patients did consume about 0.7g of ALA per day against about 1.8 in the experimental group, i.e., giving an LA to ALA ratio of about 10 to 1 in control against about 4 to 1 in the experimental group was lower than in the control group, the risk in the control group was not high compared with previous studies indication that the 10 to 1 ratio was, in theory, not so bad. Because the Mediterranean diet tested in the trial was different from the control diet in many other aspects than the LA to ALA ratio (less saturated fat, more antioxidants from various sources, more vitamins of the B group including folic acid, more vegetable proteins, and so on), the next question was to try and specify the exact role of ALA in the cardioprotection observed in the trial.

Using multivariate analyses and adjustment for several confounders, the authors found that the plasma ALA levels measured two months after randomization were significantly associated with the risk of recurrence, and in particular of fatal recurrence. It could be said, however, that it is not ALA per se that was protective but the very long-chain omega-3 fatty acids derived from ALA, eicosapentanoic and docosahexanoic acids, which were also increased in the plasma of experimental patients. These very long long-chain omega-3 fatty acids have indeed been demonstrated to prevent ventricular fibrillation (VF) and sudden cardiac death (SCD) in animal experiments and in human trial. However, in the Lyon trial, these fatty acids were not significantly (borderline non significant with docosahexanoic acid) associated with a lower risk, which suggests that ALA was the main protective factor. Also, a specific antiarrhythmic effect of ALA itself was reported in the animal studies where it was tested. It does not mean, however, that the benefits of ALA are not due, at least partly, to its conversion into very long chain omega-3 fatty acids, and further studies are required to differentiate the individual effects of each omega-3 fatty acids in the context of myocardial ischemia and ventricular arrhythmias. Earlier studies on seven Day Adventists and American nurses suggested that eating nuts was associated with a diminished risk of CHD. Potentially protective constituents of nuts include ALA, folates, magnesium , potassium, fibre, vitamin E, and arginine ratios. These ratios have been claimed to be important in the pathogenesis of CHD, the lysine –to-arginine ratio (an indirect evaluation of the consumption of animal and vegetable proteins) being potentially involved in atherogenesis and the methionine –to-arginine ratio being important for endothelial function because arginine is the precursor of NO (which protects the endothelium) and methionine is the precursor of homocysteine which is toxic for the endothelium.

INDO-MEDITERRANEAN DIET HEART STUDY

Singh et al. (122) tested an 'Indo-Mediterranean diet' in 1,000 patients in India, with existing coronary disease or at high risk for coronary disease. When compared with the control diet, the intervention diet characterized by increased intake of mustard or soyabean oil, nuts (walnuts, almonds), vegetables, fruits and whole grains-reduced the rate of fatal myocardial infarction by one-third and the rate of sudden death from cardiac causes by two-thirds. Esposito et al. (123) randomized 180 patients (99men, 81 women) with the metabolic syndrome to a Mediterranean style diet, characterized with whole grains, vegetables, fruits, nuts and olive oil versus a cardiac-prudent diet with fat intake <30%. After a follow up of two years, subjects in the intervention diet showed greater weight loss, had lower C-reactive protein, and proinflammatory cytokine levels, had less insulin resistance, as well as lower total cholesterol and triglycerides and higher HDL cholesterol. The prevalence of metabolic syndrome was reduced to one half. The Japan Public Health Centre based study (124) showed that eating more w-3 fatty acids by increased intake of fish was associated with significant reduction in cardiovascular disease and cardiac mortality.

THE INDIAN EXPERIMENTS OF INFARCT SURVIVAL

Acute myocardial infarction (AMI) is associated with hyperglycemia, hypertriglyceridemia, hyperinsulinemia, increased FFA, free radical stress, IL-6, TNF-alpha and deficiency of antioxidant vitamins and w-3 fatty acids, which appear to be responsible for complications and deaths among these patients (33, 125-137). Therefore, AMI or acute coronary syndrome (ACS) appears to be the best model to examine the effects of any intervention on various biochemical markers and associated factors during AMI. Recent studies (34-36) indicated that eating high fat, refined carbohydrate rich fast foods (western diet), can produce a similar proinflammatory state in our body, resulting in endothelial dysfunction, which may have adverse effects in patients with AMI. It is therefore, logical to avoid western diet in patients with ACS, and administer diet which is beneficial to vascular endothelium and myocardium.

There is limited evidence regarding the role of dietary intervention in patients with AMI (125-128). The aim of the Indian experiment was to determine the effects of a diet rich in w-3 fatty acids, vitamins, minerals and antioxidants (fruits, vegetables, legumes, walnuts, almonds, fish, mustered and soyabean oils) and low in refined carbohydrates, in patients with (AMI) (126-129). All patients with a diagnosis of ACS were assigned to an intervention diet (n=204) or a control diet (n=202) within 48 hours of the onset of the symptoms of AMI. The intervention group was advised to consume 600g/day of fruits, vegetables, legumes and almonds and walnuts, in a soup or semisolid form. Tomato soup, skim milk and curd (yogurt) were commonly used to mix crushed almonds and walnuts and other foods, which were grilled with mustered oil. The control group was advised a low fat diet consistent with National Cholesterol Education Program. Clinical characteristics, time elapsed from symptom onset to the index infarction, site of infraction, drug therapy and final diagnosis were comparable between the two groups. Intake of foods and selected nutrients was assessed during the 1 week and after 1 year. After 1 week, plasma lipid peroxides, vitamin C and lactate dehydrogenase levels were determined. Compared with the control groups, patients allocated to the dietary intervention consumed significantly greater amounts of fruit, vegetables, pulses, almonds, walnuts, oils and fish both during the first trial week (126) and 1 year after AMI (128). The consumption of n-3 fatty acids was also significantly greater in the intervention group than in the control group (1.8 ± 0.66 versus $0.65\pm0.4g$ day, $P<0.01$, see table 3). The consumption of proinflammatory foods, such as butter and clarified butter, refined starches and sugar were significantly greater in the control group than in the intervention group (see table 3). Plasma lipid peroxide level decreased significantly in the intervention group compared with the control group, indicating a decrease in oxidative stress which is protective against proinflammatory IL-6 and TNF-alpha as well as endothelial disfunction, although these data were not measured in our study. Lactate dehydrogenase (LDH) level increased less in the intervention group than in the control group, indicating that myocardial damage was prevented by the cardioprotective diet (see table 4). The increased intake of n-3 fatty acids from mustard and soy bean oil associated with the Mediterranean diet might be responsible for the significant reduction in the cardiac enzyme LDH and lipid peroxides in the intervention compared with the control group. Total cardiac events, including fatal and non-fatal myocardial infarctions and sudden cardiac deaths, were significantly lower in the intervention group compared with the control group, both after six weeks (127) as well as after one year (see table 5, 6) (128). These beneficial effects may be due to protection of mitochondria from damaging effects of free radicals. Effect of low omega-6/omega-3 fatty acid ratio Paleolithic Style Diet in patients with acute coronary syndromes: a randomized, single blind, controlled trial showed that a low ratio of <5.0 was associated with significant decline in cardiac events (Table 7, Figure 2, 3) (137).

Table 5. Ethnic differences in fatty acid levels in thrombocytes phospholipids and percentage of all deaths from cardiovascular disease. Modified from Simopoulos (57)

	Europe and USA %	Japan %	Greenland Eskimos %
Arachidonic acid(20:4w6)	26	21	8.3
Eicosapentaenoic acid(20:5w-3)	0.5	1.6	8.0
Ratio of w-6/w-3			
Mortality from cardiovascular	50	12	1
disease	45	12	7

Table 6. Fatty acid ratio in the diets. Modified from Simopoulos (3,57)

Subjects	w-6/w-3	
Paleolithic	0.79	Estimated
Greece prior to 1960	1.00-2.00	Current 7.10
Japan	4.00	Early 1-2
India, rural	5-6.1	Prior to 1960, 3-4
India urban	38-50	Prior to 1960, 5-10
UK	15.00	Prior to 1960,10.00
Northern Europe	15.00	Prior to 1960,10.00
USA	16.74	Prior to 1950 7-8
Slovakia	20-25	Estimated
Poland	20-25	Estimated

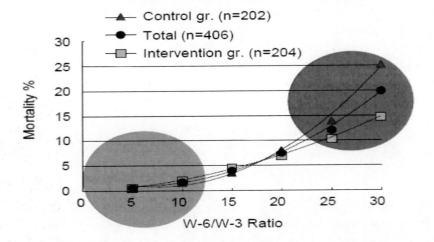

Association of W-6/W-3 Ratio of fatty acids with mortality

Figure 3. Association of w-6/w-3 ratio of fatty acids with mortality in the intervention and control groups and among total subjects. Singh et al. (137).

Table 7. Fatty acid consumption in the Paleolithic style diet group and standard diet group

Fatty acid KJ/day	Before entry All patients (n=406)	At entry Paleolithic (n=204)	Standard (n=202)	After one year Paleolithic (n=204)	Standard (n-202)
Saturated	10.0 (0.39)	7.0(0.22)	10.0(0.38)	7.2(0.24)	10.8(0.36)
Monounsaturated	9.3(0.38)	9.5(0.37)	7.6(0.26)	8.0(0.35)	10.2(0.32)
Polyunsaturated	6.7 (0.30)	8.1(0.44)	6.5(0.39)	8.6(0.39)	7.0(0.26)
W-6	6.5(0.29)	6.3(0.28)	6.3(0.29)	7.0(0.36)	6.2(0.24)
W-3	0.2(0.07)	1.8(0.13)**	0.2(0.082)	1.6(0.12)**	0. 3(0.083)
W-6/W-3 ratio	32.5(3.3)**	3.5(0.76)**	31.5(2.4)	4.4(0.56)**	20.6(2.1)
Main dietary oil	Pea nut	Mustard	Sunflower	Mustard	Sunflower

Values are mean± Standard deviation **=p<0.01, Singh et al. (77), their reference 40.

The effects of one year of treatment with fish oil (122 patients, eicosapentaenoic acid, EPA 1.08 g daily) mustard oil (120 patients, alpha-linolenic acid 2.9g daily) and no treatment (118 patients, placebo group) on the outcome of patients with suspected AMI were compared in a randomized, placebo-controlled trial) (130). Treatments were administrated within, on average 18h of onset of symptoms. Clinical characteristics, extent of cardiac damage and rise of cardiac enzymes and lipid peroxides were comparable among the three groups at study entry. After randomization, angina pectoris (18.0 and 21.6 versus 42.3%), arrhythmias (13.1 and 13.3 versus 28.7%) and poor left ventricular function (22.8 and 26.6, versus 47.4%) were significantly lower in the fish oil and mustard oil treatment groups compared with the placebo group. Sudden cardiac deaths (1.6 and 1.6 versus 6.6%), total cardiac deaths (11.4 and 13.3 versus 22.0%) non-fatal infarctions (13.0 and 15.0, versus 25.4%) and total cardiac events 24.5 and 28.2 versus 47.4%) were also significantly lower in the two intervention groups. A modest improvement in dyslipidaemia and a decrease in oxidative damage were observed in the fish oil and mustard oil groups, but not in the placebo group. On the third and the fifth day after AMI, serum glutamic oxalo-transaminase (SGOT) and LDH cardiac enzymes showed greater decline in the fish oil and mustard oil groups compared with the placebo group. These intervention trials indicate that further studies should be conducted with Columbus diet and Columbus oil (olive oil+linseed oil) in patients with AMI, to demonstrate, cytokine and endothelial function mediated mechanisms, in the pathophysiology of complications and deaths, among these patients.

RECOMMENDATIONS

There is no precise and proven, guideline for dietary advice, in patients with AMI, which may be protective against recurrent cardiac events (Table 8). A Columbus soup (tomatoes, grapes, vegetables, walnuts, almonds+linseed and olive oil) or yogurt containing, walnuts, almonds, raisins, could be prepared for ready use, for nonpharmacological intervention, among patients of AMI. Such recipes have been commonly used by us in our studies and clinical practice (126-133). These strategies can influence receptors, enzymes and nitric oxide (NO) secretion via increased intake of w-3 fatty acids (134, 135), apart from prevention of oxidation of blood lipids, which are protective. These methods are similar to dietary approaches proposed in the DASH diet used in earlier studies (15-17) in patients with multiple risk factors of CAD, indicating metabolic syndrome. The effects of diet on dyslipedimia and glucose were much better, when these dietary interventions were combined with exercise (67, 68). It is possible that high doses of EPA and DHA (3 to 4 g/day) providing low w-6/w-3 ratio of the diet, have been shown to increase systemic arterial compliance, indicating that marine omega-3 PUFAs improve endothelial function (33, 136-139). Therefore, a diet containing fish or fish oil supplements or columbus foods (eggs, chicken and oils) rich in w-3 fatty acids (25, 140) may be advised to provide protection against western diet-induced inflammation. Studies with ALA have been conflicting, with some positive and some negative studies. In a controlled trial (25), Columbus eggs showed beneficial effects on blood lipoproteins. Additionally, the omega-3 PUFAs exhibit an anti-inflammatory effect. EPA and DHA reduced tumor necrosis factor, interleukin-6, vascular cellular adhesion molecule-1, and E-selectin at relatively low doses ranging from 0.3 to 1 g/day. Although fewer studies have been performed, the results have been mixed with respect to the effect of ALA on inflammatory markers such as C-reactive protein, vascular cellular adhesion molecule- 1, E-selectin, and interleukin-6. The mechanistic studies with EPA and DHA have pointed to an antiarrhythmic effect, and data with ALA are less conclusive. Studies attempting to attribute other antiatherogenic properties to EPA, DHA, and ALA have not been consistent and many of these studies have demonstrated effects at doses much higher than those used in clinical end point trials. As a result of the previously mentioned omega-3 PUFA trials and recent epidemiologic evidence, the American Heart Association has published guidelines for the consumption of fish and fish oil, indicating that patients with CAD should try to consume a combination of EPA and DHA totaling 1 g/day. Many patients, however; do not enjoy eating fish or have concerns about pollutants. Rich sources of ALA, including canola, lin and flax seed meal and walnuts can be easily incorporated into the western diets.

Table 8. Dietary guidelines and desirable level of risk factors for populations. Modified from Indian Consensus Group, J Nutr Environ Med, 1996

Factors	Desirable Values
Energy (k calories/day)	1900-2300
Total Carbohydrate (k calories/day)	65.0
Complex Carbohydrate ((k calories/day)	55.0
Total Fat (k calories/day)	21.0
Saturated Fatty Acids (k calories/day)	7.0
Polyunsaturated Fatty Acids (k calories/day)	7.0
Polyunsaturated/Saturated Fat Ratio	1.0
n 6/n-3 Fatty Acid Ratio	1:1
Dietary Cholesterol (mg/day)	100
Whole Grains (wheat, rice, corn, legumes) (g/day)	400-500
Fruit, vegetables and nuts (g/day)	400-500
Salt (g/day)	<6.0
Brisk Walking (km/day)	9.0
Meditation/pranayam (minutes/day)	30.0
Body Mass Index (kg/m2)	
Range	19.0-23.0
Average	21.0
Waist-Hip Girth Ratio	
Male	<0.88
Female	<0.85
Serum Total Cholesterol (mg/dl) (4.42 mmol/L)	<170
Mild Hypercholesterolemia (mg/dl) (4.42-5.20 mmol/L)	170-200
Hypercholesterolemia (mg/dl) (>5.20 mmol/L)	>200
Low Density Lipoprotein Cholesterol (mg/dl) (2.32 mmol/L)	<90
Borderline High (mg/dl) (2.32-2.84 mmol/L)	90-110
High (mg/dl) (2.84 mmol/L)	>110
Triglycerides (mg/dl) (1.7 mmol/L)	<150
High Density Lipoprotein Cholesterol (mg/dl) (0.9 mmol/L)	>40 men, >50women
Blood Pressure (mmHg)	<125/85
Drug therapy in view of high risk of diabetes and CAD.	Amblodipine, ACE-I , receptor blockers and new beta-blockers? Fish oil, aspirin, statins

Columbus oil containing olive oil+linseed oil could be the best combination along with western diet, for prevention of metabolic syndrome. If clinical trials demonstrate that ALA is as effective as EPA and DHA in reducing cardiovascular events, the public health implications could be significant. The evidence supports a role for fish oil (EPA, DHA) or fish in secondary prevention, because the clinical trials have demonstrated a reduction in total mortality, CHD death, and sudden death. The evidence from these trials has indicated that EPA plus DHA supplementation in the range of 0.5 to 1.8 g/day provides significant benefit. More research is needed to determine whether the benefits of fish oil or fish extend to the world population in secondary and primary prevention.

The data on the plant-based n-3 PUFA, ALA, is very promising. However, the existing studies were small, and a large randomized controlled trial is needed before recommendations can be definitely made for CHD prevention. The data for ALA indicate, possible reductions in sudden death and nonfatal myocardial infarction, suggesting other potential cardioprotective mechanisms other than a predominately antiarrhythmic role. An urgent need exists to perform more clinical trials with ALA, because the results of such trials could have significant public health implications. Recommendations are given in table 7.

Diet and lifestyle intervention can reduce the risk for conversion of IFG/IGT to type 2 diabetes. Clinical studies, indicate that metformin or thiazolidinediones also reduce risk for type 2 diabetes in people with IFG or IGT. On the other hand, no clinical trial evidence indicates that these drugs will reduce risk for cardiovascular disease events in patients with the metabolic syndrome. Currently, metformin or thiazolidinediones are not recommended solely for the prevention of diabetes. The cost-effectiveness of this approach has not been established. When patients with type 2 diabetes concomitantly exhibit other features of the metabolic syndrome they are at particularly high risk for cardiovascular disease. Clinical trials show that high priority should be given to treatment of dyslipidaemia and hypertension. Glycaemic control to a haemoglobin A1c of less than 7% will reduce microvascular complications and could decrease risk for macrovascular disease as well. The use of lipid-altering, antihypertensive and hypoglycaemic drugs can modify insulin sensitivity and bodyweight. Metformin and thiazolidinediones improve insulin sensitivity, but have discrepant effects on body weight: metformin reduces weight whereas thiazolidinediones increase it. The increase in weight in patients treated with insulin secretagogues (sulfonylureas and repaglinide or nateglinide) and insulin results mostly from improved glycaemic control and increases in caloric intake as a result of hypoglycaemia. With the exception of nicotinic acid, lipid-altering drugs do not affect insulin sensitivity or weight, whereas the effect of antihypertensive drugs is more complex. Beta-adrenergic blockers and thiazide diuretics might decrease insulin sensitivity but less so at low doses, whereas ACE inhibitors and angiotensin II receptor antagonists have variable effects. By uncertain mechanisms, ACE inhibitors and angiotensin II receptor antagonists seem to decrease the incidence of type 2 diabetes.

Thrombogenic risk factors are characterised by elevations of fibrinogen, plasminogen activator inhibitor 1 and possibly other coagulation factors as well as lipoprotein phospholipase A2. The only available clinical approach to an increased risk for arterial thrombosis in patients with diabetes is low-dose aspirin or other antiplatelet drugs. These drugs are universally recommended unless contraindicated in patients with established cardiovascular disease. Their efficacy in patients with type 2 diabetes in the absence of cardiovascular disease has not been established through clinical trials, although they are widely recommended. In other people with the metabolic syndrome, coenzyme Q10 and aspirin prophylaxis are a therapeutic option when the risk for cardiovascular disease events is judged to be relatively high. A proinflammatory state or premetabolic syndrome is identified by elevated cytokines (e.g., TNF-alpha and interleukin 6) as well as by elevations in acute phase reactants (C-reactive protein and brinogen). An elevated concentration of C-reactive protein is widely thought to be an indicator of a proinfammatory state and to be associated with higher risk for both cardiovascular disease and diabetes.

Lifestyle therapies, especially weight reduction, moderate physical activity and alcohol intake in moderation might reduce concentrations of this cytokine and thus can mitigate an underlying inflammatory state. No specific anti-inflammatory drugs are available to treat the proinammatory state. However, several drugs used to treat other metabolic risk factors—statins, fibrates, and thiazolidinedione, and coenzyme Q10, have been reported to reduce concentrations of C-reactive proteins and cytokines. However, these agents (accept w-3 fatty acids, coenzyme Q10 or a Mediterranean diet or a DASH diet) cannot be recommended specifically to reduce a proinflammatory state independent of other risk factors (135, 144). The association between overall dietary patterns and mortality due to cardiovascular disease and other chronic diseases is not unknown. In one study (145), a population of >70 000 apparently healthy US women over the course of 18 years, was followed, assessing dietary intake repeatedly. By applying factor analysis, the authors identified two major dietary patterns. A greater adherence to the pattern labeled as prudent (characterized by a high consumption of plant foods such as vegetables, fruit, legumes, and whole grains as well as fish and poultry) was related to a 28% reduced risk of cardiovascular disease mortality and a 17% reduced risk of premature all-cause mortality. By contrast, a greater adherence to the pattern labeled as western (characterized by a high consumption of red and processed meat, refined grains, french fries, and sweets) was associated with a 22% increased risk of cardiovascular disease mortality, a 16% increased risk of cancer mortality, and a 21% increased risk of premature all-cause mortality. The observed associations were independent of known risk factors including age, smoking, physical inactivity, body mass index, and total caloric intake. NCX1.3 is more sensitive to inhibition by ALA than NCX1.1. In addition, only w-3 PUFA inhibits NCX1.1, but several classes of fatty acids inhibit NCX1.3. The differential sensitivity of NCX isoforms to fatty acids may have important implications as therapeutic approaches for hypertension, heart failure and arrhythmias.(146) Nutritional recommendations to prevent CVDs and type 2 diabetes mellitus and promote longevity may need to focus on overall dietary patterns rather than on individual nutrients. Large cohort studies, further confirms the findings of the Indian experiment, the Lyon heart study and the Indo-Mediterranean diet heart study regarding protective effects of Tsim Tsoum foods in the prevention of CVD and all cause mortality (9, 147-151).

ACKNOWLEDGMENTS

We appreciate Columbus Paradigm Institute, Belgium and Tsim Tsoum Institute, Krakow, Poland for support to write this work. We are grateful to the International College of Nutrition and International College of Cardiology for logistics and academic support.

REFERENCES

[1] Eaton B. Evolution and cholesterol. World Rev Nutr Diet 2009; 100: 46-54.

[2] De Meester F. Progress in lipid nutrition: the Columbus concept addressing chronic diseases. World Rev Nutr Diet 2009;100: 110-21.

[3] Eaton SB, Eaton SB III, Sinclair AJ, Cordain I, Mann NJ. Dietary intake of long chain polyunsaturated fatty acids during the Paleilithic period. In Simopoulos AP edition. The return of w-3 fatty acids in the food supply. Land based animal food products and their health effects. World Rev Nutr Dietetics 1998;83:12-23.

[4] American Heart Association Heart and Stroke Statistical Update, 2008. http://www. americanheart.org/downloadable/heart/ 1200078608862HS Stats%202008.final.pdf

[5] The PURE Investigators. Prevalence of a healthy lifestyle among individuals with cardiovascular disease in high-, middle- and low-income countries: The Prospective Urban Rural Epidemiology (PURE) Study. JAMA 2013;309:1613-21.

[6] Singh RB, Singh V, Kulshrestha SK, Singh S, Gupta P, Kumar R, et al. Social class and all cause mortality in the urban population of north India. Acta Cardiol 2005;60:611-7.

[7] Fedacko J, Vargova V, Singh RB, Anjum B, Takahashi T, Tongnuka M, et al. Association of high w-6/w-3 fatty acid ratio diet with causes of death due to noncommunicable diseases among urban decedents in North India. Open Nutra J 2012;5:113-23.

[8] Joshi R, Cardona M, Iyengar S et al.Chronic diseases now a leading cause of death in rural India: mortality data from Andhra Pradesh rural initiative. Int J epidemiol 2006;35:1522-9.

[9] Mohan V, Shanthirani CS, Deepa M, Deepa R, Unnikrishnan RI, Datta M. Mortality rates due to diabetes in a selected urban south Indian population. The Chennai urban population study(CUPS-16). JAPI 2006;54:113-7.

[10] Goyal A, Yusuf F. The burden of cardiovascular disease in the Indian subcontinent. Ind J Med Res 2006;124:235-44.

[11] Chaturvedi N, Fuller JH. Ethnic differences in mortality from cardiovascular disease in the UK: Do they persist in people with diabetes? J Epidemiol Community Health 1996;50:137-9.

[12] Chaturvedi N, Jarrett J, Morrish N, Keen H, Fuller JH. Differences in mortality and morbidity in African Caribbean and European people with non-insulin dependent diabetes mellitus: results of 20 year follow up of a London cohort of a multinational study. BMJ 1996;313:848-52.

[13] Forouhi NG, Sattar N, Tillin T, McKeigue PM, Chaturvedi N. Do known risk factors explain the higher coronary heart disease mortality in South Asian compared with European men? Prospective follow-up of the Southall and Brent studies, UK. Diabetologia 2006;49:2580-8.

[14] DeMeester F, Wild-type land based foods in health promotion and disease prevention: the LDL-CC:HDL-CC model. In: DeMeester F, Watson RR, eds. Wild type foods in health promotion and disease prevention. Totowa, NJ: Humana Press, 2008:3-20.

[15] Fung TT, Chiuve SE, McCullough ML, Rexrode KM, Logroscino G, Hu FB. Adherance to DASH-style diet and risk of coronary heart disease and stroke in women. Arch Intern Med 2008;168:713-20.

[16] Sack FM, Svetkey LP, Vollmer WM, Appel LJ, Bray GA, Harsha D, et al. DASH-Sodium Collaborative Research Group. Effects on blood pressure of reduced dietary sodium and the Dietary Approaches to Stop Hypertension (DASH) diet. DASH-Sodium Collaborative Research Group. N Engl J Med 2001;344:3-10.

[17] Obarzanek E, Sacks FM, Vollmer WM, Bray GA, Miller ER 3rd , Lin PH, et al. Effects on blood lipids of a blood pressure-lowering diet: the Dietary Approaches to Stop Hypertension (DASH) Trial. Am J Clin Nutr 2001;74:80-9.

[18] Katcher HI, Legro RS, Kunselman AR, et al. The effects of whole grain- enriched hypocaloric diet on cardiovascular disease risk factors in men and women with metabolic syndrome. Am J Clin Nutr 2008; 87:79-90.

[19] Zhang C, Rexrode KM, van Dam RM, Li TY, Hu FB. Abdominal obesity and the risk of all cause, cardiovascular and cancer mortality. Sixteen years of follow-up in US women. Circulation 2008 117(13):1658-67.

[20]   Harris WS, Reid KJ, Sands SA, et al. Blood omega-3 and trans fatty acids in middle aged acute coronary syndrome patients. Am J Cardiol. 2007;99:154–161.

[21]   Singh RB, Takahashi T, Nakaoka T, Otsuka K, Toda E, Shin HH, Kyu Lee M, Beeharry V, Hristova K, Fedacko J, Pella D, De Meester F,Wilson DW, Juneja LR. Nutrition in transition from Homo sapiens to Homo economicus. Open Nutra J 2013;6:6-17.

[22]   Harper CR, Jacobson TA. Usefulness of omega-3 fatty acids and the prevention of coronary heart disease. Am J Cardiol 2005;96:1521-9.

[23]   Mozaffarian D, Geelan A, Brouwer IA, et al. Effect of fish oil on heart rate in humans, a metaanalysis of randomized, controlled trials. Circulation 2005;112:1945-52.

[24]   Jiang Z, Sim JS. Consumption of polyunsaturated fatty acid eggs and changes in plasma lipids of human subjects. Nutrition 2003;9:513-8.

[25]   Sumbalova Z, Kucharaska J, Kasparova S, Mlynarik V, Bystricky P, Bozek P, et al. Brain energy metabolism in experimental chronic diabetes: effect of long term administration of coenzyme Q10 and w-3 polyunsaturated fatty acids. Biologia 2005;11:1-13.

[26]   Zarranga IGE, Schwartz ER. Impact of dietary patterns and interventions on cardiovascular health. Circulation 2006;114:961-73.

[27]   Kang JS, Wang J, Wu I et al. Fat-1 mice convert w-6 to w-3 fatty acids. Nature 2004; 427:504-5.

[28]   Drukteinis JS, Roman J, Fabsitz RR, Lee ET, Best LG, Russel M, Devereux RB. Cardiac and systemic haemodynamic characteristics of hypertension and prehypertension in adolescents and young adults. The Strong Heart Study. Circulation 2007;115:211-7.

[29]   Lacroix FCM, De Meester F. The return to wild-type fats in the diet. Brit Nutr Found Nutr Bull 2007; 32:168-72.

[30]   Eberly LE, Prineas R, Cohen JD, Vazquez G, Zhi X, Neaton JD, Kuller LH. Multiple Risk Factor Intervention Trial Research Group.Metabolic syndrome:risk factor distribution and 18 year mortality in the multiple risk factor intervention trial. Diab Care 2006;29:123-30.

[31]   Lioyd-Jones DM, Liu K, Colangilo LA, Yan LL, Klein L, Loria CM, Lewis CE, Savage P. Consistent or stable body mass index in young adulthood and longitudinal changes in metabolic syndrome components. The Coronary Artery Risk Development in Young Adult Study. Circulation 2007;115:1004-11.

[32]   Heart Disease and Stroke Statistics 2013 Update. A report from the American Heart Association. Circulation 2013;127:e6-e245.

[33]   Singh RB, Pella D, DeMeester F, Otsuka K, Chopra R. Fatty acids in the causation and prevention of metabolic syndrome. In: Watson RR, DeMeester F, eds. Wild foods and health and disease. New York: Humana Press, 2008:263-84.

[34]   Esposito K, Glugliano D. Diet and inflammation:a link to metabolic and cardiovascular diseases. Euro Heart J 2006;27:15-20.

[35]   Vogel RA. Eating,vascular biology and atherosclerosis: A lot to chew on. Euro Heart J 2006;27:13-4.

[36]   Singh RB, Pella D, Kartikey K, DeMeester F. Prevalence of obesity, physical inactivity and undernutrition, a triple burden of diseases, during transition in a middle income country. Acta Cardiol 2007;62:119-7.

[37]   Singh RB, IL Suh, Singh VP, Chaithiraphan S, Laothavorn P, Sy RG, et al. Hypertension and stroke in Asia: prevelance, control and strategies in developing countries for prevention. J Hum Hyper 2000;14:749-63.

[38]   Singh RB, Mori H, Chen J, Mendis S, Moshiri M, Shoumin Z, et al. Recommendations for the prevention of coronary artery disease in Asians: a scientific statement of the International College of Nutrition. J Cardiovas Risk 1996,3:489-94.

[39]   Singh RB, Niaz MA, Ghosh S, Beegom R, Rastogi V, Sharma JP, Dube GK. Association of trans fatty acids (vegetable ghee),and clarified butter(Indian ghee) intake with higher risk of coronary artery disease, in rural and urban populations with low fat consumption. Int J Cardiol 1996;56:289-98.

[40]   Singh RB, Sircar AR, Rastogi SS, Singh R. Dietary modulators of blood pressure in hypertension. Euro J Clin Nutr 1990;44:319-27.

[41]   Singh RB, Sircar AR, Rastogi SS, Ghose S, Singh R. Can diet modulate blood pressure and blood lipids in hypertension? J Nutr Med 1991; 2:17-24.

[42]   Singh RB, Sharma VK,Gupta RK: Nutritional modulators of lipoprotein metabolism in patients with risk factors for coronary heart disease. J Am Coll Nutr 1992;11:391-8.

[43]   Singh RB, Rastogi SS, Niaz MA, Ghosh S, Singh R. Effects of fat modified and fruits vegetable enriched diets on blood lipids in the Indian diet heart study. Am J Cardiol 1992;69:869-74.

[44]   Singh RB, Rastogi SS, Ghosh S, Singh R, Niaz MA: Effects of guava intake on serum total and high density lipoprotein cholesterol levels and on systemic blood pressure. Am J Cardiol 1992;70:1287-91.

[45]   Singh RB, Rastogi SS, Ghosh S, Niaz MA, Singh NK. The diet and moderate exercise trial (DAMET): Results after 24 weeks. Acta Cardiol 1992;48:543-57.

[46]   Singh RB, Rastogi SS, Sircar AR, Mani UV, Singh NK, Niaz MA: Effect of lifestyle changes on atherosclerotic risk factors in the Indian diet heart study. Am J Cardiol 1993;71:1283-8.

[47]   Singh RB, Otsuka K, Chiang CE, Joshi SR. Nutritional predictors and modulators of metabolic syndrome. J Nutr Environ Med 2004;14:3-16.

[48]   Singh RB, Rastogi SS, Rastogi V, Niaz MA, Madhu SV, Chen Min, Shoumin Z. Blood pressure trends, plasma insulin levels and risk factors, in rural and urban elderly populations of north India. Coro Art Dis 1997;8:463-8.

[49]   Pella D, Singh RB, Tomlinson B, Kong CW. Coronary artery disease in developing and newly industrialized countries: A scientific statement of the International College of Cardiology. In: Dhalla NS, Chocklingham A, Berkowitz, HJ, Singal PK, eds. Frontiers of cardiovascular health. Boston: Kluwer Acad, 2003:473-83.

[50]   Singh RB, Pella D, Sharma JP, Rastogi S, Kartikey K, Goel VK, Sharma R, Neki NS, Kumar A, Otsuka K. Increased concentrations of lipoprotein(a), circadian rhythms and metabolic reactions, evoked by acute myocardial infarctions, in relation to large breakfast. Biomed Pharmacother 2004;58(Suppl):116-22.

[51]   Singh RB, Pella D, Neki NS, Chandel JP, Rastogi S, Mori H, Otsuka K.. Mechanism of acute myocardial infarction study. Biomed Pharmacother 2004;58(Supple):111-5.

[52]   Singh RB, Beegom R, Verma SP, Haque M, Singh R, Mehta AS, et al. Association of dietary factors and other coronary risk factors with social class in women in five Indian cities. Asia Pac J Clin Nutr 2000;9:298-302.

[53]   Aratti P, Peluso G, Nicolai R, Calvani M. Polyunsaturated fatty acids:biochemical, nutritional and epigenetic properties. J Am Coll Nutr 2004;23:281-302.

[54]   Simopoulos AP. Is insulin resistance influenced by dietary linoleic acid and trans fatty acids? Free Radical Biol Med 1994:17;367-72.

[55]   Singh RB, Niaz MA, Beegom R, Wander GS, Thakur AS, Rissam HS. Body fat percent by bioelectrical impedence analysis and risk of coronary artery disease among urban men, with low rates of obesity:the Indian paradox. J Amer Coll Nutr 1999,18:268-73.

[56]   Pella D, Dubnov G, Singh RB, Sharma R, Berry EM, Manor O. Effects of an Indo-Mediterranean diet on the omega-6/omega-3 ratio in patients at high risk of coronary artery disease: The Indian paradox. In: Simopoulos AP, Cleland LG, eds. World Rev Nutr Diet 2003;92:74-80.

[57]   Simopoulos AP. Importance of the ratio of omega-6/omega-3 essential fatty acids:evolutionary aspects. World Rev Nutr Diet 2003;92:1-22.

[58]   Storlien LH., Jenkins AB, Chisholm DJ, Pascoe WS, Khouri S, Kraegen EW. Influence of dietary fat composition on development of insulin resistance in rats. Relationship to muscle triglyceride and omega-3 fatty acids in muscle phospholipid. Diabetes 1991;40:280-9.

[59]   Lardinois CK, Strarich GH. Polyunsaturated fats enhance peripheral glucose utilization in rats. J Am Coll Nutr 1991;10:340-5.

[60]   Axen KV, Dikeakos A, Sclafani A. High dietary fat promotes syndrome x in nonobese rats. J Nutr 2003;133:2244-9.

[61]   Hu FB van Dam RM, Liu S. Diet and risk of type II diabetes: the role of types of fat and carbohydrate. Diabetologia 2001;44:805-7.

[62]   Swinburn BA. Effect of dietary lipid on insulin action. Clinical studies. Ann NY Acad Sci.1993; 683:102-9

[63] Unsitupa M, Schwab U, Makimattila S, Karhapaa P, Sakkinen E, Maliranta H, Agren J, Penttila I. Effects of two high fat diets with different fatty acid compositions on glucose and lipid metabolism in healthy young women. Am J Clin Nutr.1994;59:1310-6.

[64] Vessby B, Unsitupa M, Hermansen K, Riccardi G, Rivellese AA, Tapsell LC, et al. Substituting dietary saturated for monounsaturated fat impairs insulin sensitivity in healthy men and women: The KANWU Study. Diabetologia 2001;44:312-9.

[65] Marshall J, Bessesen D, Hamman R. High saturated fat and low starch and fibre are associated with hyperinsulinaemia in a non-diabetic population: The san Luis Valley. Diabetologia 1997;40:430-8.

[66] Feskens EJ, Loeber JG, Kromhout D. Diet and physical activity as determinants of hyperinsulinemia: the Zutphen Elderly Study. Am J Epidemiol 1994;140:350-60.

[67] Mayer-Davis EJ, Monaco JH, Hoen HM, Carmichael S, Vitolins MZ, Rewers MJ, et al. Dietary fat and insulin sensitivity in a triethnic population: the role of obesity. The Insulin Resistance Atherosclerosis Study (IRAS). Am J Clin Nutr 1997;65:79-87.

[68] Salmeron J, Hu FB, Manson JE, Stampfer MJ, Colditz GA, Rimm EB, Willett WC. Dietary fat intake and risk of type 2 diabetes in women. Am J Clin Nutr 2001;73:1019-26.

[69] Hwalla N, Torbay N, Andari N, Adra N, Azar ST, Harbal Z. Restoration of normal insulinemia and insulin sensitivity in hyperinsulinemic normoglycemic men by a hypoenergetic high monounsaturated fat diet. J Nutr Environ Med 2004;14:29-38.

[70] Folsom AR, Ma J, McGovern PG, Eckfeldt JH. Relation between plasma phospholipid, saturated fatty acids and hyperinsulinemia. Metabolism 1996;45:223-28.

[71] Lovejoy JC, Champagne CM, Smith SR. Relationship of dietary fat and serum cholesterol ester and phospholipid fatty acids to markers of insulin resistance in men and women with a range of glucose tolerance. Metabolism 2001;50:86-9.

[72] Low CC, Grossman EB, Gumbiner B. Potentiation of effects of weight loss by monounsaturated fatty acids in obese NIDDM patients. Diabetes 1996,45:569-75.

[73] Gumbiner B, Low CC, Reaven PD. Effects of monounsaturated fatty acid-enriched hypocaloric diet on cardiovascular risk factors in obese patients with type 2 diabetes. Diab Care 1998;21:9-15.

[74] Heilbronn LK, Noakes M, Clifton PM. Effect of energy restriction , weight loss and diet composition on plasma lipids and glucose in patients with type 2 diabetes. Diabetes Care 1999;22:889-95.

[75] Ruiz-Gutierrez V, Morgado N, Prada JL. Composition of human VLDL triacylglycerol after ingestion of olive oil and high oleic sunflower oil. J Nutr 1998;128:570-6.

[76] McNamara DJ. Dietary fatty acids, lipoproteins and cardiovascular disease. Adv Food Nutr Res 1992;36:253.

[77] Montalto MB, Bensadoun A. Lipoprotein lipase synthesis and secretion: Effects of concentration ands type of fatty acids in adipocyte cell culture. J Lipid Res 1993;34:397-407.

[78] Kafatos A, Comas GE. Biological effect of olive oil in human health. In: Kiritsakis A, ed. Olive oil. Champaign, IL: Am Oil Chemists Society, 1990;157.

[79] Roche HM, Zampelas A, Knapper JME. Effect of long-term olive oil dietary intervention on postprandial triacyglycerol and factor VII metabolism. Am J Clin Nutr 1998;68:552-60.

[80] Blades B, Garg A. Mechanisms of increase in plasma triacylglycerol concentrations as a result of high carbohydrate intake in patients with non-insulin-dependent diabetes mellitus. Am J Clin Nutr 1995;62: 996-02.

[81] Kiens B, Essen-Gustausson B, Gad P, Lithell H. Lipoprotein lipase activity and intra-muscular triglyceride store after long-term high fat and high-carbohydrate diets in physically trained men. Clin Physiol 1987;7:1.

[82] Hung T, Sievenpiper JL,Marchie A. Fat verses carbohydrate in insulin resistance,obesity,diabetes and cardiovascular disease. Curr Opin Clin Nutr Metab Care 2003;6:165-76.

[83] Schulze MB. Dietary approaches to prevent the metabolic syndrome. Diab Care 2004;27:613-4.

[84] McKeown NM, Meigs JB, Liu S, Saltzman E, Wilson PWF, Jacques PF. Carbohydrate nutrition, insulin resistance, and the prevalence of the metabolic syndrome in the Framingham Offspring cohort. Diab Care 2004;27:538-46.

[85] Bazzano LA, Serdula M, Liu S. Prevention of type 2 diabetes by diet and lifestyle modification. J Am Coll Nutr 2005;24:310-9.

[86]   Pella D, Thomas N, Tomlinson B, Singh RB. Prevention of coronary artery diseases: the South Asian paradox. Lancet 2003;361:79.

[87]   The World Health Report 2004. Global strategy on diet, physical activity and health. Geneva: WHO, 2004.

[88]   Anderson CAM, Appel LJ. Dietary modification and CVD prevention: A matter of of fat. JAMA 2006;295:693-5.

[89]   Pickering TG. New guidelines on diet and blood pressure. Hypertension 2006;47:135-6.

[90]   Pereira MA, Kartashow AI, Ebbeting CB, Van Horn L, Slattery ML, Jacobs DR, Ludwig DS. Fastfood, weight gain and insulin resistance(the CARDIA Study). 15-year prospective analysis. Lancet 2005;365:36-42.

[91]   Nissen SE, Tuzcu EM, Schoenhagen P, Brown BG, Ganz P, Vogel RA, et al. Reversal Investigators. Effect of intensive compared with moderate lipid lowering therapy on progression of coronary atherosclerosis.A randomized controlled trial. JAMA 2004;291:1071-80.

[92]   Cannon CP, Braunwald E, McCabe CH, Rader DJ, Rouleau JL, Belder R, et al. Pravastatin or atorvastatin evaluation and infection therapy. Thrombolysis in myocardial infarction 22 investigators. Intensive verses moderate lipid lowering with statins after acute coronary syndromes. N Eng J Med 2004;350:1495-504.

[93]   Esposito K, Glugliano D, Nappo F, Marfella R for the Campanian Postprandial Hyperglycemia Study Group. Regression of carotid atherosclerosis by control of postprandial hyperglycemia in type 2 diabetes mellitus. Circulation 2004;110:214-9.

[94]   Ceriello A, Assaloni R, Da Ros R, Maier A, Piconi I, Quagliaro R, et al. Effect of atorvastatin and irbesarten,alone and in combination on postprandial endothelial dysfunction,oxidative stress and inflammation in type 2 diabetes patients. Circulation 2005;111:2518-24.

[95]   Boger RH. Association of asymmetric dimethylarginine and endothelial dysfunction. Clin Chem Lab Med 2003;41:1467-72.

[96]   Exposito K, Nappo F, Giugliano F, Giugliano G, Martella R, Giugliano D. Effect of dietary antioxidants on postprandial endothelial dysfunction induced by a high meat in healthy subjects. Am J Clin Nutr 2003;77:139-43.

[97]   Bowen PE, Borthakur G. Postprandial lipid oxidation and cardiovascular risk. Curr Atheroscler Rep 2004;6:477-84.

[98]   Ceriello A, Motz E. Is oxidative stress the pathogenetic mechanism underlying insulin resistance, diabetes and cardiovascular disease? The common soil hypothesis revisited. Arterioscler Thromb Vasc Biol 2004;24:816-23.

[99]   Dandona P, Aljada A, Chaudhuri A, Mohanty P, Garg R. Metabolic syndrome. A comprehensive perspective based on interactions between obesity, diabetes and inflammation. Circulation 2005;111:1448-54.

[100]   Esposito K, Nappo F, Marfella R, Giugliano G, Giugliano F, Ciotola M, et al. Inflammatory cytokine concentrations are acutely increased by hyperglycaemia in humans: role of oxidative stress. Circulation 2002;106:2067-72.

[101]   Cerietto A, Quagliaro L, Catone B, Pascon R, Piazzola M, Bais B, et al. The role of hyperglycaemia in nitrotyrosine postprandial generation. Diab Care 2002;25:1439-43.

[102]   Esposito K, Nappo F, Giugliano F, Di Palo C, Ciotola M, Barbieri M, et al. Meal modulation of circulating interleukin-18 and adiponectin concentrations in healthy subjects and in patients with type 2 diabetes mellitus. Am J Clin Nutr 2003;78:1135-40.

[103]   Tataranni PA, Ortega EA. Burning question.Does an adipokine induced activation of the immune system mediate the effect of overnutrition on type 2 diabetes. Diabetes 2005;54:917-27.

[104]   Pankow JS, Duncam BB, Schmidt MI, Ballantyne CM, Couper DJ, Hoogeveen RC, Golden SH. Atherosclerotic Risk in Community Study. Fasting plasma free fatty acids and risk of type 2 diabetes: the atherosclerotic risk in community study. Diab Care 2004;27:77-82.

[105]   Meigs JB, Hu FB, Rifai N, Manson JE. Biomarkers of endothelial dysfunction and risk of type 2 diabetes mellitus. JAMA 2004;291:1978-86.

[106] Kim F, Tysseling KA, Julie R, Pham M, Haji L, Gallis BM, et al. Free fatty acid impairment of nitric oxide production in endothelial cells is mediated by IKK? Arterioscler Thromb Vasc Biol 2005;25:989-94.

[107] Gao Z, Hwang D, Bataille F, Lfevre M, York D, Quon MJ, Ye J. Serine phosphorylation of insulin receptor substrate 1 by inhibitor kappa B kinase complex. J Biol Chem 2002;277:48115-21.

[108] Cai D, Yuan M, Frantz DF, Metendez PA, Hansen L, Lee J, Shoelson SE. Local and systemic insulin resistance resulting from hepatic activation of IKK-b and NF-kappa B. Nat Med 2005;11:183-90.

[109] Yamauchi T, Kamon J, Waki H, Terauchi Y, Kubota N, Hara K. The fat derived hormone adiponectin reverses insulin resistance associated with both lipoatrophy and obesity. Nat Med 2001;7:941-6.

[110] Lopez-Garcia E, Schulze MB, Meigs JB, Manson JE, Rifai N, Stampfer MJ, Willett WC, Hu FB. Consumption of trans fatty acids is related to plasma biomarkers of inflammation and endothelial dysfunction. J Nutr 2005;135:562-6.

[111] Pirro M, Schilaci G, Savarese G, Gemelli F, Mannarino MR, Siepi D, et al. Attenuation of inflammation with short-term dietary intervention is associated with a reduction of arterial stiffness in subjects with hypercholesterolaemia. Eur J Cardiocasc Prev Rehabil 2004;11:497-02.

[112] Lopez-Garcia E, Schulze MB, Manson JE, Albert CM, Rifai N, Willett WC, Wu FB. Consumption of (n-3) fatty acids is related to plasma biomarkers of inflammation and endothelial activation in women. J Nutr 2004;134:1806-11.

[113] Kris-Etherton PM, Lichtenstein AH, Howard BV, Steinberg D, Witztum JL for the Nutrition Committee of the American Heart Association Council on Nutrition, Physical Activity and Metabolism. Antioxidant vitamin supplements and cardiovascular disease. Circulation 2004;110:637-41.

[114] Lau DCW, Dhillon B, Yan H, Szmitko PE, Verma S. Adipokines: molecular links between obesity and atherosclerosis. Am J Physiol Heart Circ Physiol 2005;288: H2031-H41.

[115] Diamant M, Lamb HJ van de Ree MA, Endert EL, Groeneveld Y, Bots ML, Kostense PJ, Redder JK. The association between abdominal visceral fat and carotid stiffness is mediated by circulating inflammatory markers in uncomplicated type 2 diabetes. J Clin Endocrinol Metab 2005;90:1495-1501.

[116] Eche ME, Lemieux S, Weisnagei SJ, Corneau L, Nadeau A, Bergeron J. Relation of high-sensitivity C-reactive protein, interleukin-6, tumor necrosis factor alpha and fibrinogen to abdominal adipose tissue, blood pressure and cholesterol and triglyceride levels in healthy postmenopausal women. Am J Cardiol 2005;96:92-7.

[117] Pereira MA, Kartashow AI, Ebbeling CB, Van Horn L, Slattery ML, Jacobs DR Jr, Ludwig DS. Fast-food weight gain and insulin resistance (the CARDIA study): 15-year prospective analysis. Lancet 2005;365:36-42.

[118] Drapeau V.Despres JP, Bouchard C, Allard L, Fournier G, Leblance C, Tremblay A. Modifications in food-group consumption are related to long-term body-weight changes. Am J Clin Nutr 2004;80:29-37.

[119] Knoops KTB, de Groot LC, Kromhout D, Perrin AE, Moreiras-Varela O, Menotti A, van Staveren WA. Mediterranean diet, lifestyle factors and 10-year mortality in elderly European men and women. The HALE project. JAMA 2004;292:1433-39.

[120] Trichopoulou A, Costacou T, Bamia C, Trichopoulos D. Adherence to a Mediterranean diet and survival in a Greek population. N Engl J Med 2003;348:2599-08.

[121] De Lorgeril M, Salen P, Martin JL, Monjaud I, Delaye J, Mamelle N. Mediterranean diet, traditional risk factors and the rate of cardiovascular complications after myocardial infarction .Final report of the Lyon Diet Heart Study. Circulation 1999;99:779-85.

[122] Singh RB, Dubnov G, Niaz MA, Ghosh S, Singh R, Rastogi SS, et al. Effect of an Indo-Mediterranean diet on progression of coronary disease in high risk patients:a randomized single blind trial. Lancet 2002,360:1455-61.

[123] Esposito K, Marfella R, Ciotola M, Di Palo C, Giugliano G, D'Armiento M, et al. Effect of a Mediterranean-style diet on endothelial dysfunction and markers of vascular inflammation in the metabolic syndrome: a randomized trial. JAMA 2004;292:1440-6.

[124] Iso H, Kobayashi M, Ishihara J, Sasaki S, Okada K, Kita Y, et al. Intake of fish and n3 fatty acids and risk of coronary heart disease among Japanese: The Japan Public Health Center-Based (JPHC) Study Cohort I. Circulation 2006;113 195-02.

[125] Gramenzi A, Gentile A, Fasoli M, Negri E,Parazzini F.La Vecchia C. Association between certain foods and risk of acute myocardial infarction in women. BMJ 1990;300:771–3.

[126] Singh RB, Niaz MA, Agarwal P, Beegum R, Rastogi SS. Effect of antioxitant rich foods on plasma ascorbic acid, cardiac enzyme and lipid peroxide levels in patients hospitalized with acute myocardial infarction. J Am Diet Assoc 1995;95:775-80.

[127] Singh RB, Rastogi SS, Verma R, Bolaki L, Singh R, Ghosh S. An Indian experiment with nutritional modulation in acute myocardial infarction. Am J Cardiol 1992; 69:897-85.

[128] Singh RB, Niaz MA, Kartik C.Can omega-3 fatty acids provide myocardial protection by decreasing infarct size and inhibiting atherothrombosis? Eur Heart J 2001;3(suppl D):62-9.

[129] Singh RB, Niaz MA, Sharma JP, Kumar R, Rastogi V, Moshiri M. Randomized, double blind, placebo controlled trial of fish oil and mustard oil in patients with suspected acute myocardial infarction: The Indian Experiment of Infarct Survival-4. Cardiovasc Durg Ther 1997;11:485-91.

[130] GISSI-Prevenzione Investigators.Dietary supplementation with n-3 polyunsaturated fatty acids and vitamin E after myocardial infarction:results of the GISSI prevenzione trial. Lancet 1999;354:447-55.

[131] Robinson R.The fetal origins of adult disease. BMJ 2001;322:375.

[132] Kumar SG, Das UN, Kumar KV, Tan BKH, Das NP. Effects of n-6 and n-3 fatty acids on the proliferation and secretion of TNF and IL-2 by human lymphocytes in vitro. Nutr Res 1992;12:815-20.

[133] Endres S, Ghorbani R, Kelley VE. The effect of dietary supplementation with n-3 polyunsaturated fatty acids on the synthesis of interleukin-1 and tumor necrosis factor by mononuclear cells. N Engl J Med 1989;320:265-8.

[134] Borovikova LV, Ivanova S, Zhang M. Vagal nerve stimulation attenuates the systemic inflammatory response to endotoxin. Nature 2000;405:458-62.

[135] Burr ML, Fehily AM, Gilbert JF. Effects of changes in fat, fish and fibre intakes on death and myocardial infarction: Diet and Reinfarction Trial (DART). Lancet 1989;ii:757-61.

[136] Wang H,Yu M, Ochani M, et al. Nicotinic acetylecholine receptor alpha-7 subunit is an essential regulator of inflammation. Nature 2003;421:384-8.

[137] Singh RB, Fedacko J, Vargova V, Pella D, Niaz MA, Ghosh S. Effect of low W-6/W-3 fatty acid ratio paleolithic style diet in patients with acute coronary syndromes: A randomized, single blind, controlled trial. World Heart J 2012;4:71-84.

[138] Harper CR, Jacobson TA. Usefulness of omega-3 fatty acids and the prevention of coronary heart disease. Am J Cardiol 2005;96:1521-9.

[139] Mozaffarian D, Geelan A, Brouwer IA, et al. Effect of fish oil on heart rate in humans, a meta analysis of randomized, controlled trials. Circulation 2005;112:1945-52.

[140] Whiteworth JA. World Health Organization (WHO)/International Society of Hypertension (ISH) statement on management of hypertension. J Hypertens 2003;21:1983-92.

[141] Singh RB. Prevalence and prevention of hypertension, diabetes mellitus and coronary artery disease in India: A scientific statement of the Indian Society of Hypertension, International College of Nutrition and International College of Cardiology. World Heart J 2010;2: 31-44.

[142] Singh RB, Wilczynska A, Fedacko J, Pella D, De Meester F. Pranayama: The power of breath. Int J Disabil Hum Dev 2009;8: 141-53.

[143] Singh RB, De Meester F, Pella D, Watson RR, Basu TK. Globalization of dietary wild foods protect against cardiovascular disease: A scientific statement from the International College of Cardiology, Columbus Paradigm Institute and International College of Nutrition. Open Nutra J 2009;2:42-5.

[144] Drukteinis JS, Roman J, Fabsitz RR, Lee ET, Best LG, Russel M, Devereux RB. Cardiac and systemic haemodynamic characteristics of hypertension and prehypertension in adolescents and young adults. The Strong Heart Study. Circulation 2007;115:221-7.

[145] Heidemann C, Schulze MB, Franco OH, van Dam RM, Mantzoros CS, Hu FB. Dietary patterns and risk of mortality from cardiovascular disease, cancer, and all causes in a prospective cohort of women. Circulation 2008;118:230-7.

[146] Ander BP, Hurtado C, Raposo CS, et al. Differential sensitivities of the NCX1.1 and NCX1.3 isoforms of the Na+—Ca2+ exchanger to á-linolenic acid. Cardiovasc Res 2007;73:395–403.

[147] Singh RB, Rastogi SS, Verma R, Laxmi B, Singh R, Ghosh S, Niaz MA. Randomized, controlled trial of cardioprotective diet in patients with acute myocardial infarction: results of one year follow up. BMJ 1992;304:1015-9.

[148] Singh RB, Fedacko J, Pella D, De Meester F, Moshiri M, Aroussy WE. Superfoods dietary approaches for acute myocardial infarction. World Heart J 2010;2:45-52.

[149] Singh RB, De Meester F, Wilczynska A. The Tsim Tsoum approaches for prevention of cardiovascular diseases. Cardiol Res Prac 2010; doi:10.4061/2010/824938.

[150] de Lorgeril M, Renaud S, Mamelle N, Salen P, Martin JL, Monjaud I, Guidollet J, Touboul P, Delaye J. Mediterranean alpha-linolenic acid-rich diet in secondary prevention of coronary heart disease. Lancet 1994;343(8911):1454-9. Erratum in: Lancet 1995;345 (8951):738.

[151] Renaud S, de Lorgeril M, Delaye J, Guidollet J, Jacquard F, Mamelle N, et al. Cretan Mediterranean diet for prevention of coronary heart disease. Am J Clin Nutr 1995;61(6 Suppl):1360S-7.

In: Food, Nutrition and Eating Behavior
Editors: Joav Merrick and Sigal Israeli

ISBN: 978-1-62948-233-0
© 2014 Nova Science Publishers, Inc.

Chapter 11

ANTIDIABETIC POTENTIAL OF THE GENUS CASSIA

Amritpal Singh, MD Ayurveda, Sanjiv Duggal, M Pharmacy, Sushma Devi and Navdeep Bharti*

Department of Dravyaguna, Shri Dhanwantry Ayurvedic College, Chandigarh and
Lovely School of Applied Medical Sciences, Department of Pharmaceutical Sciences,
Lovely Professional University, Phagwara, India

Diabetes mellitus is characterized by hyperglycemia, altered metabolism of lipids, carbohydrates and proteins. Type-2 diabetes constitutes 90% of the total diabetics in most countries with nearly 80% of the burden in developing countries. Insulin and other oral hypoglycemic drugs are most widely used for the diabetes, but they also have various side effects. Many medicinal plants have been found to be successfully used to manage diabetes. Plants belonging to genus Cassia are used extensively in various parts of the world against a wide range of ailments. Scientific studiers done on various species of Cassia, demonstrates their potential in the treatment of diabetes mellitus. This review summarizes the potential of Cassia species plants reported to possess antidiabetic activity.

INTRODUCTION

Diabetes mellitus is a metabolic disorder; it consists of a group of disease characterized by hyperglycemia, altered metabolism of lipids, carbohydrates and proteins (1). The pathophysiology of the diabetic mellitus involves decrease in the circulating concentration of insulin (insulin deficiency) and a decrease in the response of peripheral tissues to insulin (insulin resistance). These abnormalities lead to alterations in the metabolism of carbohydrates, lipids, ketones, and amino acids; the central feature of the syndrome is hyperglycemia (2).

It is estimated that there has been an explosive increase in the diabetes in the last two to three decades. Diabetes has become a major health concern worldwide with over 190 million suffering from disease, now with a potential to have 324 million by 2025. Type-2 constitutes

* Correspondence: Amritpal Singh, 2101, Ph-7, Mohali Distt, Mohali 160062, India. E-mail: amritpal2101@yahoo.com.

90% of the total diabetics in most countries with nearly 80% of the burden in developing countries. The World Health Organization has predicted that the major burden will occur in the developing countries. There will be a 42% increase from 51 to 72 million in the developed countries and 170% increase from 84 to 228 million, in the developing countries (3).

Particularly in India, there are currently 50 million people with diabetes, which are projected to increase by 90 million in the 2030. The fear of diabetic epidemic looms with statements in the press that read, as "Every fifth Indian and every fifth diabetic will be an Indian". The fact confirmed by reports from the World Health Organization (WHO) shows that India has the largest number of diabetic subjects in the world (4).

Insulin and other oral hypoglycemic drugs are most widely used for the diabetes but they also have various side effects like hypoglycemia, weight gain (sulphonyl urea), lactic acidosis with bigunoids and of these drug cause liver and renal damage. In spite of the introduction of new hypoglycemic agents, diabetes and the related complications continue to be a major medical problem. However, allopathic treatment for diabetes helps to control the disease to an extent but regular medication and constant medical supervision always leads to non patient compliance (4). This has been the rationale for the development of new antidiabetic drugs, includes drugs from herbal plants. Many indigenous Indian medicinal plants have been found to be successfully used to manage diabetes (5-7).

This review summarizes the features of cassia species plants reported to possess antidiabetic activity. Plants belonging to Cassia species are used extensively in various parts of the world against a wide range of ailments, the synergistic action of its metabolite being probably responsible for the plants beneficial effects. Cassia invites attention of researchers worldwide for its pharmacological activities ranging from antidiabetic to other various diseases. Cassia is a large genus of around 500 species of flowering plants in the family Fabaceae and is widely distributed throughout Asia including India, Mauritius, China, East Africa, South Africa, America, Mexico, West Indies and Brazil (8).

CASSIA AURICULATA LINN

C auriculata, commonly known as 'Tanner's Cassia'. It grows abundantly all over India (9). It is reported to possess antidiabetic, hypoglycemic and antihyperglycemic (10-12), anticancer (13), antibacterial (14), hypolipidemic (15), antioxidant (16), hepatoprotective (17), antispasmodic (18) and antipyretic (19) activities.

Flowers of C auriculata contain ß-sitosterol, kaempferol and proanthocyanidin dimer. Leaves of the plant are reported to contain keto alcohols, ß-sitosterol, kaempferol and emodin. Pod husk contains ß-sitosterol, chrysophanol, emodin, rubiadin and nonacosan-6-one (20).

Dinex, a poly herbal formulation prepared from the mixture of the aqueous extracts of C auriculata in combination with Eugenie jabalona, Gymnema sylvesre, Momordica charantia, Azadirachia indica, Aegle marmelos, Withania somnifera and curcuma longa. It showed significant (p<0.05) hypoglycaemic activity in both normal and diabetic animal (21).

Diasulin a, poly herbal drug prepared from C auriculata, Coccinia indica, Curcuma longa, Emblica officinalis, Gymnema sylvestre, Momordica charantia, Scoparia dulcis, Syzigium cumini, Tinospora cardifolia and Trigonella foenum showed significant (p<0.05) effect in lowering blood glucose and increasing plasma insulin level in alloxan diabetic rats and decrease in the content of cholesterol, triglycerides, free fatty acids and phospholipids at dose 200 mg/kg b.wt p.o. for 30 days when compared with diabetic control rats with normal rats (22).

Administration of aqueous extract of C auriculata flowers at 0.15, 0.30 and 0.45 g/kg b. wt p.o. for 30 days, suppressed the elevated blood glucose and lipid levels in diabetic rats. The antihyperlipidaemic and antidiabetic activity of aqueous extract of C auriculata flowers at doses of 0.45 g/kg was at par with glibenclamide (23).

An exploratory study showed that chronic administration of the ethanol: water (1:1) leaf extract of C. auriculata in alloxan induced diabetic rats; significantly ($p<0.01$) reduced the serum glucose level. The extract was found to inhibit the body weight reduction induced by alloxan administration.24 Aqueous extract of leaves, stems, flowers and roots of Cassia auriculata demonstrated antidiabetic activity at 250 mg/ kg b. wt p.o. in alloxon induced diabetic rat (10).

A study reported that ethanol and methanol extract of C. auriculata leaves and flowers significantly ($p<0.001$) controlled the increase in blood glucose levels in alloxan induced diabetic rats. The antihyperglycemic effect was attributed to the stimulation of the insulin secretion from the ß cells or regeneratation of the same (25).

Hydromethanolic, n-butanol and ethyl acetate fractions of C. auriculata flowers showed significant ($p<0.001$) reduction in blood glucose level in Alloxon treated rats. However, n-butanol fraction was highly effective and results are comparable with reference drug phenformin. Alloxon treated rats showed substantial weight loss as compare to treated group rats (26).

In yet another study, aqueous extract of C. auriculata significantly suppressed the elevated glucose and lipid levels at doses of 150, 300,500 mg/kg b.wt p.o. for 30 days in diabetic rats and also demonstrated anti-nociceptive activity in mice and 500mg/kg was found comparable to the standard reference drugs (27).

CASSIA TORA LINN

C tora is popularly known as sickle senna, sickle pod, coffee pod or foetid cassia. The seeds of the plant are rich in chrysophanic acid and anthraquinone glucosides, glucoobtusifolin and glucoaurantioobtusifolin. Pods are reported to contain sennosides (20).

An investigational study reported that 10% of C tora in diet lowered plasma glucose level, and this effect was as acute as seen even at the first week of feeding. The butanolic fraction of the methanol extract decreased plasma glucose levels, and the decrease was shown at the 4th day of feeding (28). Emodin and obtusifolin isolated from an ethyl acetate soluble extract of the seeds of C tora exhibited a significant ($p<0.05$) in vitro inhibitory activity against advanced glycation end products (29).

The serum glucose level in the C tora seeds butanol fraction group shows a slower uprising in the glucose curve and the postprandial rise of glucose was significantly ($p<0.05$) reduced and delayed after loading maltose orally and decrease fasting serum glucose level in diabetic rats. C tora seeds butanol fraction does not influence the insulin secretion from the pancreas of the normal rats, but in the diabetic rats the insulin secretion was significantly ($p<0.05$) stimulated from the pancreas (30).

In a study 15 type II diabetic subjects were given C tora fiber supplement consisting of 2 g of soluble fiber extracted from C tora. 200 mg of a-tocopherol, 500 mg of ascorbic acid, and 300 mg of maltodextrin, C. tora supplements moderately (P<0.1) decreased the serum total cholesterol, serum triglycerides levels and low-density lipoprotein-cholesterol. But there were no effect on fasting blood glucose, hemoglobin, blood urea nitrogen, creatinine, and activities of serum aspartate aminotransferase and alanine aminotransferase (31).

CASSIA FISTULA LINN

C fistula is medicinal plant belonging to family Fabaceae. It is commonly known as 'Aragbadh'. In English it is called Indian laburnum. Leaves of the drug contain sennosides A and B. Bark and heartwood are reported to contain leucoanthocyanidin, fistucacidin, barbaloin and rhein. Stem-bark contains lupeol, ß-sitosterol and hexacosanol (20).

Administration of hexane extract of C fistula bark were evaluated in streptozotocin induced diabetic rats at the doses of 0.15, 0.30 and 0.45 g/kg b.wt for 30 days. The extract demonstrated significant antihyglycemic and antilipidemic effects, which were attributed to antioxidant and polyphenol content present in the extract (32).

CASSIA KLEINII W AND A

C kleinii is an herb which grows as a weed and commonly cultivated. It is commonly known as malam-todda-vadi (20).

In a study, leaf and root water suspension of C kleinii significantly (p<0.05) increased tolerance for glucose at a dose of 500 mg/kg b.wt.p.o. The hypoglycemic effect of alcoholic extract of the leaf of C kleinii was found to be effective at a dose 200 mg/kg b.wt.p.o in the fasted rats. As well as the alcoholic extract exhibited concentration dependent antihyperglycemic effect in glucose loaded rats. The alcoholic extract was found to be effective as insulin (5 U/kg) in lowering glucose level in alloxon induced diabetic rats (33).

In streptozotocin induced diabetic rats, the alcoholic extract of the C. kleinii leaf at dose 200 mg/kg b wt. p.o. showed significant antidiabetic property as evident from body weight, serum glucose, lipids, cholesterol and urea, and liver glycogen levels. The effect of alcoholic extract was found to be comparable with glibenclamide. The antihyperglycemic activity was found predominately in the chloroform fraction of the alcoholic extract at dose 25 mg/kg b.wt p.o (34).

CASSIA GLAUCA LAM

Bark and leaves are used in diabetic and gonorrhea in the folklore medicine (35).

Acetone extract of C glauca leaf extract caused significant (p<0.01) reduction in blood glucose level in fasted diabetic rats. Further fraction I of acetone extract showed maximum reduction in fasting blood sugar and significantly (p<0.01) improvement in the level of hepatic enzyme aspartate transaminase, alanine transaminase, creatine kinase and lactate dehydrogenase at a dose 100 mg/kg b.wt p.o. in diabetic rats 15 days after treatment (36).

Cassia alata Linn

The plant contains xanthone known as cassioolin and anthraquinones; including chrysophanol, emodin, rhein and emodin (20). The ethyl acetate extract of C. alata leaves was found to be hypoglycemic at doses 5mg/20g mice. It decreased the blood sugar level of mice by 58.3% (37).

CASSIA MARGINATA ROXB, C RENIGERA WALL EX BENTH AND C OBTUSIFOLIA LINN

Animals were fed with diets containing protein isolates of C marginata, C renigera and C obtusifolia seeds respectively for ten days. They were found to have a marked lowering effect on blood and liver cholesterol levels. Maximum lowering effect on total blood cholesterol level was observed to be 26.88% by C marginata seed proteins. The proteins of C renigera seed had lowering value of 22.5% while the proteins of C obtusifolia seed had a minimum lowering effect of 21.47% (P<0.01).

CONCLUSIONS

The genus Cassia definitely holds promise of providing potent drug for diabetes mellitus. Several species subjected to antidiabetic investigations; in animal models, have reported favorable results. C auriculata, single and in combination with other herbs, has shown potent antidiabetic and antihyperlipidaemic activities. Considering in account, the drug-resistance and cost-effectiveness, the genus Cassia can be exploited for clinical studies for justifying antidiabetic claims.

REFERENCES

[1] Satyavati GV, Neeraj T, Madhu S. Indigenous plant drugs for diabetes mellitus. J Ethnopharmacol 1989;12:23-8.

[2] Davis SN. Insulin, oral hypoglycemic agents, and the pharmacology of the endocrine pancreas. In: Brunton LL, ed. Goodman & Gilman's. The pharmacological basis of therapeutics, 11th ed. New York: McGraw-Hill, 2000:1411.

[3] King H, Aubert RE, Herman WH. Global burden of diabetes, 1995-2025: Prevalence, numerical estimates, and projections. Diabetic Care 1998;21:1414-43.

[4] Garg M, Garg C. Scientific alternative approach in diabetes-An overview. Pharmacognosy Rev 2008;2:284-301.

[5] Nagarajan S, Jain HC, Aulakh GS. Indigenous plants in the control of diabetes. New Delhi: Publ Inform Dir CSIR, 1987:586.

[6]   Rajasekharan S, Tuli SN. 'Vijaysar' (Petrocarpus marsupium) in the treatment of 'Madhumeha' (diabetes mellitus): a clinical trial. J Res Indian Med Yoga Homeopathy 1976;9:76-8.

[7]   Anjali P, Manoj KM. Some comments on diabetes and herbal therapy. Ancient Sci Life 1995;1:27-9.

[8]   Mazumder PM, Percha V, Farswan M, Upaganlawar A. Cassia: A wonder gift to medical sciences. Int J Comm Pharmacy 2008;1:16-38.

[9]   Joshi SG. Textbook of medicinal plants. New Delhi: IBH Publ, 2000:119.

[10]   Devi PU, Selvi S, Selvam K. Chinnaswamy P. Antidiabetic and hypoglycemic effect of Cassia auriculata in alloxan induced diabetic rats. Int J Pharmacol 2006;2:601-7.

[11]   Pari L, Latha M. Effect of Cassia auriculata flowers on blood sugar levels, serum and tissue lipids in streptozotocin diabetic rats. Singapore Med J 2002;43:617-21.

[12]   Abesundara KJM, Mastsui T, Matsumoto K. Glucosidase inhibitory activity of some Sri Lanka plant extracts, one of which, Cassia auriculata, exerts a strong antihyperglycemic effect in rats comparable to the therapeutic drug acarbose. J Agricultural Food Chemistry 2004;52:2541-5.

[13]   Prasanna R, Harish CC, Pichai R, Sakthisekaran D, Gunasekaran D. Anti-cancer effect of Cassia auriculata leaf extract in vitro through cell cycle arrest and induction of apoptosis in human breast and larynx cancer cell lines. Cell Biol Int 2009;33:127-34.

[14]   Girish HV, Satish S. Antibacterial activity of important medicinal plants on human pathogenic bacteria-a comparative analysis. World Appl Sci J 2008;5:267-71.

[15]   Gupta SA, Sharma SB, Bansal SK, Prabhu KM. Antihyperglycemic and hypolipidemic activity of aqueous extract of Cassia auriculata L. leaves in experimental diabetes. J Ethnopharmacol 2009;123: 499-503.

[16]   Kumaran A, Karunakaran RJ. Antioxidant activity of Cassia auriculata flowers. Fitoterapia 2007;78:46-7.

[17]   Kumar RS, Ponmozhi M, Viswanathan P, Nalini N. Effect of Cassia auriculata leaf extract on lipids in rats with alcoholic liver injury. Asia Pacific J Clin Nutr 2002;11:157-63.

[18]   Dhar ML, Dhar MM, Dhawan BN, Mehrotra BN, Ray C. Screening of Indian plants for biological activity. Indian J Exp Biol 1968; 6:232-47.

[19]   Vedavathy S, Rao K.N. Antipyretic activity of six indigenous medicinal plants of Tirumala hills. J Ethnopharmacol 1991;33:193-6.

[20]   Aolkar LV, Kakkar KK, Chakre OJ. Second supplement to glossary of Indian medicinal plants with active principles. Part 1 (A-K). New Delhi: Natl Inst Sci Comm Inform Resources, CASIR, 1981:176-80.

[21]   Mutalik S, Chetana M, Sulochana B, Devi PU, Udupa N. Effect of Dianex, a herbal formulation on experimentally induced diabetes mellitus. Phytother Res 2005;219:409-15.

[22]   Saravanan R, Pari L. Antihyperlipidemic and antiperoxidative effect of Diasulin, a polyherbal formulation in alloxan induced hyperglycemic rats. BMC Complement Altern Med 2005;5:1-8.

[23]   Pari L. Latha M. Antihyperglycaemic effect of Cassia auriculata in experimental diabetes and its effects on key metabolic enzymes involved in carbohydrate metabolism. Clin Exp Pharmacol Physiol 2003;30:38-43.

[24]   Sabu MC, Subburaju T. Effect of Cassia auriculata Linn on serum glucose level, glucose utilization by isolated rat hemidiaphragm. J Ethnopharmacol 2002;80:203-6.

[25]   Kalaivani A, Umamaheswari A, Vinayagam A, Kalaivani K. Anti-hyperglycemic and antioxidant properties of cassia auriculata leaves and flowers on alloxan-induced diabetes. Pharmacol Online 2008;3:32.

[26]   Surana SJ, Ghokhle SB, Jadhav SB, Sawant RL, Wadekar JB. Antihyperglycemic activity of various fractions of Cassia auriculata Linn. in alloxon induced diabetic rats. Indian J Pharmaceutical Sci 2008;70:227-9.

[27]   George M, Ramaswamy JL. Effect of cassia auriculata extract on nociception, experimental diabetes and hyperlipidemia in mice and rats. Highland Med Res J 2007;5:11-9.

[28]   Lim SJ, Han HK. Hypoglycemic effect of fractions of Cassia tora extract in Streptozotocin-induced diabetic rats. J Korean Soc Food Sci Nutr 1997;13:23-9.

[29] Jang DS, Lee GY, Kim YS, Lee YM, Kim CS, Yoo JL et al. Anthraquinones from the seeds of Cassia tora with inhibitory activity on protein glycation and aldose reductase. Biol Pharmaceutical Bull 2007;30:2207-10.

[30] Patil UK, Saraf S, Dixit VK. Hypolipidemic activity of seeds of Cassia tora Linn. J Ethnopharmacol 2004;90:249-52.

[31] Cho SH, Kim TH, Lee NH et al. Effects of Cassia tora fiber supplement on serum lipids in Korean diabetic patients. J Med Food 2005;8:311-8.

[32] Nirmala A, Eliza J, Rajalakshmi M, Priya E, Daisy, P. Effect of hexane extract of Cassia fistula barks on blood glucose and lipid profile in Streptozotocin diabetic rats. Int J Pharmacol 2008;4:292-6.

[33] Babu V, Gangadevi T, Subramoniam A. Antihyperglycemic activity of Cassia kleinii leaf extract in glucose fed normal rat and alloxon induced diabetic rats. Indian J Pharmacol 2002;34:409-15.

[34] Babu V, Gangadevi T, Subramoniam A. Antidiabetic activity of ethanol extract of Cassia kleinii leaf in streptozotocin induced diabetic rats and isolation of an active fraction and toxicity evaluation of the extract. Indian J Pharmacol 2003;35:290-6.

[35] Warrier PK. Indian medicinal plants. Chennai: Orient Longman, 2002:3-30.

[36] Farswan M, Mazumder PM, Percha V. Protective effect of Cassia glauca Linn on the serum glucose and hepatic enzyme level in streptozotocin induced NIDDM in rats. Indian J Pharmacol 2009;41:19-22.

[37] Villaseñor IM, Canlas AP, Pascua MP, Sabando MN, Soliven LA. Bioactivity studies on Cassia alata Linn. leaf extracts. Phytother Res 2002;1:93-6.

[38] Singh KN, Chandra V, Earthwal KC. Effects of proteins of cassia marginata, cassia renigera and cassia obstusifolia wild leguminous seeds on blood and liver cholesterol in young albino rats. Indian J Pharmacy 1976;9:149-52.

In: Food, Nutrition and Eating Behavior
Editors: Joav Merrick and Sigal Israeli

ISBN: 978-1-62948-233-0
© 2014 Nova Science Publishers, Inc.

Chapter 12

PAINFUL DIABETIC NEUROPATHY

Nabil Majid, MD, MPH, FACP, FACPE[*]
Mercy General Hospital, Sacramento, California, US

Painful diabetic neuropathy affects the quality of life and has no curative therapy. It manifests mainly as burning, pins and needles sensation starting in the feet and progresses upwards. It has established metabolic and vascular pathophysiologic mechanisms. Recent studies try to combine these mechanisms in one big scheme. The diagnosis is mainly clinical. Electrophysiologic studies and skin biopsy plays a supportive role. The physician needs also to exclude other etiologies, commonly encountered in diabetics, such as neuropathies from alcoholism, vitamin B12 deficiency, and uremia among others. Although many screening tests were introduced over the decades, the tuning fork test is still the simplest and widely used. The treatment is multidisciplinary. While tight glycemic control is the main pillar of prevention, drugs are the only proven treatment. Duloxetine and pregabalin are the only FDA approved medications for PDN. Generally, antidepressants and anticonvulsants are the most commonly used. Rational polypharmacy has recently emerged as a necessary way to decrease the effective dose of the prescribed drugs while benefiting from its synergistic outcome. This way we can spare the patient an array of unpleasant side effects. These are the main reason behind medical noncompliance. Lifestyle modifications produce subjective well being. Physical and occupational therapy help patients cope with pain among other benefits. Finally, several authoritative medical associations have published guidelines for therapeutic approach to PDN. It cannot be overemphasized that the approach needs to be individualized.

INTRODUCTION

There are more than 14 million people in the United States with diabetes mellitus (1). Half of them develop peripheral neuropathies after 25 years of follow-up (2). Risk factors for diabetic neuropathy itself have not yet been ascertained, but may include increased age, duration of

[*] Correspondence: Nabil Majid, MD, MPH, FACP, FACPE, Mercy General Hospital,1888 Spaletta Way, Sacramento, CA 95835, United States. E-mail: majid_nabil@msn.com.

diabetes, lipotoxicity and glucotoxicity, genetic susceptibility, inflammation and oxidative stress (1, 3, 4).

Up to 25% of individuals with diabetes develop painful diabetic neuropathy (PDN), suffering spontaneous pain, allodynia (pain from stimuli which are not normally painful, the pain may occur somewhere other than the area that is being stimulated), hyperalgesia (increased sensitivity to pain stimulation), and burning. Decreased physical activity, increased fatigue, and mood and sleep problems can result (5).

It has been established that glycemic control can prevent complications such as neuropathy, cardiovascular disease, stroke, blindness, and renal failure. In conjuncture, periodic foot care, by both the primary physician and a podiatrist, is essential in preventing lower extremities' complications that can lead to amputation.

Further, amputation can be prevented by identifying at risk individuals and the specific factors placing them at risk; protecting of the foot against the adverse effects of external forces (pressure, friction, and shear) by prescribing special diabetic shoes, for instance; and reducing the incidence of diabetic foot ulcers through educational programs that teach patients the techniques of foot-inspection and the merits of seeking early medical attention (6).

This article will review the manifestations, pathophysiology, diagnosis (including various screening tests), complications, monitoring, and different treatment options of PDN.

MANIFESTATIONS

There are many forms of diabetic neuropathy including large-fiber neuropathy, small-fiber neuropathy, proximal motor neuropathy, acute mononeuropathies, and pressure palsies (see figure 1) (5). Although, as mentioned below, there are a continuous range of manifestations to this disease, small-fiber form manifesting as burning, pins and needles and loss of sensation is still the most frequently encountered in clinical practice. Also, it is important to note that the major neurotransmitter in small unmyelinated C fibers is substance P. This fact has a therapeutic implication and will be mentioned later.

The most common type though is distal symmetric polyneuropathy which can be due either to large-fiber or small-fiber neuropathies or both. It may affect sensory, motor, or sensorimotor neurons (3). In fact the earliest signs of damage to the sensory fibers translate into loss of light touch and temperature sensation and impaired pain (small fiber damage), and later, loss of vibration sensation and altered proprioception (large fiber injury). On the other hand, the earliest signs of damage to the motor fibers manifest as decreased or absent ankle reflexes. The loss of other reflexes and local or widespread motor weakness are later findings.

Proximal motor neuropathy (the term was recently changed to diabetic polyradiculopathy) typically affects older patients who have coexisting peripheral polyneuropathy and weakness or even atrophy in the distribution of one or more contiguous nerve roots with frequent territorial expansion. It usually happens as diabetes injures the nerve roots at one or more thoracic or high lumbar levels with subsequent axonal degeneration and frequent contralateral, cephalad, or caudal extension.

Diabetic Mononeuropathy mostly attacks the cranial nerves (III-VI). There, it can cause diplopia, ptosis, or unilateral pain. It usually spears the papillary function. The facial nerve can also be affected and leads to Bell's-Palsy-like signs and symptoms. Peripherally, diabetic mononeuropathy (also called pressure palsies) commonly affect the median, ulnar, and peroneal nerves and leads to paresthesias, pain, and even foot drop (in case of the involvement of the latter) (7).

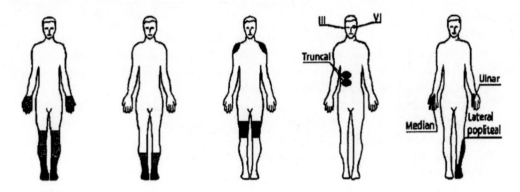

Large fiber Neuropathy	Small fiber Neuropathy	Proximal motor Neuropathy	Acute mono Neuropathies	Pressure Palsies
Sensory loss: 0→ +++ (Touch, vibration) Pain: + → +++ Tendon reflex: N → ↓↓↓ Motor deficit 0 → +++	Sensory loss: 0 → + (thermal , allodynia) Pain: + → +++ . Tendon reflex: N → ↓ Motor deficit: 0	Sensory loss: 0 → + Pain: + → +++ Tendon reflex: ↓↓ Proximal Motor deficit: + → +++.	Sensory loss: 0 → + Pain: + → +++ Tendon reflex: N Motor deficit: + → +++	Sensory loss in Nerve distribution: + → +++ Pain: + → ++ Tendon reflex: N Motor deficit: + → +++

N: normal.

+: mild, ++: moderate, +++: severe.

↓: mildly depressed, ↓↓: moderately depressed, ↓↓↓: severely depressed.

Figure 1. Classifications of PDN.

It is been estimated that at the time of their initial presentation 10-18% of newly diagnosed diabetics have an evidence of nerve damage. This finding and others support the recent conclusion that impaired glucose metabolism, during the pre-diabetes status, can lead to neuropathic manifestations (7).

The classic peripheral neuropathy presentation, the stocking-glove parasthesia, usually starts in the feet and ascends centrally. As it reaches the calf, it begins in the hands and spread to the wrists. This cephalad direction in damage stretch confirms the notion that longer axons are damaged early in the process. Later, motor involvement appears as neuropathy becomes more severe.

It is interesting to know that pre-diabetics can present with intensely painful feet. Pre-diabetes is an indication of an insulin-resistance state and a risk factor for type 2 diabetes. It is defined by the American Diabetes Association as fasting serum glucose between 100 and 125 mg/dl or serum glucose between 140 and 199 mg/dl on an oral glucose tolerance test. This information signifies the role of screening for diabetes mellitus through fasting blood glucose, a glucose tolerance test, and even measuring Hemoglobin A1c in every case presents with painful neuropathy.

PATHOPHYSIOLOGY

There is mounting evidence to support the combined metabolic and ischemic theories behind diabetic neuropathy. Eventually, the resultant damage overwhelms the nerve repair mechanism (8).

The proponents of the metabolic theory stress out that the systemic accumulation of advanced glycosylation end products, the accumulation of the intraneuronal sorbitol, and the impaired resistance to microvascular and neuronal oxidative stress are the three primary metabolic mechanisms that lead to diabetic neuropathy.

The accumulation of advanced glycosylation end products leads to microvascular injury. Chronic hyperglycemia encourages the excess glucose to binds to amino acids on circulating and tissue proteins. Although this nonenzymatic process is reversible early in the course, later it forms irreversible advanced glycosylation end products via Amadori rearrangement; i.e., the catalyzed isomerization of the resulting glycosylamines (9).

The accumulation of sorbitol causes an increase in intraneuronal osmolality and eventually interferes with cellular metabolism. Aldose reductase plays an essential role in the formation of sorbitol. This fact explains the benefit aldose reductase inhibitors provides to some patient with diabetic neuropathy in recent studies (10).

Also, hyperglycemia causes the accumulation of highly reactive oxygen radicals. In the context of lack of antioxidants, these radicals lead to oxidative stress and peripheral nerve damage in animal and vitro models of diabetes (11).

Endothelial dysfunction, thickened endoneural blood vessel walls, and vascular occlusions are the three ischemic mechanisms that lead to diabetic neuropathy according to the ischemic theory. Clinical evidence supports this observation. Patient with advanced diabetic neuropathy were found to have reduced endoneural oxygen tension in the sural nerves (12). Further, microvascular embolization resembling vasculitis were detectable in the nerves of type 2 diabetics with neuropathy.

Recent literature tried to combine the two theories (metabolic and ischemic) in one big scheme to explain the development of diabetic neuropathy. It was observed that ischemia itself has metabolic consequences that can be exacerbated by insulin deficiency and hyperglycemia (13). Furthermore, metabolic interventions (e.g., the use of aldose reductase inhibitors) have improved nerve conduction and corrected nerve blood flow in diabetic animals (14). In another study, oxygen free radicals were found to abolish the endothelial relaxation mechanism in diabetic rat aorta. This conclusion was reached after the observation that endothelium-dependent relaxation by acetylcholine was reduced by 50%. The endothelium-independent relaxation by nitroglycerin and papaverine were not affected, however (15).

Clinically, diabetic neuropathy is characterized by axon "dying back." It affects the longer myelinated and unmyelinated sensory axons first, with relative sparing of motor axons (16-18). Therefore, it manifests as distal parasthesia that seems to spread centrally. The spinal cord also appears to be affected; it's unclear however whether this happens through a primary or a secondary process (19).

DIAGNOSIS

The neuropathic pain is defined as pain initiated or caused by a primary lesion or a dysfunction in the nervous system (19). Both clinical exam and electrophysiological studies are essential to make the diagnosis of PDN and rule out other diseases. A skin biopsy can also be used to help the diagnosis and follow up on the progression.

The examiner needs to pay a special attention to the quality (e.g., burning, shooting, or electric), intensity, and duration of spontaneous pain as well as its location (20). Pain typically occurs symmetrically in the feet and ankles (i.e., glove and stocking distribution). Patients may also have dysesthesias and paresthesias, such as crawling, itching, numbness, and tingling. Sensory loss may also be reported. Pain quality and intensity can be estimated with the Neuropathic Pain Scale, the Neuropathic Pain Questionnaire, and other scales (20). An assessment of global function, sleep, psychological comorbidity, and other issues should be undertaken to determine the effect of diabetic neuropathy on the patient's quality of life, using a neuropathy-specific tool such as the Norfolk QOL-DN (21).

Electrophysiologically, both nerve conduction studies and electromyography can show abnormalities. Although non-specific, when taken in the context of a history of diabetes, the presence of other diabetic complications (retinopathy, nephropathy...etc.), and with the exclusion of other common etiologies such as drug side-effects, infections, and heavy-metal poisoning (as I will discuss later) the diagnosis become more compelling (22).

The nerve conduction velocities are mildly reduced and the sensory nerve potentials are often diminished in amplitude. Focal slowing of conduction velocity can be seen in susceptible nerves (median, ulnar, and peroneal) especially in cases of long-standing diabetes. Electromyography can detect denervation in distal muscles, scattered axonal degeneration, and regenerating nerve sprouts (23).

Skin biopsy is a safe, almost painless, and cheap technique for evaluating small nerve fibers. The density of these fibers can be measured easily using bright field microscopy in sections cut from the specimen and appropriately immunostained. Skin biopsy can also be repeated within the same nerve territory to evaluate the natural progression of the neuropathy. The positive predictive value of skin biopsy in diagnosing small fiber neuropathy is estimated at 93%; specificity is 97% and sensitivity ranges from 69% to 82% (24).

SCREENING TESTS

Both the San Antonio Consensus (19) and the Mayo Clinic criteria are thorough, lengthy, and complex. They include symptoms scoring, quantitative examinations and electrophysiologic measurements. Therefore, they are more suitable for research purposes and may not be as practical in routine clinical practice. Therefore, two simpler, clinician-friendly screening tests were developed to tackle this inconvenience: one from the United Kingdom (20) and other from the University of Michigan (22).

Still the Tuning Fork test is one of the oldest and simplest screening tests for peripheral neuropathy. However, it screens only for vibration sensation, hence, large myelinated fibers involvement. The problem with these scoring systems lays in their validity and reproducibility. For instance, the inter-examiner and intra-examiner validity of the Rochester

Diabetic Neuropathy Study was limited at best even among highly qualified specialists. This fact was mainly a result of inter-examiner differences in scoring symptoms severity regardless of the system used; be it the Neuropathy Symptom Score or the Neuropathy Symptom Profile (21). Therefore, the diagnosis of diabetic neuropathy is one in which the physician needs to consider all clinical and laboratory findings in order to exclude other diagnoses. Despite of all their shortcomings, the following scoring test are common medical practice due to their simplicity and inclusiveness.

United Kingdom screening test

This test tries to create a neuropathy score based on patient complaints (symptoms) and physicians findings (physical examination) (20). Ask the following questions to score the patient's symptoms:

Question	Max Score	Answer	points
What is the sensation felt?	2	burning, numbness, or tingling in the feet	2
		fatigue, cramping, or aching	1
What is the location of symptoms?	2	feet	2
		calves	1
		elsewhere	0
Have the symptoms ever awakened you at night?	1	yes	1
		no	0
What is the timing of symptoms?	2	worse at night	2
		present day and night	1
		present only during the day	0
How are symptoms relieved?	2	walking around	2
		standing	1
		sitting or lying or no relief	0

The total symptom score can be interpreted as follows:

Total Score	Interpretation
0 to 2	normal
3 to 4	mild neuropathy
5 to 6	moderate neuropathy
7 to 9	severe neuropathy

The physical findings can be scored as follows:

Exam	Max Score	Finding	points
Achilles tendon reflex	4	absent	2 points for each foot
		present with reinforcement	1 point for each foot
		Normal	0 points for each foot
Vibration sense	2	Absent or reduced	1 point for each foot
		Normal	0 points
Pin prick sensation	2	Absent or reduced	1 point for each foot
		Normal	0 points
Temperature sensation	2	Absent or reduced	1 point for each foot
		Normal	0 points

The total physical findings score can be interpreted as follows:

Total Score	Interpretation
0 to 2	normal
3 to 5	mild neuropathy
6 to 8	moderate neuropathy
9 to 10	severe neuropathy

A score of at least 8 puts the patient at higher risk to develop a diabetic foot ulcer.

Michigan neuropathy screening score

This is a simple screening test to diagnose diabetic neuropathy in outpatient clinics. (22) During the patient interview the following questions are addressed:

Exam	Max Score	Finding	points
Dermatologic findings	2	dry skin, callus, fissure, infection or deformities	1
		ulcer	1
		Normal	0
Vibration sense on the dorsum of the great toe	2	Absent	1
		Reduced	0.5
Achilles tendon reflex	2	Absent	0.5
		Normal	0

A score of at least 3 carries 95% specificity and 80% sensitivity in diagnosing diabetic neuropathy. It's important to know that this test has been validated against the more rigorous San Antonio Consensus Criteria. This fact puts an easy, readily available, valid test in the hands of healthcare allies involved in the diabetic patient care.

Tuning fork test

Using the 128 Hz tuning fork to test for vibration sensation (or the lack thereof), this test is quick, simple, and reliable (25). In its most common form, the examiner places the tuning fork at the dorsal aspect of the base of the great toe. If the patient feels no vibration, he gets a score of 2 points. The test is then terminated. However, if the patient feels the vibration, the examiner quickly moves the tuning fork to the dorsal bony prominence of the patient's wrist. There, the patient compares the strength of the vibration with that of the great toe. A score of 0 is given in the event of lack of difference in the strength of the vibration. Otherwise, the patient scores 1.

A score of 0 indicates the absence of neuropathy.
A score of 1 indicates mild to moderate neuropathy
A score of 2 indicates severe neuropathy.

Of course there are other methods of using the tuning fork to assess vibration sensation; of particular interest are the on-off method and the timed method.[26] In the former, the patient is asked to report the perception of both the start and the cessation of vibration on dampening when the fork is applied to the bony prominence of the dorsum of the first toe just proximal to the nail bed. The test is repeated twice on each toe (total of 4 tests). One point is scored for each time the start of vibration is not felt. Another point is scored when the cessation of vibration on dampening is not felt (a maximum of 8 points)

The timed method refers to comparing the period the patient feels the vibration of a tuning fork when placed on the dorsum of the first toe to that of the examiner (as a reference) when the fork is placed on the dorsal aspect of the distal phalanx of the examiner's thumb (26).

Table 1. Clinical manifestations and initial work up for common pain syndromes similar to PDN (5)

Condition	Key characteristics and differentiating features
Claudication	• Intermittent pain that is worsened by walking and remits with rest; other signs/symptoms suggest arterial insufficiency • The causing pathology is peripheral arterial occlusion with underlying atherosclerosis • Patients with diabetes are at higher risk and may present with normal extremities and absent foot pulses • Doppler ultrasonography confirms clinical diagnosis of arterial occlusion
Morton's neuroma	• Benign neuroma formation on third plantar interdigital nerve • Generally unilateral • More frequent in women • Pain elicited when pressure is applied with the thumb between the first and fourth metatarsal heads
Osteoarthritis	• the pain is usually gradual in onset and in 1 or 2 joints • Morning stiffness, diminished joint motion, and flexion contractures are characteristic • Pain worsens with exercise and improves with rest • Diagnosis is confirmed by x-ray
Radiculopathy	• Parasthesias, muscle weakness, and/or absent reflexes along the path of the affected nerve root(s). A result of diabetes, arthritis, or a metastatic disease • Pain can occur in thorax, extremities, shoulder, or arm, depending on site of lesion Neurologic examinations and imaging can localize lesion site
Charcot's neuroarthropathy	• May result from osteopenia due to increased blood flow following repeated minor trauma in individuals with diabetic neuropathy • Warm to hot foot with increased blood flow • Decreased warm sensory perception and vibration Clinical exam and xray of the affected foot can confirm the diagnosis
Plantar fasciitis	• Pain in the plantar region of the foot • Tenderness along the plantar fascia when ankle is dorsiflexed • Shooting or burning in the heel with each step • Worsening pain with prolonged activity • Often associated with calcaneal spur on radiography Clinical diagnosis by exclusion. Xray helps rule out other etiologies
Tarsal tunnel syndrome	• Caused by entrapment of the posterior tibial nerve •Pain and numbness radiate from beneath the medial malleolus to the sole • Clinical examination includes percussion, palpation for possible soft tissue matter, nerve conduction studies, magnetic resonance imaging

DIFFERENTIAL DIAGNOSIS

Table 2. Differential diagnosis of PDN

Distal symmetrical polyneuropathy
Metabolic
Uremia
Folic acid/cyanocobalamin deficiency
Hypothyroidism
Acute intermittent porphyria
Toxic
Alcohol
Heavy metals (lead, mercury, arsenic)
Industrial hydrocarbons
Various drugs
Infectious or inflammatory
Sarcoidosis
Leprosy
Periarteritis nodosa
Other connective-tissue diseases (eg, systemic lupus erythematosus)
Other
Dysproteinemias and paraproteinemias
Paraneoplastic syndrome
Leukemias and lymphomas
Amyloidosis
Hereditary neuropathies
Pains and paresthesias without neurologic deficit
Early small-fiber sensory neuropathy
Psychophysiologic disorder (eg, severe depression, hysteria)
Femoral neuropathy (sacral plexopathy)
Degenerative spinal-disc disease
Intrinsic spinal-cord-mass lesion
Equina cauda lesions
Coagulopathies
Cranial neuropathy
Carotid aneurysm
Intracranial mass
Intracranial hypertension
Mononeuropathy multiplex
Vasculidites
Amyloidosis
Hypothyroidism
Acromegaly
Coagulopathies
Medications [63]
isoniazide
hydralazine
Antineoplastic drugs such as paclitaxel (Taxol)
Antimacrobials such as metronidazole (Flagyl), dapsone, and nitrofurantoin (Macrobid)
Amiodarone

A slue of other diseases can cause neuropathy that is, at least clinically, indistinguishable from those occur in diabetes. Top on the list one can find alcohol abuse, uremia, vitamin B12 deficiency, hypothyroidism, and rarely chronic inflammatory demyelinating polyneuropathy (CIDP) (27) (tables 1 and 2).

The following laboratory tests can rule in or out most of other causes of neuropathies that maybe present concomitantly with diabetes: urinalysis, complete blood count, comprehensive metabolic panel, lipid profile, prothrombin and partial thromboplastin time, c-reactive protein, erythrocytes sedimentation rate, the levels of vitamin B12, methylmalonic acid, homocysteine, folate, vitamin B1, vitamin B6, protein and immunofixation electrophoresis, antinuclear antibodies, rheumatoid factor, thyroid function test , HIV test, hepatitis B and C tests, Alcohol level, and heavy-metal levels (such as lead, mercury, and arsenic) if clinical suspension is high (28).

MONITORING

The American Diabetes Association practice statement, published in 2005 (27), demands from practitioners to screen their patients for neuropathy at the time of the diagnosis of type 2 diabetes and annually thereafter. For those with type 1 diabetes, the initial screening test can be postponed until the 5th anniversary of making the diagnosis, and then be performed annually thereafter. The initial screening test should include a detailed history. It should focus on the following physical examination points:

- Pinprick
- Temperature
- Vibration with a tuning fork (as I described above)
- Pressure by applying a monofilament at the of the great toes bilaterally (see figure 2)

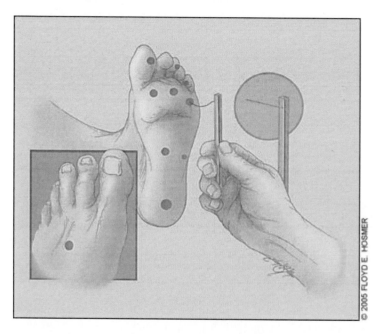

Figure 2. How to use the microfilament to screen for pressure sensation in diabetics.

Table 3. Medications, doses, titration schemes, NNT, and time to effects in PDN (28)

Medication	Usual effective dosage range	Titration scheme	NNT (95% CI) to achieve 50% pain reduction	Time to effect
Tricyclic antidepressants				
Amitriptyline	100–150 mg/day (150 mg at bedtime or 75 mg twice daily)	Day 1: 12.5 mg/day Days 2–7: 25 mg/day Week 2: 50 mg/day Week 3: 75 mg/day Week 4: 100 mg/day Weeks 5–8: 150 mg/day	2.1 (1.8–2.6)[30]	6–8 weeks
Nortriptyline	100–150 mg/day (50 mg three times daily)	Day 1: 12.5 mg/day Days 2–7: 25 mg/day Week 2: 50 mg/day Week 3: 75 mg/day Week 4: 100 mg/day Weeks 5–8: 150 mg/day	Cannot calculate NNT; similar to desipramine	6 weeks
Imipramine	150 mg/day (75 mg twice daily)	Week 1: 25 mg twice daily Week 2: 50 mg twice daily Week 3: 75 mg twice daily	2.1 (1.8–2.6)[30]	4 weeks
Desipramine	200–250 mg/day (250 mg daily or 125 mg twice daily)	Week 1: 50 mg/day Week 2: 100 mg/day Week 3: 200 mg/day Week 4: 250 mg/day	2.5 (1.9–3.6)[30]	6 weeks
Other antidepressants				
Venlafaxine	150–225 mg/day (75 mg three times daily or extended release formulation daily)	Week 1: 37.5 mg/day Week 2: 75 mg/day Week 3: 150 mg/day Week 4: 225 mg/day	5.5 (3.4–14)[30]	4–6 weeks
Duloxetine	60–120 mg/day (60 every day or twice a day)	Week 1: 10 mg/day Week 2: 20 mg/day Week 3: 60 mg/day Week 4: 120 mg/day	4 (3–9)[82]	4 weeks
Antiepileptics				
Carbamazepine	600 mg/day (200 mg three times daily)	Weeks 1–2: 100 mg three times daily Week 3: 200 mg three times daily	2.3 (1.6-3.9)[30]	4 weeks
Lamotrigine	200–400 mg/day (200 mg twice daily)	Week 1: 25 mg/day Week 2: 50 mg/day Week 3: 100 mg/day Week 4: 200 mg/day Week 5: 400 mg/day	4.0 (2.1–42)[30]	6–8 weeks
Valproate	1,000–1,200 mg/day (500 mg twice daily or 400 mg three times daily)	Week 1: 600 mg/day Week 2: 1,200 mg/day	2.5 (1.8–4.1)[30]	4 weeks
Topiramate	300–400 mg/day (200 mg twice daily)	Week 1: 25 mg/day Week 2: 50 mg/day Week 3: 75 mg/day Week 4: 100 mg/day Week 5: 150 mg/day Week 6: 200 mg/day Week 7: 300 mg/day Week 8: 400 mg/day	7.4 (4.3–28)[30]	12 weeks
Gabapentin	2,400–3,600 mg/day (1,200 mg three times daily or 900 mg four times daily)	Week 1: 300 mg at bedtime Week 2: 300 mg twice daily Week 3: 300 mg three times daily Week 4: 600 mg three times daily Week 5 : 900 mg three times daily	3.9 (3.2–5.1) for doses ≥ 2,400 mg/day[30]	4 weeks
Pregabalin	300–600 mg/day (300 mg twice daily or 200 mg three times daily)	Week 1: 150 mg/day Week 2: 300 mg/day Week 3: 600 mg/day (Dosed twice or three times daily)	4.2 (3.4–5.4)[30]	4–6 weeks
Others				
Capsaicin cream	0.075% four times daily	No titration needed	6.7 (4.6–12)	8 weeks
Tramadol	200–400 mg/day (100 mg four times daily)	Week 1: 50 mg/day Week 2: 100 mg/day Week 3: 150 mg/day Week 4: 200 mg/day Week 5: 300 mg/day Week 6: 400 mg/day	3.5 (2.4–6.4)[30]	6 weeks
Mexilitine	450–675 mg/day (225 mg three times daily)	Week 1: 225 mg/day Week 2: 450 mg/day Week 3: 675 mg/day	2.2 (1.3–8.7)[30]	1–4 days

CI— Ninety-five percent confidence interval. **NNT**— Number-Needed-to-Treat (is the number of patients needed to be treated to prevent one bad outcome. It is the inverse of the absolute risk reduction).

Nabil Majid

Table 4. Side-effects, contraindications, and recommended monitoring for the commonly used medications in treating PDN (28)

Medication	Adverse events	Contraindications for use	Recommended monitoring
Tricyclic antidepressants			
Amitriptyline	Dry mouth, sedation, dizziness, confusion, orthostatic hypotension, constipation, urinary retention, blurred vision, weight gain, arrhythmias	Cardiovascular disease; with or within 14 days use of MAO inhibitors; concurrent use of cisapride	Blood pressure and heart rate before and during initiation; weight; EKG before and during initiation; mental status
Nortriptyline	Dry mouth, sedation, dizziness, confusion, orthostatic hypotension, constipation, urinary retention, blurred vision, weight gain, arrhythmias	Cardiovascular disease; with or within 14 days use of MAO inhibitors; pregnancy	Blood pressure and heart rate before and during initiation; weight
Imipramine	Dry mouth, sedation, dizziness, confusion, orthostatic hypotension, constipation, urinary retention, blurred vision, weight gain, arrhythmias	Acute recovery phase of myocardial infarction; with or within 14 days use of MAO inhibitors; pregnancy	Blood pressure and heart rate before and during initiation; weight; EKG in older adults; mental status
Desipramine	Dry mouth, sedation, dizziness, confusion, orthostatic hypotension, constipation, urinary retention, blurred vision, weight gain, arrhythmias	Acute recovery phase of myocardial infarction; with or within 14 days use of MAO inhibitors	Blood pressure and heart rate before and during initiation; weight; EKG before and during initiation; mental status
Other antidepressants			
Venlafaxine	Headache, nausea, sedation, constipation, diarrhea, dizziness, dry mouth, sexual dysfunction, hypertension, seizures Rare: SIADH (syndrome of inappropriate antidiuretic hormone secretion), hyponatremia	With or within 14 days use of MAO inhibitors	Blood pressure; cholesterol; heart rate
Duloxetine	Nausea, somnolence, dizziness, dry mouth, constipation, sweating, weakness, headache, diarrhea	Hepatic insufficiency of any degree; substantial alcohol use; creatinine clearance < 30 ml/min; with or within 14 days use of MAO inhibitors; uncontrolled narrow angle glaucoma; caution in patients with delayed gastric emptying	Blood pressure; mental status; liver enzymes
Antiepileptics			
Carbamazepine	Agitation, dry mouth, sedation, ataxia, nausea, vomiting, blurred vision, confusion, fatigue, nystagmus Rare: aplastic anemia	Hypersensitivity to TCAs; bone marrow depression; with or within 14 days of MAO inhibitor use; pregnancy	Complete blood count with platelet count, reticulocytes, serum iron, lipid panel, liver function tests, urinalysis, BUN, serum carbamazepine levels, thyroid function tests, serum sodium; ophthalmic exams (pupillary reflexes); observe patient for excessive sedation, especially when instituting or increasing therapytional pacemaker
Lamotrigine	Dizziness, ataxia, sedation, headache, blurred vision, diplopia, nausea, confusion, nystagmus, rhinitis Rare: aplastic anemia, toxic epidermal necrolysis	Use with caution with valproic acid	Serum levels of concurrent antiepileptics; hypersensitivity reactions, especially rash
Valproate	Dizziness, somnolence, alopecia, insomnia, nausea, diarrhea, vomiting, thrombocytopenia, tremor, weakness Rare: aplastic anemia, pancreatitis, toxic epidermal necrolysis	Hepatic dysfunction, urea cycle disorders, pregnancy; concurrent use with topiramate	Liver enzymes; complete blood count with platelet count
BUN, blood urea nitrogen; MAO, monoamine oxidase.			
Topiramate	Dizziness, ataxia, psychomotor slowing, memory problems, speech difficulties, serum bicarbonate decreased, nausea, migraine, weight loss, anorexia Significant: metabolic acidosis (hyperchloremic, non-anion gap), nephrolithiasis, hyperthermia, central nervous system effects, secondary angle closure glaucoma. Must be tapered to avoid withdrawal.	Use with caution in hepatic and renal impairment; concurrent use with valproic acid	Hydration status; electrolytes prior and periodically during treatment; acute acidosis, complications of chronic acidosis (nephrolithiasis, osteomalacia); ammonia for unexplained lethargy; symptoms of acute glaucoma
Gabapentin	Somnolence, dizziness, ataxia, nausea, dry mouth, constipation, nystagmus, leucopenia, weight gain	Cautiously in patients with severe renal dysfunction	Serum levels of concomitant antiepileptic therapy
Pregabalin	Peripheral edema, dizziness, somnolence, ataxia, tremor, blurred vision, diplopia, weight gain. Rare: rhabdomyolysis, acute renal failure, prolong PR interval, thrombocytopenia. Must be tapered to avoid withdrawal.	Cautiously in patients with congestive heart failure, hypertension; concurrent use of thiazolidinedione	Degree of sedation; symptoms of myopathy or ocular disturbance; weight gain/edema; creatine phosphokinase; skin integrity (in diabetic patients)
Others			
Capsaicin cream	Localized burning and itching, cough, sneezing	Open wounds	Skin breakdown
Tramadol	Nausea, sedation, constipation, headache, dry mouth, urinary retention, confusion, tremor, seizures	Substantial alcohol use	Respiratory rate, blood pressure, heart rate; signs of tolerance or abuse
Mexilitine	Dyspepsia, dizziness, tremor, ataxia, insomnia, diarrhea, constipation, headache, nervousness, hepatotoxicity, arrhythmia Rare: agranulocytosis, toxic epidermal necrolysis	History of cardiogenic shock; second- or third-degree atrioventricular block (unless with functional pacemaker)	EKG prior to and during therapy; complete blood count with platelets; liver enzymes

In addition to the above, the annual screening test should include a careful evaluation of the ankle reflexes. Noteworthy, patient's education is key in preventing complications (as I will mention below). The patient must be encouraged to perform daily feet inspection even if he's asymptomatic. A referral to podiatry can be made at the discretion of the primary physician.

TREATMENT

Although clinicians have been using an array of medications to treat diabetic neuropathy, only Duloxetine (Cymbalta) and pregabalin (Lyrica) are formally approved by the FDA for this sole purpose. Other agents that are being used widely or tried experimentally are antiepileptics, tricyclic antidepressants, topical remedies, local anesthetics, opioids, nutraceuticals, dietary supplements, antioxidants, vasodilators, antiarrhythmias, and acupuncture. The patient expectations need to be realistic. All these therapies will not modify the disease state. Also, the patient needs to understand that there is no cure for PDN. However, the symptoms can be managed to a tolerable level. Table 3 lists the most commonly used drugs in treating PDN along with effective doses, titration schedules, number-needed-to-treat, and duration to effect. Table 4 lists the most commonly encountered side-effects for these medications, their contraindications, and recommended monitoring (28).

FDA APPROVED TREATMENTS

Duloxetine (Cymbalta)—is indicated for the treatment of major depressive disorder (MDD), management of pain associated with diabetic neuropathy, and treatment of generalized anxiety disorder (GAD). It is a selective serotonin and norepinephrine reuptake inhibitor. In its approval for duloxetine use in treating PDN, the FDA depended on an established record of safety and efficacy. Two 12 weeks randomized control trials that recruited almost 800 patients confirmed that duloxetine has a relatively rapid onset and a prolonged effect (29,30). Patients receiving higher dose manifested more intolerable side effects. The two cons of these studies were short duration and small size. Further, there is no head-to-head comparison of duloxetine with any other treatment for PDN.

Pregabalin (Lyrica)—is indicated for the management of pain associated with diabetic neuropathy, management of postherpetic neuralgia, fibromyalgia, and as an adjunctive therapy for partial seizure disorder in adults. Although related to gabapentin, pregabalin exerts no influence over the GABA or benzodiazepine receptors. Yet, it is still considered a Schedule IV drug that can be a habit forming. A daily dose of 300-600 mg can result in a sustained symptomatic relief within one week. This was established in a recent randomized control study of more than 330 patients (31). It is customary to start a low dose of 150 mg/day and titrate up to an effective dose within 1-2 weeks. Pregabalin is usually given three times a day.

Antiepileptics—other antiepileptics that have been tried in treating diabetic neuropathy with variable degrees of benefits were:

1. **Gabapentin (Neurontin)**—is indicated as an adjunct therapy for partial seizures in adult and pediatric patients older than three years of age and for the management of postherpetic neuralgia (PHN) in adults. Gabapentin can significantly improve quality of life (32-34). Several recent studies showed that it was effective in reducing pain perception and improving quality of sleep. Both factors were conducive to improved mood as well. Gabapentin can be as effective as amitriptyline yet more tolerable. In addition, it became more affordable since it started getting distributed in a generic form. Typically, the effective dose is 900-1,800 mg/day in three divided doses.

2. **Lamotrigine**—was evaluated in two small, short-term studies one of them was placebo-controlled, randomized and double-blinded (35). Both suggested that the medicine is superior to placebo. Effective doses range between 50mg to 400 mg daily.

3. **Carbamazepine**—is FDA approved for trigeminal neuralgia and may also be appropriate for PDN (36). Two small randomized, blinded, placebo-control studies suggested that carbamazepine can be effective in doses between 200-600 mg daily in relieving muscular pains, shooting pains, burning, numbness, cutaneous hyperalgesia, cramps, and tingling (37). Larger, long-term studies are needed to confirm these findings.

4. **Valproic acid**—the results of two short-term randomized trials were contradictory. One showed significant pain control with 1200 mg daily (without electrophysiological benefits) (38). The other could not prove that valproic acid was superior over placebo (39).

5. **Topiramate**—using identical methods, three simultaneous, placebo-controlled studies of topiramate for PDN did not show significance (40). Topiramate, however, reduced body weight. This can be a beneficial effect in type 2 diabetes especially if it can be found to be effective in relieving neuropathic pain in certain diabetic subgroups.

Antidepressants

Several studies have compared the tricyclic antidepressants (TCA) in a head-to-head style and relative to placebo and serotonin reuptake inhibitors (SSRI) (41-43). All in all, the TCA were superior to both placebo and SSRI in terms of pain relief. However, no relation between the symptomatic improvement and the dose was noted. This implies that the clinician should titrate up the dose to produce maximal clinical response with minimal side effects. Moreover, the side-effects can be a detrimental factor in your choice between different TCAs. For example, desipramine had somewhat fewer side effects than amitriptyline, particularly dry mouth. Therefore, it is better tolerated in the elderly.

Heart disease is prevalent in diabetics in general and those with neuropathy in particular. Caution must be exerted when using TCA especially in the elderly. In fact, both amitriptyline and nortriptyline are contraindicated in patients with established cardiac history. After consulting with a cardiologist, you may try doxepin, trazodone (44) or paroxetine (45) instead.

A recent multi-center, double-blinded, randomized, placebo-controlled study was conducted to evaluate the benefit of venlafaxine ER in painful diabetic neuropathy. It included 244 adults with metabolically stable type 1 or 2 diabetes. The study concluded that venlafaxine ER appears effective and safe in relieving pain associated with diabetic neuropathy. NNT values for higher dose venlafaxine ER are comparable to those of tricyclic antidepressants and the anticonvulsant gabapentin (31).

Topical remedies

When it is applied to the skin, capsaicin cream has been found to deplete substance P—the neurotransmitter of pain. Initially, it produces a burning sensation. Shortly thereafter, it converts into a cooling feeling. It has long been used topically to relieve many kinds of pain including arthritic and neuropathic. Thirteen out of 16 randomized controlled trials involving a total of 1,535 people found capsaicin to be more effective than placebo in relieving pain and improving daily tasks (46). The combination of TCA and capsaicin was also found to be effective in several studies (47). A recommended starting dose is 0.025% cream applied four times a day. If this dose is ineffective, a 0.075% cream can be used. Many of the unpleasant local effects subside with continuous use.

Local anesthetics

Lidocaine patches 5% are approved for the relief of pain associated with postherpetic neuralgia. Like any other topical treatment, cutaneous absorption is minimal, estimated at 3%. Therefore, multiple patches applied several times a day maybe needed to achieve the desirable effect. In fact, one study showed that using up to four patches per day can be helpful in relieving PDN pain (48, 49).

Opioids

It is common practice to use narcotics for PDN. Several short-term studies (8 days to 8 weeks) showed that narcotics can decrease neuropathic pain. It is still controversial at best, however, whether narcotics can improve quality of life (31). The main problem with these medications is tolerance and dependency. Both problems are subtle and can cause disruptive behaviors on the long run that add to the complexity of managing chronic pain.

Vasodilators

As a vasodilator, nitric oxide (NO) controls neural blood flow. Recent evidence, suggests that diabetes may impair the metabolism of NO, the fact that can be conducive to the pathogenesis of PDN. A short-term, double-blinded, randomized, placebo-controlled, cross-over study, which recruited 22 patients, showed that isosorbide dinitrate spray, a drug that induces NO generation, can relieve PDN burning perception.[50] The treatment, which consisted of spraying the affected area before bedtime, was extremely well tolerated, with only two patients complaining of transient headache. Relief was provided throughout the night and subsequent day until the next treatment. However, this study did not discuss whether the findings made any difference in quality of life and daily activities. Further it was relatively brief and small, but the results suggest great potential benefit with little risk for severely afflicted patients. Isosorbide dinitrate is not currently available in the United States

Antiarrhythmias

Mexiletine—originally indicated for the management of serious ventricular arrhythmias, it is being used for PDN as an investigational agent. It's a type Ib antiarrhythma medication. The evidence behind its efficacy for painful diabetic neuropathy was extrapolated from one study that demonstrated moderate pain relief with intravenous lidocaine (51). Mexiletine is the oral analogue of lidocaine and is thought to exert its analgesic and antiarrhythmic effects by membrane-stabilizing Na^+-channel antagonism. Doses up to 675 mg/day were well tolerated. Cardiac patients were excluded in all studies. Clearance from a cardiologist is then recommended before initiating the therapy. Also, it's better be left as an alternative agent for patients with extreme, refractory symptoms and no cardiac risk.

Nutraceuticals

Alpha-lipoic acid is a potent antioxidant. Being both water- and fat-soluble adds to its efficacy. It thought to work by improving the underlying pathophysiology of neuropathy, and hence reduce pain. Several short-term, prospective, placebo-controlled studies (52,53) have examined its benefit in PND and found it to be better than placebo at all doses studied especially at 600 mg daily where it was associated with the least side effects (nausea, vomiting, vertigo). This therapy is recommended when the patient shows intolerance to the more potent therapies such as antiepileptics and antidepressants.

Dietary supplements

Acetyl L-carnitine was evaluated in two randomized trials. They produced contradictory results. One showed a benefit the other did not. To further the confusion, the benefit was shown at 1000 mg three times a day dose but not at 500 mg (54, 55).

Acupuncture

Different kinds of acupuncture were tested head to head to find whether they have any benefit in relieving painful PDN. A pilot study evaluated the clinical and mechanistic effects of two styles of acupuncture, Traditional Chinese Medicine (TCM) and Japanese acupuncture. Despite its small cohort and short-term, the study suggested superior benefit of TCM over the

Japanese acupuncture. No evident changes were observed in glucose control or heart rate variability in either group (56).

Electrical stimulation

Two types of electrical stimulation were evaluated in short term, randomized, single-blinded trials for the treatment of refractory PDN; they are transcutaneous electrical nerve stimulation (TENS) and percutaneous electrical nerve stimulation (PENS). As the terms imply, the former uses non invasive method to deliver the electrical pulse, while the latter stimulates via needles.

One trial that tested TENS recruited 31 patients with symptoms and signs of peripheral neuropathy. They were randomized to the electrotherapy or sham treatment (control) group. Patients received treatment to their lower extremities for 30 min daily for four weeks at home. Nine patients from the sham-treatment group participated for a second period, during which all of them received the active electrotherapy. The study concluded that the transcutaneous electrotherapy ameliorated the pain and discomfort associated with peripheral neuropathy (57).

The trial that evaluated PENS involved 50 adult patients with type 2 diabetes and peripheral neuropathic pain of the lower extremities for more than six months duration. They were randomly assigned to receive active PENS or sham treatments (needles only) for three weeks. Each series of treatments was administered for 30 min three times a week according to a standardized protocol. After a 1-week washout period, all patients were subsequently switched over to the other modality.

The study concluded that PENS can be a useful non-pharmacological therapeutic modality for treating PDN in some patients. In addition to relieving neuropathic pain, PENS therapy improved physical activity tolerance, the feeling of well-being, and the quality of sleep. Therefore, it may help reduce the need for oral non-opioid analgesic medications (58).

Rational polypharmacy

This concept stems out from the notion that, when used in combinations, several drugs of different mechanism of action can work synergistically to provide better pain relief than monotherapy. This can be achieved at lower doses of these drugs, thus fewer side effects.

One recent study has evaluated the use of lidocain 5% patches with gabapentin for neuropathic pain including PDN. It concluded that the use of peripherally acting analgesics can further improve mood, walking ability, and other daily activities when combined with gabapentin (59).

Non-pharmacological therapy

Physical therapy may be a useful adjunct to other therapy, especially when muscular pain and weakness are a manifestation of the patient's neuropathy. The physical therapist can instruct the patient in a general exercise program to maintain his or her mobility and strength. The patient also should be educated on independent pain management, relaxation strategies, balance training, and fall prevention. Aquatic therapy, brace assessment, orthotic or prosthetic training, and walking aid assessment and implementation can all be helpful.

Occupational therapy is necessary in cases where there is severe loss of functional status. Recreational therapy can help the patient with performance of community activities. Many patients with chronic disease, especially elderly patients, become isolated and are at risk for comorbid conditions such as depression.

PREVENTION

Tight glycemic control

The most important approach for the prevention of diabetic neuropathy is optimal glucose control. In the Diabetes Control and Complications Trial (DCCT), tight glycemic control have resulted in a 60% reduction in the risk of developing clinical neuropathy over 10 years by maintaining the hemoglobin A1c around 7% for both types of diabetes. However, no clinical data is available to suggest similar benefit in the elderly, the very young, or in patients with advanced complications (7). Whether glycemic control can also treat PDN is not as well established. Having said that, the DCCT found at 5-year follow-up, that nerve conduction studies have improved in the tight glycemic control group. The clinical significance of this finding is not known yet (60).

Lifestyle modifications

The European Diabetes (EURODIAB) Prospective Complications Study (61) concluded that diabetic neuropathy is associated with potentially modifiable cardiovascular risk factors, including a raised triglyceride level, a high body-mass index, smoking, and hypertension. The Japan Diabetes Complications Study (61) found only central obesity can impose a statistically significant risk on diabetics to develop neuropathy. Lifestyle modifications, however, that target other habits as well are important to help the patient live with the disease. Therefore, following the American Diabetes Association dietary guidelines, regular exercise, smoking cessation, reducing alcohol consumption, maintaining good bodily hygiene, proper uninterrupted sleep, and relaxation exercises should be part of a comprehensive multidisciplinary plan to prevent the progression of diabetic neuropathy and assist the patient cope with the pain.

GUIDELINES

There is still no general consensus in this field between different authoritative medical societies on the optimal medical treatment for PDN. The American Diabetes Association recommends treatment in sequential steps as follows (27):

1. Exclude non-diabetic etiologies
2. Stabilize glycemic control
3. Antidepressant drugs
4. Anticonvulsants
5. Alpha-lipoic acid
6. Opioid or opioid-like drugs
7. Consider pain clinic referral

Based on positive results from randomized, controlled trials and the expert clinical opinion, in 2003, the members of the faculty of the Fourth International Conference on the Mechanisms and Treatment of Neuropathic Pain recommended the following as first-line medications: gabapentin, 5% lidocaine patch, opioid analgesics, tramadol, and tricyclic antidepressants (5).

However, in 2006 a panel of pain specialist from New York University School of Medicine produced guidelines for the treatment of PDN based on the strength of the scientific evidence and number of supportive studies. They divided the drugs into three lines (62,63):

1. First Line— supported by evidence from two or more randomized clinical trials, were duloxetine, pregabalin, controlled-release oxycodone, and tricyclic antidepressants
2. Second Line—supported by evidence from one randomized clinical trial, were carbamazepine, gabapentin, lamotrigine, tramadol, and extended-release venlafaxine
3. Third Line—Topical therapies, supported by evidence from one randomized clinical trial or evidence from studies of other painful neuropathies, included capsaicin and lidocaine

A new literature review has found that anticonvulsants and antidepressants are still the most commonly used options to manage diabetic neuropathy. Oral tricyclic antidepressants and traditional anticonvulsants are better for short term pain relief than newer generation anticonvulsants. Evidence of the long term effects of oral antidepressants and anticonvulsants is still lacking. Further studies are needed on opioids, N-methyl-D-aspartate antagonists, and ion channel blockers. (50)

CONCLUSION

Painful diabetic neuropathy affects the quality of life and has no curative therapy. It manifests mainly as burning, pins and needles sensation starting in the feet and progresses upwards. It has established metabolic and vascular pathophysiologic mechanisms. Recent studies try to combine these mechanisms in one big scheme. The diagnosis is mainly clinical. Electrophysiologic studies and skin biopsy plays a supportive role.

The physician needs also to exclude other etiologies, commonly encountered in diabetics, such as neuropathies from alcoholism, vitamin B12 deficiency, and uremia among others. Although many screening tests were introduced over the decades, the tuning fork test is still the simplest and widely used.

The treatment is multidisciplinary. While tight glycemic control is the main pillar of prevention, drugs are the only proven treatment. Duloxetine and pregabalin are the only FDA approve medications for PDN. Generally, antidepressants and anticonvulsants are the most commonly used. Rational polypharmacy has recently emerged as a necessary way to decrease the effective dose of the prescribed drugs while benefiting from its synergistic outcome. This way we can spare the patient an array of unpleasant side effects. These are the main reason behind medical noncompliance.

Lifestyle modifications produce subjective well being. Physical and occupational therapy help patients cope with pain among other benefits. Finally, several authoritative medical associations have published guidelines for therapeutic approach to PDN. It cannot be overemphasized that your approach needs to be individualized, however.

REFERENCES

[1]   Schmader KE. Epidemiology and impact on quality of life of postherpetic neuralgia and painful diabetic neuropathy. Clin J Pain 2002;18:350–4.

[2]   Pirart J. Diabetes mellitus and its degenerative complications: a prospective study of 4,400 patients observed between 1947 and 1973. Diabetes Care 1978; 1: 168–188, 252–63.

[3]   Vinik A, Mehrabyan A. Diabetic neuropathies. Med Clin North Am 2004;88:947–99.

[4]   Ziegler D, et al. Oxidative stress and antioxidant defense in relation to the severity of diabetic polyneuropathy and cardiovascular autonomic neuropathy. Diabetes Care 2004;27:2178–83.

[5]   Vinik A. Use of antiepileptic drugs in the treatment of chronic painful diabetic neuropathy. J Clin Endo Metab 2005;90(8):4936-45.

[6]   Sanders LJ. Diabetes mellitus. Prevention of amputation. J Am Podiatr Med Assoc 1994;84(7):322-8.

[7]   Aring AM, et al. Evaluation and prevention of diabetic neuropathy. Am Fam Physician 2005;71:2123-8, 2129-30.

[8]   Kilo S, Berghoff M, Hilz M, Freeman R. Neural and endothelial control of the microcirculation in diabetic peripheral neuropathy. Neurology 2000;54(6):1246-52.

[9]   Singh R, Barden A, Mori T, Beilin L. Advanced glycation end-products: a review. Diabetologia 2001;44(2):129-46.

[10]   Hotta N, et al. Long-term clinical effects of epalrestat, an aldose reductase inhibitor, on diabetic peripheral neuropathy: 3-year, multicenter, comparative aldose reductase inhibitor-Diabetes Complications Trial. Diabetic Care 2006; 29(7):1538-44.

[11]   Vincent AM, et al. Short-term hyperglycemia produces oxidative damage and apoptosis in neurons. FASEB J. 2005;19(6):638-40.

[12]   Newrick PG, et al. Sural nerve oxygen tension in diabetes. Br Med J (Clin Res Ed) 1986;293:1053.

[13]   Stevens MJ. The aetiology of diabetic neuropathy: the combined roles of metabolic and vascular defects. Diabet Med 1995l;12(7):566-79.

[14]   Yasuda H, et al. Effect of prostaglandin E1 analogue TFC 612 on diabetic neuropathy in streptozotocin-induced diabetic rats. Comparison with aldactose reductase inhibitor ONO 2235. Diabetes 1989;38(7): 832-8.

[15]   Pieper GM, et al. Oxygen free radicals abolish endothelium-dependent relaxation in diabetic rat aorta. Am J Physiol 1988;255(4 pt 2):H825-33.

[16]   Partanen, J, et al. Natural history of peripheral neuropathy in patients with non-insulin-dependent diabetes mellitus. N Engl J Med 1995;333:89.

[17]   Davies, M, et al. The prevalence, severity, and impact of painful diabetic peripheral neuropathy in type 2 diabetes. Diabetes Care 2006;29:1518.

[18]   Mulder DW, et al. The neuropathies associated with diabetes mellitus. A clinical and electromyographic study of 103 unselected diabetic patients. Neurology 1961; 11(4) Pt 1:275.

[19]   Consensus statement: Report and recommendations of the San Antonio conference on diabetic neuropathy. American Diabetes Association American and Academy of Neurology. Diabetes Care 1988;11:592.

[20]   Young, MJ, et al. A multicentre study of the prevalence of diabetic peripheral neuropathy in the United Kingdom hospital clinic population. Diabetologia 1993; 36:150.

[21]   Dyck, PJ, et al. The Rochester Diabetic Neuropathy Study: Design, criteria for types of neuropathy, selection bias, and reproducibility of neuropathic tests. Neurology 1991;41:799.

[22]   Feldman, EL, et al. A practical two-step quantitative clinical and electrophysiological assessment for the diagnosis and staging of diabetic neuropathy. Diabetes Care 1994;17:1281.

[23]   Rowland LS, ed. Merritt's textbook of neurology, 8th ed. Philadelphia, PA: Lea Febiger, 1989.

[24]   Lauria G, Lombardi R. Skin biopsy: a new tool for diagnosing peripheral neuropathy. BMJ 2007;334(7604):1159-62.

[25]   Meijer, JW, et al. Back to basics in diagnosing diabetic polyneuropathy with the tuning fork!. Diabetes Care 2005;28:2201.

[26]   Perkins BA, et al. Simple screening tests for peripheral neuropathy in the diabetes clinic. Diabetes Care 2001;24:250-6.

[27]   Boulton, AJ, et al. Diabetic neuropathies: a statement by the American Diabetes Association. Diabetes Care 2005;28:956.

[28]   Huizinga MM, et al. Painful diabetic neuropathy: A management-centered review. Clin Diabetes 2007;25:6-15.

[29]   Goldstein DJ, et al. Duloxetine vs. placebo in patients with painful diabetic neuropathy. Pain 2005;116:109.

[30]   Wernicke, JF, et al. A randomized controlled trial of duloxetine in diabetic peripheral neuropathic pain. Neurology 2006;67:1411.

[31]   Eisenberg E, McNicol ED, Carr DB. Efficacy and safety of opioid agonist in the treatment of neuropathic pain of nonmalignant origin systematic review and meta-analysis of randomized controlled trials. JAMA 2005;293(24):3043-52.

[32]   Backonja, M, et al. Gabapentin for the symptomatic treatment of painful neuropathy in patients with diabetes mellitus. A randomized controlled trial. JAMA 1998;280:1831.

[33]   Morello, CM, et al. Randomized double-blind study comparing the efficacy of gabapentin with amitriptyline on diabetic peripheral neuropathy pain. Arch Intern Med 1999;159:1931.

[34]   Rowbotham, M, et al. Gabapentin for the treatment of postherpetic neuralgia: a randomized controlled trial. JAMA 1998;280:1837.

[35]   Eisenberg E, et al. Lamotrigine in the treatment of painful diabetic neuropathy. Eur J Neurol 1998:167–73.

[36]   Dworkin RH, et al. Advances in neuropathic pain: diagnosis, mechanisms, and treatment recommendations. Arch Neurol 2003;60:1524-34.

[37]   Rull JA, et al. Symptomatic treatment of peripheral diabetic neuropathy with carbamazepine (Tegretol): double blind crossover trial. Diabetologia 1969;215-8.

[38]   Kochar DK, et al. Sodium valproate in the management of painful neuropathy in type 2 diabetes: a randomized placebo controlled study. Acta Neurol Scand 2002; 248-52.

[39]   Otto M, Bach FW, Jensen TS, Sindrup SH. Valproic acid has no effect on pain in polyneuropathy: a randomized, controlled trial. Neurology 2004;62(2):285-8.

[40]   Thienel U, Neto W, Schwabe SK, Vijapurkar U. Topiramate in painful diabetic polyneurophathy: findings from three double-blind placebo-controlled trials. Acta Neurol Scand 2004;110(4):221-31.

[41]   Max, MB, et al. Amitriptyline relieves diabetic neuropathy pain in patients with normal or depressed mood. Neurology 1987;37:589.

[42]   Max, MB, et al. Effects of desipramine, amitriptyline, and fluoxetine on pain in diabetic neuropathy. N Engl J Med 1992;326:1250.

[43]   Kvinesdal, B, et al.. Imipramine treatment of painful diabetic neuropathy. JAMA 1984;251:1727.

[44]   Wong, MC, et al. Effects of treatments for symptoms of painful diabetic neuropathy: systematic review. BMJ 2007;335:87.

[45]   Davis, JL, et al. Peripheral diabetic neuropathy treated with amitriptyline and fluphenazine. JAMA 1977;238:2291.

[46]   Capsaicin Study Group. Effect of treatment with capsaicin on daily activities of patients with painful diabetic neuropathy. Diabetes Care 1992;15:159.

[47]   Mason, L, et al. Systematic review of topical capsaicin for the treatment of chronic pain. BMJ 2004;328:991.

[48]   Ackerman WE, et al. The management of oral mexiletine and intravenous lidocaine to treat chronic painful symmetrical distal diabetic neuropathy. J Ky Med Assoc 1991;89:500.

[49]   Gidal B, Blington Rl. New and emerging treatment options for neuropathic pain. Am J Man Care 2006;12:S 269-78.

[50]   Yuen KC, et al. Treatment of chronic painful diabetic neuropathy with isosorbide dinitrate spray: a double-blind placebo-controlled cross-over study. Diabetes Care 2002;25:1699.

[51]   Carroll I. Intravenous lidocaine for neuropathic pain: Diagnostic utility and therapeutic efficacy. Curr Pain Headache Rep 2007;11(1):20-4.

[52]   Ruhnau, KJ, et al. Effects of 3-week oral treatment with the antioxidant thioctic acid (alpha-lipoic acid) in symptomatic diabetic polyneuropathy. Diabet Med 1999;16:1040.

[53]   Ziegler, D, et al. Treatment of symptomatic diabetic polyneuropathy with the antioxidant alpha-lipoic acid: a meta-analysis. Diabet Med 2004;21:114.

[54]   Quatraro, A, et al. Acetyl-L-carnitine for symptomatic diabetic neuropathy. Diabetologia 1995;38:123.

[55]   Sima AA, et al. Acetyl-L-carnitine improves pain, nerve regeneration, and vibratory perception in patients with chronic diabetic neuropathy: an analysis of two randomized placebo-controlled trials. Diabetes Care 2005;28:89.

[56]   Ahn AC, et al. Two styles of acupuncture for treating painful diabetic neuropathy--a pilot randomised control trial. Acupunct Med 2007;25(1-2):11-7.

[57]   Kumar, D, Marshall, HJ. Diabetic peripheral neuropathy: amelioration of pain with transcutaneous electrostimulation. Diabetes Care 1997;20:1702.

[58]   Hamza MA, et al. Percutaneous electrical nerve stimulation: a novel analgesic therapy for diabetic neuropathic pain. Diabetes Care. 2000;23(3):365-70.

[59]   White WT, et al. Lidocaine patch 5% with systemic analgesics such as gabapentin: a rational polypharmacy approach for the treatment of chronic pain. Pain Med 2003;4(4):321-30.

[60]   Diabetes Control and Complications Trial Research Group. Effect of intensive diabetes treatment on nerve conduction in the Diabetes Control and Complications Trial. Ann Neurol 1995;38:869-80.

[61]   Tesfaye S, Chaturvedi N, Eaton SE, Ward JD, Manes C, et al. Vascular risk factors and diabetic neuropathy. N Eng J Med 2005;352:1925-7.

[62]   Kajdasz DK, et al. Duloxetine for the management of diabetic peripheral neuropathic pain: evidence-based findings from post hoc analysis of three multicenter, randomized, double-blind, placebo-controlled, parallel-group studies. Clin Ther 2007;29(Suppl):2536-46.

[63]   Argoff CE, et al. Consensus guidelines: treatment planning and options. Diabetic peripheral neuropathic pain. Mayo Clin Proc 2006;81(4 Suppl):S12-25.

[64]   Adams RD, Victor M, Ropper AH, eds. Principles of neurology, 6th ed. Nw York: McGraw-Hill, 1997:1323-5.

SECTION 4: EATING BEHAVIORS

In: Food, Nutrition and Eating Behavior
Editors: Joav Merrick and Sigal Israeli

ISBN: 978-1-62948-233-0
© 2014 Nova Science Publishers, Inc.

Chapter 13

FRIENDSHIP, MEDIA, EATING BEHAVIOR AND PHYSICAL ACTIVITY IN ADOLESCENTS

Eveline JM Wouters* and Rinie Geenen
Department of Allied Health Professions,
Fontys University of Applied Sciences,
Eindhoven and Department of Clinical and Health Psychology,
Utrecht University, Utrecht, The Netherlands

ABSTRACT

The worldwide obesity epidemic is a complex problem, resulting from the interaction of individual metabolic, genetic, and psychological factors with meso- and macro environmental factors. Adolescents, with their rapid changes in body composition, together with their shift in orientation from the direct family to the peer-related environment, are particularly vulnerable to unhealthy changes in lifestyle, and peers seem to play an important role in shaping the behavior of adolescents. Adolescents tend to mimic their peers' behavior related to both food choices as well as to physical activity. This influence of peers depends on environmental circumstances such as availability of snacks, and it is affected by individual psychological and demographic factors as well as by macro-environmental factors such as cultural and social norms, legislation, food distribution, and media and advertising. Rapidly expanding sources of influence on health behavior are media such as television, the internet, and smartphones. These media may enhance overweight and a sedentary lifestyle. However, potentially these media could be used to monitor and influence snacking behavior and physical activity for the better. An example of the use of new technology to enhance health behavior is the 'Wii' home video game. Using insights from social psychology, thoughtful choice architecture can be established to nudge adolescents to choose what is best for them without restricting freedom of choice and to help them with really implementing healthy intentions. A challenge for the coming decade is to develop 'Apps' aimed to decrease adolescent obesity while making use of social networks.

---

* Correspondence: Eveline JM Wouters, PhD, MD, MSc. Department of Allied Health Professions, Fontys University of Applied Sciences, Th. Fliednerstraat 2, 5631 BN, room 0.214, Eindhoven, The Netherlands. E-mail: e.wouters@fontys.nl.

INTRODUCTION

The obesity epidemic is a major and complex problem, resulting from the interaction of environmental, metabolic, genetic and psychological factors (1). To date, 17% of children and adolescents in the US are diagnosed to be obese (2). This high prevalence in obesity has already been observed since 2007, but notably, within the group of obese children and adolescents, there is a relative increase in prevalence of obesity in the subgroup of adolescents (12-19 years) (2, 3).

Many adolescents have unhealthy diets and sedentary behavior (4). This not only bears implications at this age, but many of these behaviors are maintained during later periods of life. What was learned during adolescence has often become a habit in adult life (5). Dieting as a single intervention in adolescence, hardly ever leads to successful weight loss. Moreover, unhealthy dieting during adolescence (both in boys and girls), leads to weight gain and obesity later in life, as well as to substantially enhanced risk of developing eating disorders (6). Therefore, the recognition and prevention of these behaviors and their determinants is very important.

Adolescents, with their rapid changes in body composition, together with their shift in orientation from the direct family to the peer-related environment, are particularly vulnerable to unfavorable changes in life style. Food and exercise habits tend to change substantially in this period, as compared to earlier childhood. Besides their parents, also peers come to play an important role in what they do or what they like. Adolescents, compared to other age groups, have a stronger need to belong to a group and to be accepted by their peers (7).

In this paper, the literature on the influences of peers on eating- and exercise behavior is reviewed and the specific role of modern media in this context is discussed.

INFLUENCE OF SOCIAL NETWORKS IN ADOLESCENCE

Social networks are of great importance in adolescence (7). Many parents perceive with some anxiety that the peers of their youngsters can become very important and influential in developing all kinds of maladaptive or unhealthy behavior. Social learning theory specifies that peers may influence each other by observing, modeling, and imitating individuals in their environment (8). General learning theory suggests that behavior can be shaped by selective reinforcement and punishment by peers.

With respect to unhealthy behavior, there is convincing evidence for peer influence on smoking behavior (9). Having friends who smoke or friends who approve of smoking predicts the probability of adolescents to start smoking (9). Also other unhealthy habits, such as alcohol and drug abuse, are influenced by peers (10, 11). The better the perceived quality of the friendship, the more adolescents are apt to conform to the substance use of their peers (10).

Smoking and substance use represent addictions that, after having acquired the habit, are difficult to stop. Behavior that is less related to specific substances but that shares the compulsive nature of addictions and that can be related to the onset of obesity (in a direct or indirect way), is disordered eating such as bulimia. In bulimia, peers (both girls and boys) select each other for personality traits (related to self-esteem and perfectionism), and the socialization process influences the development of similar bulimic symptoms (12). Especially the maintenance of the bulimic behavior appears influenced by peers, because after loosening up of the friendships, bulimia symptoms tend to diminish. Also in anorexia, mostly studied in girls, peers are influential and both peers and media play an important role in the thin beauty ideal of many girls (13).

Thus, unhealthy, harmful habits can be partly attributed to the influence of peers in adolescence. Considering the increase of adolescent obesity, it is useful to gain knowledge on comparable peer influences on the development and persistence of obesity. In adults, obesity has been found to spread in social networks (14). As adolescents tend to create new and strong social networks, it is an obvious assumption that peers are important for the development of overweight and obesity.

INFLUENCE OF SOCIAL NETWORKS ON EATING BEHAVIOR IN ADOLESCENTS

Both observational and experimental studies indicate that children and adolescents model their peers' behavior related to both healthy and unhealthy food choices as well as to physical activity and sports participation (15). In this section the factors that influence eating behavior will be discussed.

Peers and parents

In research of obesity, common eating behavior is measured with variables such as daily fruit- and vegetable intake, regular consumption of breakfast, frequency of fast food restaurant visits, and calorie dense snack intake. The influence of peers varies between these variables. For instance, breakfast consumption, as compared to calorie dense snack intake, is more strongly associated with parental behavior than with peer influence. However, several food-related habits tend to run in friendship groups. For instance, peers influence each other more strongly with respect to eating in fast food restaurants (15). Moreover, snacking, defined as the intake of high caloric food and high energy soft drinks, is rather similar within peer groups of adolescents (16). Also, while hanging out with friends, the tendency to snack is stronger than without friends (17).

Moderators of peer influence on eating behavior

The relation between snacking and friends' influence is not one-to-one. Multiple factors determine snacking in interaction. First of all, the physical environment affects the influence of peers on eating behavior. If snacks are easily available in the environment, for instance, in the shops near school (18) or within school itself (16), the influence of peers is stronger.

Second, individual factors play a role. In the adult population, personality factors such as low conscientiousness (19), high impulsivity and low self-control (20) are associated with unhealthy snacking. Likely, similar personality factors influence snacking in young people.

Third, demographic factors should be taken account of. The influence of friendship groups on snacking is not similar for girls and boys. In boys, peer group snacking is somewhat stronger than in girl peer groups (16), whereas in girls, dieting within peer groups during adolescence, which is related to higher risk for developing obesity in later life, is more common (21, 22). There is also a difference between adolescents related to education level. Peer group effects on snacking are stronger in adolescents with lower education levels (16). Besides reinforcement by peers, punishment may affect eating behavior. In girls, more than in boys, peer group teasing and comments about the body appearance of overweight and obese adolescents, influence unhealthy dieting in an unfavorable manner, strengthening the effect in girls already overweight (23).

Environmental influence

There is no single determinant of unhealthy behavior. Just like other health behavior, unhealthy eating is determined by individual (personal) factors, meso-environmental factors, which can be divided into social environmental (family and peers) and physical environmental components (like availability in the community such as shops and school canteens). In addition, macro-environmental factors play a role. Cultural and social norms, legislation, food distribution as well as media and advertising, are amongst these latter factors (24). This framework that summarizes several levels of influence, and that positions individual influences central, and environmental (interpersonal and physical factors) next, is illustrated in figure 1.

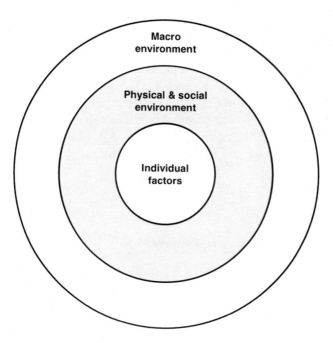

Figure 1. Factors influencing obesity-related behavior.

Up till now, many of the efforts to reduce the obesity epidemic have been directed at the individual level. Individual therapy, preferably multidisciplinary interventions including diet and physical exercise, combined with psychological support, are now common treatment. The observation that also the direct physical environment plays a role, has additionally led to interventions in communities, especially school-based interventions (25).

None of these interventions paid much attention to the role of friendship groups as a risk factor for developing and maintaining unhealthy eating habits. Comparable to the relatively late addition of psychological support to dieting and exercise in the individual treatment of overweight, this is a treatment direction that is, at the moment, still largely underdeveloped. There is ample evidence that groups of school friends have rather similar body mass indices, fast food consumption patterns and body image concerns, dieting habits, and eating disorders (26).

This indicates the potential effectiveness of school based interventions addressing the role of these friendships. Future interventions should pay more attention to this opportunity to restrict the obesity epidemic.

INFLUENCE OF SOCIAL NETWORKS ON EXERCISE BEHAVIOR IN ADOLESCENTS

Physical activity and exercise are, next to healthy diets, important in the onset and maintenance of weight loss in obesity treatment (27-29). Moreover, physical activity improves physical and mental health (30-33). Physical exercise, as a means to reduce overweight and obesity, could be especially indicated in people for whom exercising is easier than stopping superfluous eating (34).

Exercise behavior

Exercise has positive effects on physical and mental health in adolescents and the reversed effect is observed for sedentary behavior (35, 36). For adolescents, the effects of exercise can generalize to multiple dimensions of functioning. For instance adolescents who are physically active achieve better results at school (37). Despite all these favorable effects, many adolescents, even after having been physically active in childhood, stop exercising in adolescence (38, 39).

Comparable to the change in eating behavior (figure 1), reasons for the decrease of physical activity in puberty have been sought in individual factors (physical changes and maturation) and social and physical environmental factors (38). As an example of individual factors, the decrease in physical activity among adolescents is more prominent in girls (40, 41) and in lower income families (42).

Physical activity of individuals is closely linked to physical activity patterns of their peers (43). Possibly, self-esteem is a mediator of the association between physical activity of individuals and their peers (42).

Environmental influence on exercise behavior

Regarding the physical environment, the lack of possibilities and opportunities to exercise, and lack of safety in the neighborhood may hamper physical activity (44-46). Comparable to the availability of healthy instead of unhealthy food, being physically active at a regular basis needs appropriate facilities in the neighborhood.

As for eating behavior, peers have been found to play a prominent role in the physical activity patterns of adolescents. Adolescents more often befriend with adolescents with comparable amounts of physical activities and, consecutively, mimic each other's activities (47). By participation in sport activities, adolescents improve self-esteem and get positive social feedback (48). Peers represent role models who may reinforce being physically active by giving encouragement and social support. Therefore, interventions to improve physical activities in adolescents should include and optimize peer support for being successful (49). Preferably, these interventions should start before the onset of puberty, because the effect of friends is counteracted by the effect of age: in case of low baseline physical activity at the start of puberty, the net activity is generally also low during later years.

THE ROLE OF MEDIA

An influence of social networks in children and adolescents not only occurs through face-to-face contacts, but also through media such as television, the internet (e.g., Facebook, twitter), and smartphones. To date, over 900 million persons use Facebook worldwide (50). The rapidly expanding new media may impact on overweight for the worse by reinforcing a sedentary life. However, potentially these media could be used to monitor and influence snacking behavior and physical activity for the better.

Regarding the impact of media, children and youth are a special audience, because they are developmentally vulnerable and because they have always been among the earliest adopters and heaviest users of entertainment technology (51). As in face-to-face contacts, media play a role in the macro environment as well as in the more proximal social environment of adolescents, and media may influence factors related to eating and dieting, as well as energy expenditure and physical exercise.

Media and eating behavior

The role of the media in childhood overweight and obesity as a push factor has been well studied. Especially the influence of commercials of food products on children watching television has been widely established. It has, for instance, been shown that exposure to television food commercials increases the preference for energy-dense foods, particularly in children who watch more television (52). Such an impact appears stronger for boys than for girls (53).

Food markets often advertise unhealthy products specifically directed at youth. Adolescents are such an important group for industry, because people tend to use the brands they used in adolescence lifelong. The psychological mechanisms by which the influence of marketing works is widely accepted, as well as the favorable results of interventions aimed at prohibition on food advertisements during daytime, pointing at the importance of governmental policies and strategies (54, 55). In some countries bans on "unhealthy" advertisements have now been established (56, 57).

The association between media use and obesity is small, but consistent (58, 59). Thus, media use is clearly one of several factors that may impact on obesity. The American Academy of Pediatrics policy statement regarding the prevention of pediatric overweight and obesity identifies limiting television and videogame use to no more than 2 hours per day as an important strategy for preventing obesity among children and adolescents (60). However, in order to decrease the total of screen hours, especially the role of the meso-environment appears important. More clearly than policy makers, parents, peers and teachers can play a role in restricting the amount of hours that adolescents watch a screen.

Media and physical exercise

For physical exercise, the influence of media as part of the macro environment is also twofold, but slightly different from the role of media with respect to food. Watching television (or other screens) is directly and importantly related to sedentary behavior and lack of physical activity, and the number of spent hours of television watching is an important predictor of overweight and obesity (36).

Physical exercise can also be enhanced by modern media. Home video games like 'Wii' are so popular in adolescents, because they do not experience it as physical effort, but especially because the game is fun (61). In overweight and obese adolescents, playing 'exergames' in a cooperative way is more effective in being physically active and losing weight, than playing competitive exercises (62-65). Playing together and being with peers, is part of the success of these games.

Next to these games, there is a growing availability of Apps about weight-related behavior in electronic phones and tablets. In 2011, already over 2000 Apps about health and fitness were available, most of them assisting the user in logging their calorie intake and physical activity (58). However, most of the Apps are not developed for adolescents, and the effectiveness of these interventions is not yet evaluated (58).

Current and future media use

There is popular and scholarly consensus that today's adolescents, in particular, have widely adopted the use of digital media for daily life activities (58). Thus, to have an impact on daily activities of adolescents, digital media could be used. Indeed, apart from the potentially unfavorable role of mass media toward eating behavior in children and adolescents, there is also growing evidence that media can be used to prevent unhealthy behavior or to encourage or support positive changes in health behaviors (66). To create a supportive environment against obesity, policy with respect to control of unhealthy advertisement is needed along with promotion of health education.

Policymakers, employers, insurance companies, researchers, and health care providers have developed an increasing interest in using principles from behavioral economics and psychology to persuade people to change their health-related behaviors, lifestyles, and habits (67). For instance, subtle techniques have been developed to "nudge" people toward particular decisions or behaviors. Thoughtful "choice architecture" can be established to nudge adolescents to choose what is best for themselves without restricting freedom of choice (68). An example of a nudge is the development of piano stairs that make music when climbing the stairs as an alternative to using moving staircases (69). Another nudge is the tough image that was chosen for Coca-Cola Zero to tempt youth to drink this light drink instead of the calorie-dense cola. Thus, commercial techniques that have been shown to be successful to promote unhealthy products in children and adolescents can also be used to promote healthy behavior. The new media offer the opportunity to nudge children and adolescents towards healthy eating behavior and physical activity.

A new challenge is also to develop Apps to help adolescents to translate intentions in implementation intentions or action plans specifying where, with whom, and at what time, what particular health behavior will be performed. Such action plans contribute to really acting on one's intentions (70, 71). In complex behavior, it is also important to specify why a habitual, unhealthy response should be replaced with an alternative healthy response in a critical situation. In a study of the efficacy of implementation intentions to replace unhealthy snacks with healthy snacks, by linking different types of cues for unhealthy snacking (if-part) to healthy snacking (then-part), implementation intentions specifying motivational (why) cues decreased unhealthy snack consumption whereas the classic specification of where and when did not (72).

Media and social interaction

Thus, media play a role in the meso- and macro environment of adolescents both as a threat and an opportunity to influence health behavior. The popularity amongst adolescents of social media such as Facebook is most easily understood in the light of social processes. Social media offer the possibility to connect to friends in an easy way, and to be together with friends almost all the time. Presence with friends is very important in weight-related behavior (73). The potential of social media in the intervention or prevention of weight-related behavior (eating and exercise), has not yet been subject of study. For alcohol consumption in adolescents, more research results are available. Social norms and adolescents' beliefs about their friends' alcohol consumption are important determinants of alcohol consumption (74). Profiles and pictures showing alcohol drinking peers influence the attitudes towards alcohol use in friends on Facebook (75). Likewise, it can be expected that social interaction on Facebook can influence other more or less harmful health behavior. Knowing that peer influence and social media play an important role in health (including weight-related) behavior is a first step in prevention and intervention. The next, most difficult step is to offering solutions or opportunities to use these networks to promote health.

A future area of research and intervention for health care workers is to use social networks in order to influence the health behavior of adolescents. Apart from Facebook, there are many other local social network media. An example of patient social networks is Patients Like Me. These networks offer an opportunity to give health messages and to integrate patient-healthcare interaction within more general social networks. One of the problems of web users is the effort it takes to manage different sources (that is, to have profiles and to keep records), if one is using different social media. Recently, this problem has been addressed for patients, resulting in easier communication between patients and physicians (76). Future research should evaluate the benefits of social networks and effort should be put in linking up and translating lifestyle sites to popular social networks.

CONCLUSION

The global epidemic of overweight and obesity results from individual factors and from meso- and macro environmental factors. Adolescents are especially vulnerable to unhealthy changes in life style. One major influence on health behavior in this age group is represented by friends in peer groups. Young people tend to select and mimic each other with respect to both eating behavior and physical exercise. Peer groups are a close and important source of influence on health behavior and social media strengthen this influence. New research and interventions should take account of the influence of the peer group and social media.

REFERENCES

[1]   Wadden TA, Stunkard AJ. Handbook of obesity treatment. New York: Guilford, 2004.
[2]   Ogden CL, Carroll MD, Kit BK, Flegal KM. Prevalence of obesity and trends in body mass index among US children and adolescents, 1999-2010. JAMA 2012;307(5):483-90.
[3]   Whittle CR, Yarnell JW, Stevenson M, McCay N, Gaffney BP, Shields MD, et al. Is dieting behaviour decreasing in young adolescents? Public Health Nutr 2011, Available on CJO2011 doi:10.1017/S1368980011002965.
[4]   Eaton DK, Kann L, Kinchen S, Shanklin S, Flint KH, Hawkins J, et al. Youth risk behavior surveillance - United States, 2011. MMWR Surveill Summ 2012;61(4):1-162.
[5]   Larson NI, Neumark-Sztainer DR, Story MT, Wall MM, Harnack LJ, Eisenberg ME. Fast food intake: longitudinal trends during the transition to young adulthood and correlates of intake. J Adolesc Health 2008;43(1):79-86.
[6]   Neumark-Sztainer D, Wall M, Guo J, Story M, Haines J, Eisenberg M. Obesity, disordered eating, and eating disorders in a longitudinal study of adolescents: how do dieters fare 5 years later? J Am Diet Assoc 2006;106(4):559-68.
[7]   Coleman JC. Friendship and the peer group in adolescence. New York: Wiley, 1980.
[8]   Bandura A. Social foundations of thought and action: a social cognitive theory. Englewood Cliffs, NJ, US: Prentice Hall, 1986.
[9]   Gritz ER, Prokhorov AV, Hudmon KS, Mullin Jones M, Rosenblum C, Chang CC, et al. Predictors of susceptibility to smoking and ever smoking: a longitudinal study in a triethnic sample of adolescents. Nicotine Tob Res 2003;5(4):493-506.
[10]   Urberg KA, Degirmencioglu SM, Pilgrim C. Close friend and group influence on adolescent cigarette smoking and alcohol use. Dev Psychol 1997;33(5):834-44.
[11]   Urberg KA, Luo Q, Pilgrim C, Degirmencioglu SM. A two-stage model of peer influence in adolescent substance use: individual and relationship-specific differences in susceptibility to influence. Addict Behav 2003;28(7):1243-56.
[12]   Zalta AK, Keel PK. Peer influence on bulimic symptoms in college students. J Abnorm Psychol 2006;115(1):185-9.
[13]   Bell C, Cooper MJ. Socio-cultural and cognitive predictors of eating disorder symptoms in young girls. Eat Weight Disord 2005;10(4):e97-e100.
[14]   Christakis NA, Fowler JH. The spread of obesity in a large social network over 32 years. N Engl J Med 2007;357(4):370-9.

[15] Ali MM, Amialchuk A, Heiland FW. Weight-related behavior among adolescents: the role of peer effects. PloS One 2011;6(6):e21179.

[16] Wouters EJ, Larsen JK, Kremers SP, Dagnelie PC, Geenen R. Peer influence on snacking behavior in adolescence. Appetite 2010;55(1):11-7.

[17] Savige G, Macfarlane A, Ball K, Worsley A, Crawford D. Snacking behaviours of adolescents and their association with skipping meals. Int J Behav Nutr Phys Act 2007;4:36.

[18] Bibeau WS, Saksvig BI, Gittelsohn J, Williams S, Jones L, Young DR. Perceptions of the food marketing environment among African American teen girls and adults. Appetite 2012;58(1):396-9.

[19] O'Connor DB, Conner M, Jones F, McMillan B, Ferguson E. Exploring the benefits of conscientiousness: an investigation of the role of daily stressors and health behaviors. Ann Behav Med 2009;37(2):184-96.

[20] Churchill S, Jessop DC. Reflective and non-reflective antecedents of health-related behaviour: exploring the relative contributions of impulsivity and implicit self-control to the prediction of dietary behaviour. Br J Health Psychol 2011;16(2):257-72.

[21] Schutz HK, Paxton SJ. Friendship quality, body dissatisfaction, dieting and disordered eating in adolescent girls. Br J Clin Psychol 2007;46(1):67-83.

[22] Hutchinson DM, Rapee RM. Do friends share similar body image and eating problems? The role of social networks and peer influences in early adolescence. Behav Res Ther 2007;45(7):1557-77.

[23] Thompson JK, Shroff H, Herbozo S, Cafri G, Rodriguez J, Rodriguez M. Relations among multiple peer influences, body dissatisfaction, eating disturbance, and self-esteem: a comparison of average weight, at risk of overweight, and overweight adolescent girls. J Pediatr Psychol 2007;32(1):24-9.

[24] Story M, Neumark-Sztainer D, French S. Individual and environmental influences on adolescent eating behaviors. J Am Diet Assoc 2002;102(3 Suppl):S40-51.

[25] Verstraeten R, Roberfroid D, Lachat C, Leroy JL, Holdsworth M, Maes L, et al. Effectiveness of preventive school-based obesity interventions in low- and middle-income countries: a systematic review. Am J Clin Nutr 2012;96(2):415-38.

[26] Fletcher A, Bonell C, Sorhaindo A. You are what your friends eat: systematic review of social network analyses of young people's eating behaviours and bodyweight. J Epidemiol Community Health 2011;65(6):548-55.

[27] Catenacci VA, Wyatt HR. The role of physical activity in producing and maintaining weight loss. Nat Clin Pract Endocrinol Metab 2007;3(7):518-29.

[28] Ross R, Janssen I, Dawson J, Kungl AM, Kuk JL, Wong SL, et al. Exercise-induced reduction in obesity and insulin resistance in women: a randomized controlled trial. Obes Res 2004;12(5):789-98.

[29] Villanova N, Pasqui F, Burzacchini S, Forlani G, Manini R, Suppini A, et al. A physical activity program to reinforce weight maintenance following a behavior program in overweight/obese subjects. Int J Obes (Lond) 2006;30(4):697-703.

[30] Annesi JJ, Whitaker AC. Weight loss and psychologic gain in obese women-participants in a supported exercise intervention. Perm J 2008;12(3):36-45.

[31] Mathus-Vliegen EM, Basdevant A, Finer N, Hainer V, Hauner H, Micic D, et al. Prevalence, pathophysiology, health consequences and treatment options of obesity in the elderly: a guideline. Obes Facts 2012;5(3):460-83.

[32] Taylor CB, Sallis JF, Needle R. The relation of physical activity and exercise to mental health. Public Health Rep 1985;100(2):195-202.

[33] Khan KM, Thompson AM, Blair SN, Sallis JF, Powell KE, Bull FC, et al. Sport and exercise as contributors to the health of nations. Lancet 2012;380(9836):59-64.

[34] Skender ML, Goodrick GK, Del Junco DJ, Reeves RS, Darnell L, Gotto AM, et al. Comparison of 2-year weight loss trends in behavioral treatments of obesity: diet, exercise, and combination interventions. J Am Diet Assoc1996;96(4):342-6.

[35] Biddle SJ, Asare M. Physical activity and mental health in children and adolescents: a review of reviews. Br J Sports Med 2011;45(11):886-95.

[36] Tremblay MS, LeBlanc AG, Kho ME, Saunders TJ, Larouche R, Colley RC, et al. Systematic review of sedentary behaviour and health indicators in school-aged children and youth. Int J Behav Nutr Phys Act 2011;8:98.

[37] Rasberry CN, Lee SM, Robin L, Laris BA, Russell LA, Coyle KK, et al. The association between school-based physical activity, including physical education, and academic performance: a systematic review of the literature. Prev Med 2011;52 Suppl 1:S10-20.

[38] Duncan SC, Duncan TE, Strycker LA, Chaumeton NR. A cohort-sequential latent growth model of physical activity from ages 12 to 17 years. Ann Behav Med 2007;33(1):80-9..

[39] Kimm SY, Glynn NW, Kriska AM, Fitzgerald SL, Aaron DJ, Similo SL, et al. Longitudinal changes in physical activity in a biracial cohort during adolescence. Med Sci Sports Exerc 2000;32(8):1445-54.

[40] Chung AE, Skinner AC, Steiner MJ, Perrin EM. Physical activity and BMI in a nationally representative sample of children and adolescents. Clin Pediatr (Phila) 2012;51(2):122-9.

[41] Slater A, Tiggemann M. Gender differences in adolescent sport participation, teasing, self-objectification and body image concerns. J Adolesc 2011;34(3):455-63.

[42] Veselska Z, Madarasova Geckova A, Reijneveld SA, van Dijk JP. Socio-economic status and physical activity among adolescents: the mediating role of self-esteem. Public Health 2011;125(11):763-8.

[43] Frisen A, Bjarnelind S. Health-related quality of life and bullying in adolescence. Acta Paediatr 2010;99(4):597-603.

[44] Heath GW, Parra DC, Sarmiento OL, Andersen LB, Owen N, Goenka S, et al. Evidence-based intervention in physical activity: lessons from around the world. Lancet 2012;380(9838):272-81.

[45] Gordon-Larsen P, Nelson MC, Page P, Popkin BM. Inequality in the built environment underlies key health disparities in physical activity and obesity. Pediatrics 2006;117(2):417-24.

[46] Cohen DA, Ashwood JS, Scott MM, Overton A, Evenson KR, Staten LK, et al. Public parks and physical activity among adolescent girls. Pediatrics 2006;118(5):e1381-9.

[47] de la Haye K, Robins G, Mohr P, Wilson C. How physical activity shapes, and is shaped by, adolescent friendships. Soc Sci Med. 2011;73(5):719-28.

[48] Kahn JA, Huang B, Gillman MW, Field AE, Austin SB, Colditz GA, et al. Patterns and determinants of physical activity in U.S. adolescents. J Adolesc Health 2008;42(4):369-77.

[49] Garcia AW, Pender NJ, Antonakos CL, Ronis DL. Changes in physical activity beliefs and behaviors of boys and girls across the transition to junior high school. J Adolesc Health 1998;22(5):394-402.

[50] Facebook statistics 2012 Accessed Aug 29 2012 URL: http://www.socialbakers.com/countries/continents.

[51] Schmidt ME, Anderson DR. The impact of television on cognitive development and educational achievement. N. Pecora JPM, E.A. Wartella, editor. Mahaw (NJ): Lawrence Erlbaum Associates, 2006.

[52] Boyland EJ, Harrold JA, Kirkham TC, Corker C, Cuddy J, Evans D, et al. Food commercials increase preference for energy-dense foods, particularly in children who watch more television. Pediatrics 2011;128(1):e93-100.

[53] Chernin A. Overweight and obesity in America's children: causes, consequences, solutions: section two: media and culture: The effects of food marketing on children's preferences: testing the moderating roles of age and gender. Ann Am Acad Pol Soc Sci 2008;615:102-18.

[54] Harris JL, Pomeranz JL, Lobstein T, Brownell KD. A crisis in the marketplace: how food marketing contributes to childhood obesity and what can be done. Annu Rev Public Health 2009;30:211-25.

[55] Jones SC, Mannino N, Green J. 'Like me, want me, buy me, eat me': relationship-building marketing communications in children's magazines. Public Health Nutr 2010;13(12):2111-8.

[56] Ben-Sefer E, Ben-Natan M, Ehrenfeld M. Childhood obesity: current literature, policy and implications for practice. Int Nurs Rev 2009;56(2):166-73.

[57] Strasburger VC. Children, adolescents, obesity, and the media. Pediatrics 2011;128(1):201-8.

[58] Vandewater EA, Denis LM. Media, social networking and pediatric obesity. Pediatr Clin North Am 2011;58:1509-19.

[59] Marshall SJ, Biddle SJ, Gorely T, Cameron N, Murdey I. Relationships between media use, body fatness and physical activity in children and youth: a meta-analysis. Int J Obes Relat Metab Disord 2004;28(10):1238-46.

[60] Krebs NF, Jacobson MS. Prevention of pediatric overweight and obesity. Pediatrics 2003;112(2):424-30.

[61]   Lyons EJ, Tate DF, Komoski SE, Carr PM, Ward DS. Novel approaches to obesity prevention: effects of game enjoyment and game type on energy expenditure in active video games. Diabetes Sci Technol 2012;6(4):839-48.

[62]   Staiano AE, Abraham AA, Calvert SL. Motivating effects of cooperative exergame play for overweight and obese adolescents. J Diabetes Sci Technol 2012;6(4):812-9.

[63]   Staiano AE, Abraham AA, Calvert SL. Adolescent Exergame Play for Weight Loss and Psychosocial Improvement: A Controlled Physical Activity Intervention. Obesity (Silver Spring) 2012, doi: 10.1038/oby.2012.143.

[64]   Staiano AE, Abraham AA, Calvert SL. Competitive versus cooperative exergame play for African American adolescents' executive function skills: short-term effects in a long-term training intervention. Dev Psychol 2012;48(2):337-42.

[65]   Johnston JD, Massey AP, Marker-Hoffman RL. Using an alternate reality game to increase physical activity and decrease obesity risk of college students. J Diabetes Sci Technol 2012;6(4):828-38.

[66]   Wakefield MA, Loken B, Hornik RC. Use of mass media campaigns to change health behaviour. Lancet 2010;376(9748):1261-71.

[67]   Blumenthal-Barby JS, Burroughs H. Seeking better health care outcomes: the ethics of using the "nudge". Am J Bioeth 2012;12(2):1-10.

[68]   Thaler RH, Sunstein CR. Nudge: Improving decisions about health, wealth, and happiness. New York: Penguin Books, 2009.

[69]   TheFunTheory.com. Piano stairs 2009. Accessed Sept 7 2012. URL: http://www.youtube.com/watch?v=2lXh2n0aPyw.

[70]   Gollwitzer PM. Implementation intentions: Strong effects of simple plans. Am Psychol 1999;54:493-503.

[71]   Hommel B, Musseler J, Aschersleben G, Prinz W. The Theory of Event Coding (TEC): a framework for perception and action planning. Behav Brain Sci 2001;24(5):849-78; discussion 78-937.

[72]   Adriaanse MA, de Ridder DT, de Wit JB. Finding the critical cue: implementation intentions to change one's diet work best when tailored to personally relevant reasons for unhealthy eating. Pers Soc Psychol Bull 2009;35(1):60-71.

[73]   Salvy SJ, Roemmich JN, Bowker JC, Romero ND, Stadler PJ, Epstein LH. Effect of peers and friends on youth physical activity and motivation to be physically active. J Pediatr Psychol 2009;34(2):217-25.

[74]   Lewis MA, Neighbors C. Social norms approaches using descriptive drinking norms education: a review of the research on personalized normative feedback. J Am Coll Health 2006;54(4):213-8.

[75]   Litt DM, Stock ML. Adolescent alcohol-related risk cognitions: the roles of social norms and social networking sites. Psychol Addict Behav 2011;25(4):708-13.

[76]   Sahama T, Liang J, Iannella R. Impact of the social networking applications for health information management for patients and physicians. Stud Health Technol Inform 2012;180:803-7.

In: Food, Nutrition and Eating Behavior
Editors: Joav Merrick and Sigal Israeli

ISBN: 978-1-62948-233-0
© 2014 Nova Science Publishers, Inc.

Chapter 14

HYPERINSULINEMIA AND OVARIAN HYPERANDROGENEMIA AMONG PRE-PUBERTAL AND EARLY PUBERTAL OBESE GIRLS

Rasha T Hamza, MD*, Sherine M Abdel-Fattah, MD, Ahmed S Abdel-Aziz, MA and Amira I Hamed, MD

Departments of Pediatrics and Clinical Pathology, Faculty of Medicine,
Ain Shams University, Cairo, Egypt

ABSTRACT

There are very few data on hyperandrogenemia (HA) in early puberty in obese girls, a critical time when the complex interactions among the hypothalamus, pituitary and ovary are being developed. Also, hyperinsulinemia (HI) was suggested to augment ovarian androgen production via its actions as a co-gonadotropin with luteinizing hormone (LH). In this chapter we explore the hypothesis that pre-pubertal and early pubertal obesity is associated with HA and HI and to relate the degree of HA & HI to body mass index (BMI). Methods: Fifty obese patients were compared to 50 age-, sex- and pubertal stage-matched controls regarding history, anthropometric measurements, Tanner staging and morning fasting serum total testosterone, insulin and LH. Results: Serum testosterone and insulin were significantly higher in cases than controls (3.14 ± 0.88 vs 0.18 ± 0.60 ng/ml and 20.9 ± 4.7 vs 8.17 ± 1.10 µU/ml respectively, $p=0.001$) and in early pubertal than pre-pubertal cases (3.40 ± 86 vs 1.8 ± 0.4ng/ml, $p=0.029$ and 19.20 ± 5.10 vs 12.3 ± 0.7µU/ml, $p=0.031$, respectively) with 40% and 50% of cases having HA and HI respectively. Also, both testosterone and insulin correlated positively with BMI standard deviation score (SDS) in pre-pubertal ($r=+0.88$ and $+0.81$ respectively, $p<0.0001$) and early pubertal cases ($r=+0.97$ and $+0.92$ respectively, $p<0.0001$) and with each other ($r=+0.86$, $p<0.0001$). There is an association between obesity and each of HA and HI among pre-pubertal and early pubertal obese girls, and both correlate positively with BMI. Further studies are warranted regarding the interaction between obesity-HA-HI triad.

---

* Correspondence: Professor Rasha Tarif Hamza, MD, 36 Hisham Labib street, off Makram Ebeid street, Nasr City, 11371 Cairo, Egypt. E- mail: rashatarif_2000@hotmail.com.

INTRODUCTION

Excess bodyweight is the sixth most important risk factor contributing to the overall burden of disease worldwide. About 1.1 billion adults and 10% of children are now classified as overweight or obese. Although the prevalence of childhood obesity has now reached epidemic proportions, it was under recognized and under treated by pediatric primary care providers (1).

Previous studies have suggested an association between adiposity and elevated androgens in late pubertal girls. However, there are very few data on early puberty, a critical time when the complex interactions among the hypothalamus, pituitary and ovary are being developed. Moreover, confirmatory data are unavailable, and it remains unclear what mechanisms underlie this relationship in peripubertal girls (2). A British study found 33% of obese children and adolescents of different ethnicities to have evidence of insulin resistance syndrome (IRS) as defined by 3 or more of: obesity, abnormal glucose homoeostasis, dyslipidemia, and hypertension (3). Hyperinsulinemia (HI) was suggested to enhance androgen production in adult women with or without polycystic ovary syndrome (PCOS) since HI augments ovarian androgen production via its actions as a co-gonadotropin with luteinizing hormone (LH) (2).

With this background, we were stimulated to explore the hypothesis that pre-pubertal and early pubertal obesity is associated with hyperandrogenemia (HA) and HI and to relate the degree of HA & HI to BMI.

OUR STUDY

This cross sectional case-control study was conducted on 50 female children and adolescents with simple obesity (BMI of ≥97th centile) diagnosed according to the reference ranges of Sempe, 1991 (4). Patients were recruited from the Pediatric Outpatient Clinic, Children`s Hospital, Faculty of Medicine, Ain Shams University, Cairo, Egypt during the period from the beginning of May 2008 till the end of August 2009. Their ages ranged between 7 and 14 years with a mean age of 10.2±1.9 years. Obese patients were further subdivided into two groups according to their Tanner pubertal stage: pre-pubertal group (20 girls in Tanner stage I) and early pubertal group (30 girls of whom 20 were in Tanner stage II and 10 were in Tanner stage III). Obese girls due to causes other than simple obesity (e.g., syndromic obesity) were excluded from the study.

Obese girls were studied in comparison to 50 healthy age-, sex-, and pubertal stage-matched girls serving as controls. Their ages ranged between 7 and 13.5 years with a mean age of 10.8±1.4 years. The latter had average BMI`s and BMI SDS`s according to normal age- and sex- specific reference ranges (4, 5). They were also subdivided into two groups according to their Tanner pubertal stage: pre-pubertal group (22 girls in Tanner stage I) and early pubertal group (28 girls of whom 16 were in Tanner stage II and 12 were in Tanner stage III).

None of the participants were taking medications known to affect the reproductive axis or body weight, and none had used hormonal medications for 90 days prior to study. Also, none of them had any chronic systemic illness or endocrine disorder that could lead to obesity or HA or could affect pubertal development. All studied children were subjected to:

1) Medical history laying stress on menstrual irregularities where subjects were considered to have irregular menses if they were at least 2 years post menarche and had an average inter-menstrual length of more than 45 days (6).
2) Physical examination with special emphasis on:
   - Measurement of weight and height. Standard deviation scores (SDS`s) of weight for height and height for age were calculated according to the norms of Sempe et al. (7).
   - BMI was calculated using the formula: weight (in kg)/height2 (in meters). Obesity was defined if the BMI was above the 97th percentile (4). SDS of BMI was calculated from the age- and sex- specific reference values (5).
   - Tanner pubertal breast staging according to Marshall and Tanner (8). Both palpation and observation of breasts were employed by a single examiner at each time point (to differentiate glandular from fatty tissue).
   - Hirsutism which was defined by the presence of excessive body hair
   - distributed in an androgen-dependent pattern (9) with a modified Ferriman-Gallwey score of 8 or more (10).
3) Hormonal measurements:
   - Sample: 5 ml of blood were withdrawn from each patient in the morning (between 8:00 – 10:00 am) after 8 hours fasting then separated in aliquots and stored at -70 degrees Celcius until assayed.
   - Morning fasting total testosterone was assayed with the chemiluminescent immunometric assay using the Immulite 2000 apparatus (11). Kits of assay were manufactured by DRG International with a detection limit of 0.083 ng/ml. Reference age-, sex- and pubertal stage- matched values ranged between 0.10 to 1.22 ng/ml. Serum total testosterone concentrations above the 95th percentile of the age-, sex- and pubertal stage- matched group of healthy girls defined biochemical HA.
   - Morning fasting serum insulin was measured with the chemiluminescent immunometric assay using the Immulite 2000 apparatus (11). Kits of assay were manufactured by BioSource Company with a detection limit of 0.15 µIU/ml. Reference age- and sex- matched values ranged between 5 to 19 µIU/ml. HI was defined as a fasting insulin of ≥20 µIU/ml.
   - Morning fasting serum LH was measured with the chemiluminescent immunometric assay based on direct sandwich technique using the Immulite 2000 apparatus using commercial kits (Diagnostic Products Corp-Med lab, Los Angeles, CA) [11]. The detection limit of kits is 0.8 µIU/ml. Reference age- and sex- matched values in girls up to 10 years ranged between 0.08 to 3.9 µIU/ml, in follicular phase: 0.5 to 10.5ml µIU/ml and in midcycle: 18.4 to 61 µIU/ml.

The results were analyzed using the Statistical Package for the Social Science (SPSS) version number 10, Echosoft corp; USA, 2005. Description of quantitative variables was in the form of mean±standard deviation and range while that of qualitative variables was in the form of frequency and percentage. Student's t-test of 2 independent samples was used to compare 2 quantitative variables in parametric data while Mann Whitney test was used instead of students t-test in non parametric data. Spearman correlation coefficient test was used to rank different variables against each other either directly or indirectly. A p value of <0.05 was considered significant.

FINDINGS

Obese patients had significantly higher anthropometric measurements (weight, height, BMI, and their SDS`s), serum total testosterone and serum insulin than controls with a non significant difference between the 2 groups regarding serum LH (see table 1).

Table 1. Clinical and laboratory data among studied cases and controls

Variable	Cases (n= 50)	Controls (n=50)	t/z#	p
Age (years)	10.2 ± 1.9 (7 – 14)	10.8 ± 1.4 (7 – 13.5)	1.30	0.52
Weight (kg)	64.6 ± 13 (45-80)	40.8±5.4 (28-48)	6.92	0.01*
Weight SDS	+3.12 ± +0.2 (+2.9 to +4.4)	+0.25± +0.96 (+0.03 to +1.29)	6.21#	0.020*
Height (cm)	145.5 ± 4.6 (129 – 152)	135.7 ± 1.77 (125 – 145)	4.64	0.040*
Height SDS	+3.04 ± +2.1 (-0.6 to +4.0)	+1.20 ± +0.58 (-0.06 to +1.88)	3.12#	0.041*
BMI (kg/m^2)	31.1 ± 3.6 (26 – 41)	19.4 ± 1.77 (16 – 22)	7.50	0.001**
BMI SDS	+3.94 ± +0.68 (+3.2 to +5.8)	+0.92 ± +0.52 (+0.30 to +1.60)	10.41#	0.0001***
Serum L.H (mIU/ml)	4.7 ± 2.4 (1.5 – 17.3)	4.1 ± 2.9 (1.0 -22.0)	1.55	0.41
Serum total testosterone (ng/ml)	3.14 ± 0.88 (1.4 – 5.9)	0.18 ± 0.60 (0.44 – 1.4)	7.74	0.001**
Serum insulin (µU/ml)	20.9 ± 4.7 (11.2 – 29.4)	8.17 ± 1.10 (3.10 – 16.8)	8.26	0.001**

Results are expressed as mean± SD and range, *p<0.05, **P<0.01, ***P<0.001.
SDS: standard deviation score, BMI: Body mass index, LH: Luteinizing hormone.

Table 2. Anthropometric measurements and laboratory data among pre-pubertal cases and controls

Variable	Pre-pubertal cases (n= 20)	Pre-pubertal controls (n=22)	t/z#	p
Weight (kg)	54.4 ± 5.7 (45 – 63)	32.2 ± 3.2 (28 – 38)	7.20	0.004**
Weight SDS	+3.10 ± +0.1 (+2.9 to +3.2)	+0.19 ± +0.52 (+0.03 to +1.0)	6.30#	0.031*
Height (cm)	135.4 ± 5.4 (129 – 148)	128.1 ± 1.20 (125 - 135)	3.30	0.040*
Height SDS	+2.7 ± +0.2 (-0.6 to +3.0)	+0.92 ± +0.21 (-0.06 to +1.18)	5.31#	0.035*
BMI (kg/m^2)	29.4 ± 3.2 (26 – 33.5)	18.30 ± 1.52 (16 – 21)	8.51	0.001**
BMI SDS	+ 3.7 ± +0.1 (+3.20 to +3.9)	+1.19 ± +0.25 (+0.30 to +1.46)	6.11#	0.035*
Serum L.H (mIU/ml)	3.3 ± 1.7 (1.5 – 8.0)	2.8 ± 1.7 (1.0 – 6.0)	1.20	0.59
Serum total testosterone (ng/ml)	1.8 ± 0.4 (1.4 – 3.9)	0.11 ± 0.65 (0.44 – 1.1)	3.76	0.047*
Serum insulin (μU/ml)	12.3 ± 0.7 (11.20 – 19.80)	4.0 ± 0.3 (3.10 – 11.81)	6.85	0.038*

Results are expressed as mean± SD and range, *p<0.05, **P<0.01, ***P<0.001.
SDS: standard deviation score, BMI: Body mass index, LH: Luteinizing hormone.

All anthropometric measurements, serum total testosterone and insulin were significantly higher among pre-pubertal cases than controls with a non significant difference between the 2 groups regarding serum LH (see table 2).

All anthropometric measures, serum total testosterone and insulin were significantly higher among early pubertal cases than controls with a non significant difference between the 2 groups regarding serum LH (see table 3).

All anthropometric measures and laboratory parameters were significantly higher among early pubertal than pre-pubertal obese cases (see table 4).

Frequency of menstrual irregularities and/or hirsutism among obese cases: Of the 50 studied cases, 3(6%) had menstrual irregularities, and 2 (4%) had hirsutism and only 1 case (2%) had both complaints. All cases of menstrual irregularities and hirsutism were observed in the early pubertal group.

Frequency of HA and HI among obese cases: Of the 50 studied cases, 20(40%) had HA [among whom 6(30%) were pre-pubertal and 14(70%) were early pubertal]; while 25(50%) had HI [among whom 7(28%) were pre-pubertal and 18(72%) were early pubertal].

Table 3. Anthropometric measurements and laboratory data among early pubertal cases and controls

Variable	Early pubertal cases (n= 30)	Early pubertal controls (n=28)	t/z#	p
Weight (kg)	72.10 ± 8.0 (64 – 80)	38.20 ± 1.6 (35 – 48)	11.10	0.0001***
Weight SDS	+3.98 ± +0.01 (+3.5 to +4.4)	+0.48 ± +0.20 (+0.21 to +1.29)	6.90#	0.039*
Height (cm)	148.10 ± 5.5 (142.5 – 152)	139.9 ± 0.66 (136.5 -145)	4.11	0.038*
Height SDS	+3.7 ± +2.6 (+1.9 to +4.0)	+1.42 ± +0.38 (+0.15 to +1.88)	5.23#	0.030*
BMI (kg/m^2)	36.5 ± 3.1 (28.8 – 41.0)	19.43 ± 0.81 (16.8 – 22.0)	6.46	0.035*
BMI SDS	+4.85 ± +0.5 (+3.35 to +5.8)	+1.32 ± +0.21 (+0.90 to +1.60)	5.45#	0.0035**
Serum L.H (mIU/ml)	10.1 ± 4.2 (5.4 – 17.3)	8.7 ±1.3 (6.4 – 22)	1.80	0.36
Serum total testosterone (ng/ml)	3.4 ± 0.86 (2.3 – 5.90)	0.82 ± 0.16 (0.25 – 1.40)	7.23	0.001**
Serum insulin (μU/ml)	19.20 ± 5.10 (13.5 – 29.4)	4.2 ± 0.1 (3.9 – 16.8)	9.87	0.0001**

Results are expressed as mean± SD and range, *p<0.05, **P<0.01, ***P<0.001,
SDS: standard deviation score, BMI: Body mass index, LH: Luteinizing hormone.

Relation between Tanner breast staging and each of age, anthropometric measurements and hormonal profile among obese cases: Among studied cases, there were significant positive correlations between Tanner breast staging and each of age (r=+0.60, p=0.045), weight (r=+0.65, p=0.041), weight for height SDS (r=+0.68, p=0.01), height (r=+0.62,p=0.046), height for age SDS (r=+0.69, p=0.01), BMI (r=+0.69, p=0.01), BMI SDS (r=0.75, p=0.001), serum total testosterone (r=+0.893, p<0.0001), serum insulin (r=+0.51, p=0.048) and serum LH (r=+0.65, p=0.041).

Correlations between different hormonal parameters among obese cases:

Among studied cases, there were significant positive correlations between serum total testosterone and each of fasting serum insulin (r=+0.86, p<0.0001) and serum LH (r=+0.82, p<0.0001).

Correlation between hormonal profile and anthropometric measurements among obese cases: Among pre-pubertal cases, serum total testosterone correlated positively with each of weight (r=+0.61, p=0.046), weight for height SDS (r=+0.56, p=0.041), BMI (r=+0.78, p=0.001), BMI SDS (r=+0.88, p<0.0001, figure 1) with a non significant correlation with each of height (r=+0.88, p=0.96) and height for age SDS (r=+0.12, p=0.59). Similarly, serum insulin correlated positively with each of weight (r=+0.69, p<0.01), weight for height SDS (r=+0.40, p=0.05), BMI (r=+0.85, p<0.0001), BMI SDS (r=+0.81, p<0.0001) with a non significant correlation with each of height (r=+0.04, p=0.79) and height for age SDS (r=+0.01, p=0.88). On the other hand, there were non significant correlations between serum LH and all anthropometric measurements (p>0.05).

Table 4. Anthropometric measurements and laboratory data among pre-pubertal versus early pubertal cases

Variable	Pre-pubertal cases (n= 20)	Early pubertal cases (n=30)	t/z#	p
Weight (kg)	54.4 ± 5.7 (45 – 63)	72.10 ± 8.0 (64 – 80)	6.44	0.012*
Weight SDS	+3.10 ± +0.1 (+2.9 to +3.2)	+3.98 ± +0.01 (+3.5 to +4.4)	3.29#	0.049*
Height (cm)	135.4 ± 5.4 (129 – 148)	148.10 ± 5.5 (142.5 – 152)	4.52	0.039*
Height SDS	+2.7 ± +0.2 (-0.6 to +3.0)	+3.7 ± +2.6 (+1.9 to +4.0)	3.25#	0.045*
BMI (kg/m^2)	29.4 ± 3.2 (26 – 33.5)	36.5 ± 3.1 (28.8 – 41.0)	3.53	0.047*
BMI SDS	+ 3.7 ± +0.1 (+3.20 to +3.9)	+4.85 ± +0.5 (+3.35 to +5.8)	3.23#	0.041*
Serum L.H (mIU/ml)	3.3 ± 1.7 (1.5 – 8.0)	10.1 ± 4.2 (5.4 – 17.3)	7.41	0.001**
Serum total testosterone (ng/ml)	1.8 ± 0.4 (1.4 – 3.9)	3.4 ± 0.86 (2.3 – 5.90)	5.73	0.029*
Serum insulin (μU/ml)	12.3 ± 0.7 (11.20 – 19.80)	19.20 ± 5.10 (13.5 – 29.4)	4.92	0.031*

Results are expressed as mean± SD and range, *p<0.05, **P<0.01, ***P<0.001.
SDS: standard deviation score, BMI: Body mass index, LH: Luteinizing hormone.

Among early pubertal cases, serum total testosterone correlated positively with each of weight (+0.64, p=0.043), weight for height SDS (r=+0.67, p=0.042), BMI (r=+0.87, p<0.0001), BMI SDS (r=+0.97, p<0.0001), height (r=+0.62, p=0.047) and height SDS (r=+0.67, p=0.042). Serum insulin correlated positively with each of weight (r=+0.76, p=0.01), weight for height SDS (r=+0.70, p=0.01), BMI (r=+0.85, p<0.0001) and BMI SDS (r=+0.92, p<0.0001) with non significant correlations with each of height (r=+0.18, p=0.62) and height SDS (r=+0.31, p=0.62).Similarly, serum LH correlated positively with each of weight (r=+0.67, p=0.045), weight for height SDS (r=+0.51, p=0.05), BMI (r=+0.59, p=0.05) and BMI SDS (r=+0.61, p=0.04) with non significant correlations with each of height (r=+0.16, p=0.52) and height SDS (r=+0.13, p=0.41).

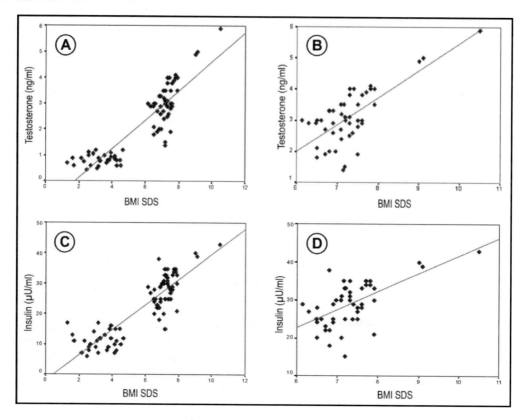

Figure 1. Correlations between BMI SDS and each of serum total testosterone in prepubertal (figure 1A) and early pubertal cases (figure 1B); and serum insulin in prepubertal (figure 1C) and early pubertal cases (figure 1D).

DISCUSSION

Our study revealed significantly higher anthropometric measurements among obese girls than normal-weight ones which was supported by another study. Obesity is associated with earlier sexual maturation among adolescent girls and young female adults. In addition, some studies revealed a younger average age of pubertal onset in the overweight group compared with their normal-weight counterparts. The causal nature of this relationship remains uncertain, but it is possible that increased androgens and their enhanced aromatization to estrogens may play a role in this phenomenon. According to Frisch's well-known "critical weight (fat) hypothesis" developed in the 1970s, a certain amount or percentage of body fat is needed for the onset of menarche, i.e., heavier girls mature earlier. It was hypothesized that subcutaneous fat tissue acts as a secondary hormonal gland and adipose tissue influences the synthesis and release of hormones (e.g., estrogen), and thus promotes the onset of menarche (12). Although the causal direction of this association remains controversial, a growing body of evidence suggests that sexual maturation has a more important effect on levels of fatness than fatness does on the timing of sexual maturation. Moreover, fatness and BMI were found to be more closely correlated with maturation stage (development age) than chronological age among adolescent girls (13).

Androgen excess is the most common endocrine disorder in females during reproductive age. This is due to either an excessive androgen production by the adrenal glands and/or the ovary or increased local tissue sensitivity to circulating androgens. Androgen excess affects different tissues and organ systems, causing clinical conditions ranging from acne to hirsutism upto frank virilization (13).

Obesity is associated with HA in adult women and a similar relationship has been described in late female adolescence. There are few data on the relationship between female obesity and HA in early puberty, a critical time when the hypothalamic-pituitary-ovarian interactions governing reproduction are established across pubertal maturation (14). Obese females with HA are more prone to metabolic disturbances, such as type 2 diabetes mellitus, lipid abnormalities, and hypertension, and may therefore be at risk of developing atherosclerotic complications. In children and adolescents, a high androgenic activity is supposed to be associated with polycystic ovarian syndrome (PCOS), precocious puberty, and accelerated bone age with relative tall stature during childhood and short final height. The latter clinical features occur in obese children more frequently than in normal-weight children (15).

Our study reported significantly higher serum testosterone among obese pre-pubertal and early pubertal girls in comparison to their age-, sex- and pubertal stage- matched normal-weight girls which is consistent with the hypothesis that excessive adiposity promotes HA (12). A study conducted on obese German girls reported an association between adiposity (BMI) and serum testosterone which was similar to our results. They found the median serum testosterone concentration to be four times as great in obese pre-pubertal girls compared to normal-weight girls. This study did not evaluate potential etiological factors such as insulin or LH but interestingly suggested that testosterone decreases when obese girls lose weight (16). Also, McCartney et al. (12), found significant elevation of serum total testosterone among obese girls (either pre- or early pubertal) in comparison to normal-weight girls of the same age and pubertal stage. Similar associations between adiposity and elevated androgens were previously observed in older adolescent girls (late pubertal Tanner stages 4-5) by Wabitsch et al. (17). On the other hand, Sudi and associates (18) found a non significant difference in total testosterone between obese girls and controls. Moreover, a study of testosterone levels in pre-pubertal girls (aged 7-9 years) and very early pubertal girls (aged 10-11years) suggested that total testosterone was approximately 40-50% higher in obese girls compared with age-matched normal-weight girls but this difference was not statistically significant which might be attributed to the smaller numbers of studied cases in comparison to our study (14). Also, the current series revealed that 40% of obese girls had HA which goes with the results of Viner et al. (3) who found 50% of their obese girls to have HA.

The cause of increased androgens in obesity is still under debate. Corticotropin releasing hormone (CRH), which is activated in obesity, has been suggested recently to increase adrenal androgen secretion directly. The fat-derived hormone leptin has a specific, dose-dependent role to promote the formation of adrenal androgens by stimulating 17, 20 lyase activity of cytochrome P450. Furthermore, leptin influences the synchronization of the luteinizing hormone releasing hormone (LHRH)- pulse generator. In addition, leptin acts in concert with other growth-derived signals to regulate the onset of puberty in humans.

Longitudinal studies have revealed that leptin increases before steroid hormones are secreted and might provide the brain with information on body composition and size to start pituitary, adrenal and gonadal maturation (19). However, the exact mechanisms underlying the relationship between peripubertal obesity and ovarian HA are still unknown (12).

In addition, our series revealed a significant positive correlation between serum total testosterone and each of BMI and BMI SDS among pre-pubertal and early pubertal obese girls which was confirmed by another study (16) who reported a positive correlation between BMI and serum total testosterone in obese girls aged 4- 14 years. Thus, the current study sheds light on the fact that there might be a causal relationship (or a directionality of the cause and effect) between adiposity and androgens and that the peripubertal obesity could promote HA. This is also in keeping with other studies demonstrating reduced serum testosterone levels in adult women, pre-pubertal, early pubertal and late pubertal girls together with improvement of their menstrual disorders and hirsutism with weight loss (16).

The current study also revealed that serum total testosterone was significantly higher in early pubertal than pre-pubertal cases, with 70% of cases of HA being early pubertal. In addition, our series revealed a significant positive correlation between Tanner breast staging and serum total testosterone among obese girls which was supported by McCartney et al. [12] and Reinehr et al. (16) meaning that; serum total testosterone was elevated among early pubertal girls in comparison to the pre-pubertal cases, that is, with progress of puberty.

Moreover, our study revealed significantly higher serum insulin among obese cases than controls. Also, 50% of our obese girls had HI which was correlated with a British study that found 33% of their obese children and adolescents of different ethnicities to have IRS as defined by 3 or more of: obesity, abnormal glucose homoeostasis and an increased risk of later diabetes, dyslipidemia, and hypertension (3). Cook and collegues (20) found that the IRS was present in 28.7% of their obese adolescents (BMI ≥ 95th percentile) compared to 6.8% of at-risk adolescents (BMI ≥ 85th to < 95th percentile) and 0.1% of those with a BMI below 85th percentile. In addition, the current series revealed positive correlations between serum insulin and each of BMI and BMI SDS which was supported by another study that demonstrated that BMI and its SDS were negatively correlated with insulin sensitivity index (21). Rosen and Spiegelman (22) found that insulin resistance was positively correlated with degree of obesity (BMI) and they concluded that the obesity-associated adipocyte apoptosis appears to be the primary event underlying insulin insensitivity. The subsequent cell death associated with infiltration of macrophages appears to explain the presence of chronic inflammation. Also, the release of macrophage chemoattractant protein-1 by the adipocyte plays a role in the recruitment of macrophages and proves that the infiltrating macrophages are implicated in cytokine production (22).

On the other hand, our study revealed a non significant difference in serum LH among cases and controls with a non significant correlation between LH and anthropometric measures among cases. McCartney and associates (12), reported that serum LH level was low among obese girls either pre- or early pubertal but, normalizes as pubertal development progress and which emphasizes that LH is heterogeneous and there is no fixed role for LH among obese girls especially during pre- and early pubertal periods. Previous studies have demonstrated a negative correlation between BMI and both mean LH and LH amplitude in adults with PCOS. This may confirm the marked heterogeneity of LH concentrations across puberty (23).

In the current series a significant positive correlation was demonstrated between serum total testosterone and each of serum insulin and LH which was supported by another study (16) meaning that there is a direct link between testosterone, insulin and LH. Because there is good evidence that HI promotes ovarian androgen production in adult women (2), we hypothesize that a similar mechanism may be responsible for HA in peripubertal obese girls. This was supported by the strong positive correlation between adiposity and fasting insulin in our study. Insulin acts synergically with LH and enhances its effect which disrupts the normal pituitary stimulation of ovarian follicle development, which in turn causes ovarian theca cells to increase their testosterone production and inhibits monthly ovarian follicle development. These effects together produce the twin characteristics of PCOS: HA and anovulation. Also, the fact that insulin decreases liver production of sex hormone binding globulin (SHBG) further increases the effective androgenemia as the circulating unbound portion of testosterone rises. Additionally, treatments that reduce HI generally ameliorate HA and ovulatory dysfunction in both adult and adolescent PCOS. Thus, peripubertal obesity with accompanying HI represents an attractive etiological candidate for peripubertal HA (24).

The PCOS affects approximately 7% of reproductive-aged women and thus may be the most prevalent endocrinal disorder in women. The hallmarks of PCOS are HA and ovulatory dysfunction, but it is also associated with obesity and IRS. The pathophysiology of PCOS is complex, and its etiology remains unclear. PCOS likely has a pre- or peripubertal origin in many women, because clinical manifestations frequently have a peripubertal onset (23). In PCOS, relative insensitivity to negative feedback by progesterone is likely mediated by excess androgens because it is reversed with androgen receptor blockers. Therefore, some authors propose that, in some females, obesity may play an early role in the genesis of PCOS by contributing to increased androgen production. So, follow up of obese girls is important for early detection and treatment of such problem to avoid long term complications e.g., infertility (25).

Lastly, we conclude that there is an association between obesity and each of HA and HI among pre-pubertal and early pubertal girls, and both correlate positively with BMI. In addition, insulin and LH contribute to ovarian HA in obese peripubertal adolescents. Further studies are warranted regarding the interaction between obesity-HA-HI triad.

REFERENCES

[1]   James WP, Haslam DW. Obesity. Lancet 2005;366:1197-220.

[2]   Poretsky L, Cataldo NA, Rosenwaks Z, Giudice LC. The insulin-related ovarian regulatory system in health and disease. Endocr Rev 1999;20:535–82.

[3]   Viner RM, Segal TY, Lichtarowicz-Krynska E, Hindmarsh P. Prevalence of the insulin resistance syndrome in obesity. Arch Dis Child 2005; 90:10-4.

[4]   Sempe M. Donnees de l'etude sequentielle francaise de la croissance du Centre International de l'Enfance Rolland- Cachera et Coll. Eur J Clin Nutr 1991; 45:13-21.

[5]   Cole TJ. A chart to link child centiles of body mass index, weight and height. Eur J Clin Nutr 2002;56:11-4□9.

[6]   Mitan LAP, Slap GB. Adolescent menstrual disorders: Update. Med Clin North Am 2000;84:851.

[7]   Sempe M, Pedrong G, Roy-Pernot NP. Auxologie methods et sequences. Paris: Theraplix, 1979. [French]

[8]   Marshall WA, Tanner JM. Variations in patterns of pubertal changes in girls. Arch Dis Child 1969;44:291-303.

[9]   Somani N, Harrison S, Bergfeld WF. The clinical evaluation of hirsutism. Dermatol Ther 2008;21(5):376–91.

[10]   Ferriman DM, Gallwey JD. Clinical assessment of body hair growth in women. J Clin Endocrinol 1961;21:1440–7.

[11]   Babson AL. The Immulite 2000. Automated immunoassay system. J Clin Immunoassay 1991;14:83-8.

[12]   McCartney CR, Blank SK, Prendergast KA, Chhabra S, Eagleson CA, Helm KD, et al. Obesity and sex steroid changes across puberty: Evidence for marked hyperandrogenemia in pre- and early pubertal obese girls. J Clin Endocrinol Metab 2007;92(2):430-6.

[13]   Kaplowitz PB, Slora EJ, Wasserman RC, Pedlow SE, Herman-Giddens ME. Earlier onset of puberty in girls: relation to increased body mass index and race. Pediatrics 2001;108: 347-53.

[14]   McCartney CR, Prendergast KA, Chhabra S, Eagleson CA, Yoo R, Chang RJ, et al. The association of obesity and hyperandrogenemia during the pubertal transition in girls: obesity as a potential factor in the genesis of postpubertal hyperandrogenism. J Clin Endocrinol Metab 2006;91:1714–22.

[15]   Gapstur SM, Gann PH, Kopp P, Colangelo L, Longcope C, Liu K. Serum androgen concentrations in young men: a longitudinal analysis of association with age, obesity, and race. The CARDIA male hormone study. Cancer Epidemiol Biomarkers Prev 2002;11:1041-7.

[16]   Reinehr T, de Sousa G, Roth CL, Andler W. Androgens before and after weight loss in obese children. J Clin Endocrinol Metab 2005;90:588–95.

[17]   Wabitsch M, Hauner H, Heinze E, Bockmann A, Benz R, Mayer H, et al. Body fat distribution and steroid hormone concentrations in obese adolescent girls before and after weight reduction. J Clin Endocrinol Metab1995;80:3469–75.

[18]   Sudi KM, Gallistl S, Borkenstein MH, Payerl D, Aigner R, Moller R, et al. Effect of weight loss on leptin, sex hormones, and measures of adiposity in obese children. Endocrine 2001;14:429-35.

[19]   Chan JL, DePaoli AM, Veldhuis JD, Mantzoros CS. The role of falling leptin levels in the neuroendocrine and metabolic adaptation to short term starvation in healthy men. Clin Invest 2003;111:1409-21.

[20]   Cook S, Weitzman M, Auinger P, Nguyen M, Dietz W.H. Prevalence of a metabolic syndrome phenotype in adolescent's findings from the third national health and nutrition examination survey, 1988-1994. Arch Peditr Adolesc Med 2003;157:821-7.

[21]   Strauss RS. Childhood obesity. Pediatr Clin North Am 2002;49:175–201.

[22]   Rosen ED, Spiegelman BM. Adipocytes as regulators of energy balance and glucose homeostasis. Nature 2006;444:847–53.

[23]   Gambineri A, Pelusi C, Vicennati V, Pagotto U, Pasquali R. Obesity and the polycystic ovary syndrome. Int J Obes Relat Metab Disord 2002; 26: 883-96.

[24]   Lord JM, Flight IH, Norman RJ. Insulin-sensitizing drugs (metformin, troglitazone, rosiglitazone, pioglitazone, D-chiro-inositol) for polycystic ovary syndrome. Cochrane Database Syst Rev 2009;3:DC003053.

[25]   Chhabra S, McCartney CR, Yoo RY, Eagleson CA, Chang RJ, Marshall JC. Progesterone inhibition of the hypothalamic gonadotropin-releasing hormone pulse generator: evidence for varied effects in hyperandrogenemic adolescent girls. J Clin Endocrinol Metab 2005; 90:2810–5.

In: Food, Nutrition and Eating Behavior
Editors: Joav Merrick and Sigal Israeli

ISBN: 978-1-62948-233-0
© 2014 Nova Science Publishers, Inc.

Chapter 15

SELECTIVE VISUAL ATTENTION, EYE MOVEMENTS DURING SOCIAL COMPARISONS AND EATING DISORDER RISK

Steven Riley Thomsen, PhD*, *Carie Breckenridge, BA,*
Valori Infanger, MA and Lisa Harding, MA
Department of Communication Eye Tracking Laboratory,
Brigham Young University, Provo, Utah, US

ABSTRACT

In this chapter we examine an eye-tracking system to observe the eye movements and pupillary response of a group of 109 college-age women as they viewed nine magazine advertisements containing images of ultra-thin models. Previous studies suggest that social comparisons often lead to body image disturbance, an important factor in the development of disordered eating. We hypothesized that individuals with an inclination toward making social comparisons would be more likely to selectively fixate and dwell on body parts typically associated with the assessment of body size and thinness than those less inclined to make social comparisons. Each participant viewed the advertisements at her own pace and was not prompted or specifically instructed to make social comparisons. Our findings confirm that high social comparers produce denser fixation patterns and longer total dwell times when viewing ultra-thin bodies, specifically when viewing faces, stomach, arms, and legs, than low social comparers. These findings suggest that advertisements featuring ultra-thin female images may be potentially harmful to at-risk individuals because these women may be more reflexively and instinctively drawn to them.

* Correnspondence: Steven Riley Thomsen, PhD, professor, Department of Communication, Brigham Young University, Provo, Utah, 84602, USA. E-mail: steven_thomsen@byu.edu.

INTRODUCTION

Social comparison has been described as the process of acquiring, thinking about, and reacting to social information in one's environment (1). This process reflects the human inclination to compare oneself, often through intense focus and scrutiny, to others whom an individual believes possess traits and characteristics that represent desired or valued physical and socio-cultural ideals (2, 3). While most social comparisons occur during the course of normal face-to-face interaction with members of an individual's social groups, they also are believed to occur with referents or targets with which an individual might not have direct interpersonal contact (4, 5). Richins (5), for example, argues that women are likely to compare themselves to the idealized images of beauty in women's fashion magazines because the models in the photographs represent a general social category to which all female readers belong. These comparisons can be both intentional as well as spontaneous and are believed to produce affective, cognitive and behavioral effects (1, 5). A growing body of research, for example, has demonstrated a strong association between social comparison tendencies and increased body dissatisfaction, an important factor in the etiology of disordered eating (2).

The social comparison process typically has been studied through the use self-report interviews, diaries, and surveys. Some researchers have used experimental designs in which participants were shown potential comparison referents followed by post-exposure surveys to measure mood, self-esteem, anger, or jealousy (1, 6, 7). The accuracy of these approaches, however, can be affected by several factors, including a lack of conscious awareness by participants that social comparisons are being made, a reluctance by most people to admit that they make social comparisons (social desirability), a limited ability by most people to recall comparison events, and the human inclination to aggregate facts surrounding comparison events into a single global impression (1, 8).

One approach to understanding and observing the social comparison process may be to study selective visual attention through the use of eye-tracking technology. Selective visual attention occurs as an individual places a priority on processing specific visual information entering one's environment (9). This attention can occur consciously, as the individual purposively examines an object and acquires information about it, or involuntarily, as a short-term reaction to a stimulus that might feature some form of novelty, intensity, complexity, incongruity, uncertainty, surprise, conflict, or other unique physical or semantic property (10, 11). Because eye-tracking systems record the both optokinetic movement of the human eye as it moves across a target image and the simultaneous pupillary reaction to the stimulus being viewed (12), this technique may provide researchers with insights into the activation of physiological and cognitive processes associated with visual attention and, in turn, social comparison.

Data recorded during eye tracking typically includes saccades and fixations. Saccades, sometimes referred to as the gaze path or scan path, are relatively rapid movements of the eye, which can occur as the eye jumps from one element to another, or as the eye moves in a general pattern or pathway across an image (12). A fixation represents the short period of time (usually measured in milliseconds) in which the eye stops or pauses to cognitively interpret a specific feature or element of the image (12-14). The number of fixations on a particular object, as well as the number of times the individual's visual attention returns to a specific object after having moved on to other objects (referred to as a "regression"), are believed to be indicators of both the depth and intensity of cognitive processing (12-15).

As a starting point, it is important to consider what has been learned from studies that have used eye-tracking equipment to examine how individuals view advertisements in general. Radach et al. (16), for example, described a two-stage process for viewing which includes an initial quick orientation to the advertisement followed by more detailed scanning. The first stage has been described as global processing. During this stage, the viewer makes a rapid acquisition of pictorial and textual information to determine the salience of the information to the viewer and if continued viewing is desirable. If the reaction is positive, the viewer engages in more detailed scanning. This second stage, which typically involves scanning only selected areas of the advertisement, usually lasts until the viewer believes that all critical information has been processed and understood. Recent studies have found that eye movement and fixation patterns during this second stage are influenced by advertisement size, graphics, color (16, 17), and the perceived task or viewer motive (18, 19). Hayhoe and Ballard (18) concluded that fixations occur only in the areas the viewer considers the most relevant.

These distinct patterns of eye movements when viewing advertisements also may reflect what has been described as visual attention states (20). Liechty, Pieters, and Wedel (20) argued that visual attention can be observed by examining sequences of saccades and fixation patterns. The global attention state is characterized by saccades of long amplitude and spatially sparse fixations with relatively short durations. These fixations typically occur only when scanning the central parts of the scene being viewed. The local attention state, on the other hand, is characterized by saccades of short amplitude and by spatially dense fixation patterns occurring in relatively small, specific areas of the scene being viewed. When one is initially shown an advertisement, the naturally occurring orienting phase may reflect the global attention state described by Liechty et al. (20). We believe that the more detailed scanning that follows in the second stage would be indicative of localized or task-related attention consistent with the social comparison process.

Recent research has proposed a link between attentional bias when viewing body images and increased risk for the development of anorexia or bulimia (8, 21-23). Freeman et al. (21), for example, showed their subjects (which included eating disorder patients) still images of themselves in form-fitting body leotards. They found that anorexic and bulimic patients were more likely than non-clinical controls to dwell selectively on those parts of their body with which they were the most dissatisfied, particularly the stomach and legs. Jansen et al. (8) compared the allocation of visual attention by eating-symptomatic and non-symptomatic participants to digitized pictures of their own bodies and to pictures of control bodies. Participants were asked to identify what they felt were the most ugly and most beautiful body parts in both sets of photographs. They found that participants scoring high on an eating disorder symptom checklist were more likely to fixate on their self-described ugly body parts rather than their beautiful body parts. Hewig et al. (22) examined the relationship between drive for thinness and attentional bias toward specific body parts that are commonly used to assess thinness (e.g., arms, legs, stomach) among a group of non-clinical college students (both female and male). Participants were shown pictures of male and female models in various states of dress and undress and eye movements were tracked. The researchers found a positive association between drive for thinness scores and an inclination to look longer at the waist, hips, legs, and arms of same-sex models. Roefs et al. (23) used eye-tracking to examine the relationship between body mass (BMI scores) and attentional bias. They found that higher BMI scores, combined with lower assessments of the beauty of one's own body parts, influence they way in which women attend to other women's bodies. They suggested that this would likely contribute to the negative outcomes associated with social comparisons, such as body image disturbance.

Our objective for the current study was to build upon this previous work by exploring what attentional bias, as measured via eye tracking, might tell us about the social comparison process. Specifically, we sought to identify points of increased sensory and cognitive activity as a group of college-age women viewed magazine advertisements containing images of ultra-thin models. We hypothesized that individuals with an inclination toward making social comparisons (both general and body specific) would be more likely to fixate, as measured by dwell time and total fixation count (density), on body parts typically associated with the assessment of body size and thinness. These included breasts, stomach, arms, thighs and legs. In summary, our goal was to demonstrate that the social comparison process could be empirically observed in an unprompted setting by studying the eye movement patterns of a non-clinical sample of college-age women.

OUR SAMPLE

Our sample consisted of 109 US female college students with normal or corrected-to-normal vision recruited via flyers and word of mouth from a large western university. The mean age of our participants was 21.1 (SD = 1.73). Slightly more than 92% of the students were white, 4% were Hispanic, 2% were Asian, 1% were African-American, and 1% were Native American. This is reflective of the overall racial breakdown for the university from which the sample was drawn. Each participant was given a $20 gift card in exchange for participation. Written informed consent was obtained from each subject prior to participation in the study. Originally, 117 participants volunteered for the study. Six did not show up for scheduled eye-tracking sessions and two were excluded because we were not able to accurately calibrate their eyes prior to tracking.

Participants were asked to come to two sessions in our laboratory for data collection. During the first session participants completed a survey that allowed us to measure an inclination to make social comparisons, anorexic risk, and basic demographic characteristics.

Social Comparisons Scale

We combined the five questions from the Physical Appearance Comparison Scale (PACS) (24) and the five questions from the Specific Attributes Comparison Scale (SACS) (25) to create an inclination for making social comparison measure (SCS) for this study. Internal consistency for our combined 10-item scale was strong ($\alpha = .89$). The PACS scale measures one's inclination to compare her overall appearance with that of others and the SACS measures one's inclination to compare specific body parts to those of others. Respondents were asked to indicate how frequently they engage in comparison behaviors using a five-point Likert scale from 1 ("never") to 5 ("almost always"). The statements included, "To determine if I am attractive, I compare my 'looks' to the 'looks' of others," "When I'm with others, I compare the width of my thighs to those of my peers," and "In a bathing suit, I am conscious of how my stomach looks compared to other women."

Anorexic risk

To measure anorexic risk, we used the 33-item Mizes Anorectic Cognition Scale (MACS) (26). The MACS measures the internalization of pathological beliefs and values associated with eating disorders (e.g., anorexia nervosa and bulimia nervosa). High scores are indicative of disordered thinking and high levels of risk in non-clinical or non-diagnosed populations. The scale's basic factor structure represents three specific dimensions of risk: the relationship between weight and social approval, the relationship between self-control (over-eating) and self-esteem, and rigid weight regulation. Mizes (26) has reported that the scale and its three subscales accurately differentiate between eating-disorder symptomatic and non-symptomatic groups. Internal consistency for the overall MACS measure for our study was strong ($\alpha = .93$).

Internalization of the thin ideal

We used the Social Attitudes Toward Appearance Questionnaire (SATAQ) (27) to measure the degree to which an individual's normative beliefs about beauty and physical appearance reflect the sociocultural standards presented in the media. This scale asked respondents to indicate their level of agreement with 14 statements that include, "I believe clothes look better on thin models," and "I wish I looked like a swimsuit model." Internal consistency for this scale also was very good ($\alpha = .82$).

Eye tracking procedure

Participants were asked to return one week after completing the survey for the second session. During this session eye-tracking data were collected using the Eye-Trac 6000, an integrated head-eye tracking system developed by Applied Science Laboratories. The system uses a head-mounted optical device, which is placed on the subject's head and worn like a visor. A reflective monocle was placed in front of the participant's left eye and a miniature infrared television camera was used to record the reflection of the cornea and pupil. These reflections were used to track the movement of the eyes and to record fixation points and fixation duration times.

During each eye-tracking session, participants viewed at their own pace a series of 14 full-page, full color advertisements that appeared in random order. The advertisements were shown in full color on a Dell UltraSharp 22-inch LCD flat screen monitor. Participants sat approximately 22 inches from the monitor and eye calibrations were checked and verified so that the average error in eye position was less than .5 degrees. The participants were told only that they were going to be shown a series of advertisements that they would later be asked to evaluate.

Nine of the advertisements were taken from women's beauty and fashion magazines (e.g., *In Style, Vogue, Cosmopolitan*); each included a photograph of a female model in which one or more of the major body parts could be easily viewed (face, arms, breasts, stomach, hips, and legs). Because we were concerned about how type and amount of clothing worn by the models in the stimulus advertisements might influence attentional bias, we chose a combination of images that included models that were either fully clothed or shown in their underwear. The remaining five advertisements were used as distracters and did not include images of ultra-thin models. Each participant was able to control the length of time each advertisement was shown on the screen.

Recorded variables from the eye-tracking sessions included total tracking time for each advertisement, average total fixation duration time (dwell time) for each advertisement, scan path measures, total number of fixations per advertisement and in each "look zone" (designated areas representing each individual body part: face, arms, breasts, stomach, thighs, and legs), and average dwell time for each specific look zone. Eye positions were sampled at 60 Hz.

FINDINGS

Overall, our subjects spent an average of 7.44 seconds (SD = 3.23) viewing each of the fashion advertisements (see table 1). This figure represents total tracking time and includes both total fixation and non-fixation times. An average of 5.46 seconds (SD = 2.58) per advertisement was spent fixating on the different elements combined (e.g., headlines, text, photographs). Of this time, our subjects spent an average 3.76 seconds (SD = 2.03), or 69% of their total dwell time per advertisement, fixating on the body parts of the female models.

As suggested in previous studies, photographs and images of models in women's beauty and fashion magazines are believed to be used as comparison targets by women who are inclined to make upward social comparisons (an "upward comparison" refers to the drive to compare with others believed to be "better off" or in possession of a desired trait or characteristic. This is particularly true when the comparison can be made without actual social contact). To test this assumption with our subjects, we calculated an approximate median point for our SCS measure in order to create two groups based on their inclination to make social comparisons (more versus less inclined). We then compared those least inclined to make social comparisons (N = 57) with those who were more inclined (N = 52). To test the discriminatory effectiveness of this approach, we compared the two groups' scores on several measures that would be symptomatic of body image disturbance and eating disorder risk. As anticipated, the upper SCS group (those more inclined toward social comparisons) scored significantly higher than those in the lower group (less inclined) on measures of the degree to which they have internalized socio-cultural standards of appearance (SATAQ) and risk for the development of an eating disorder (MAC and the three MAC subscales) (see table 2).

We then sought to determine if these two groups differed in the total number of fixations and total dwell time spent fixating on ultra-thin body parts. As can be seen in table 1, there were no significant differences in the total tracking and total fixation times for the entire ads between the two groups.

Table 1. A comparison of mean tracking times and mean dwell times (per advertisement)

Item	All Subjects (N = 109)		SCS Upper Group Most Inclined (N = 52)		SCS Lower Group Least Inclined (N = 57)		t
	M	SD	M	SD	M	SD	
Mean Tracking Time	7.44	3.23	7.75	3.56	7.15	2.91	.95
Mean Dwell Time	5.46	2.58	5.73	2.81	5.21	2.35	1.05
Mean Dwell Time Body Parts	3.76	2.03	4.13	2.33	3.42	1.67	1.83*
Mean Body Parts Dwell Time as % of Total Dwell Time	.69	.16	.73	.16	.68	.15	2.04*

* p < .05, (one-tailed significance level).

Table 2. Results of t-test comparisons

Measure	All Subjects (N = 109)		SCS Upper Group Most Inclined (N = 52)		SCS Lower Group Least Inclined (N = 57)		t
	M	SD	M	SD	M	SD	
SATAQ	45.56	7.39	49.83	6.46	41.67	5.93	6.85**
MAC	76.61	17.76	86.54	16.54	67.54	13.57	6.58**
Weight and Approval	15.93	4.39	17.88	4.72	14.14	3.19	4.80**
Self-Control and Self-Esteem	18.86	4.34	21.04	3.63	16.88	3.97	5.68**
Rigid Weight Regulation	41.82	10.86	47.62	10.38	36.53	8.34	6.17**

** p < .01 (one-tailed significance levels).

Table 3. A comparison of total fixations by body part look zones

Look Zone	All Subjects (N = 109)		SCS Upper Group Most Inclined (N = 52)		SCS Lower Group Least Inclined (N = 57)		t
	M	SD	M	SD	M	SD	
Face	27.52	12.65	29.81	1.04	25.42	11.46	1.83*
Stomach	6.65	4.91	7.50	5.67	5.88	3.99	1.74*
Breasts	8.72	5.63	9.19	6.40	8.29	4.85	1.32
Thighs	4.79	4.03	5.17	3.94	4.46	4.11	.96
Arms	9.15	6.25	10.75	7.00	7.68	5.11	2.63**
Legs	9.02	5.39	9.17	5.51	8.87	5.32	1.91*

* p < .05, ** p < .01 (one-tailed significance levels).

As predicted, however, those most inclined to make social comparisons had a greater number of fixations in the combined body part look zones and spent more overall time fixating in the body part look zones, including spending a greater percentage of total dwell time on body parts, than those less inclined. Each of these last three differences was statistically significant ($p < .01$).

One of our primary objectives was to determine which body parts received the greatest amount of attention from our subjects and, in particular, were the most frequent targets for social comparison, as measured by the total number of fixations (spatial density). To test this we summed the total number of fixations in each body part look zone for all of the target ads for each participant. As can be seen in Table 3, the greatest number of fixations occurred in the face look zones (M = 27.52, SD = 12.65), followed by arms (M = 9.15, SD = 6.25), legs (M = 9.02, SD = 5.39), breasts (M = 8.72, SD = 5.64), stomach (M = 6.65, SD = 4.91), and thighs (M = 4.79, SD = 4.03).

To determine if there were any statistically significant differences across the look zones, we conducted a one-way, within-subjects analysis of variance (ANOVA), using the body part look zones as the independent, within-subject repeated measures factor and the total combined fixation duration times as the dependent variable. The results indicate significant within-subject differences across the look zones (Wilks' $\Lambda = .19$, $F_{(5,\ 103)} = 9.09$, $p = .000$, multivariate $\eta^2 = .82$). Post hoc pairwise tests indicated significant differences ($p < .05$) for all comparisons except arms and chest, arms and legs, and chest and legs.

Finally, to test the hypothesis that individuals with an inclination toward making social comparisons would be more likely to fixate, as measured by total fixation count (fixation density), on body parts typically associated with the assessment of body size and thinness, we compared the two groups for each body part count. Not surprisingly, those most inclined to make social comparisons averaged more fixations in each of the look zones representing the six primary body parts (face, stomach, breasts, thighs, arms, and legs). We found statistically significant differences ($p < .05$) between the two groups for the face, stomach, arms and legs look zones (see table 3).

The data in table 3 indicate that the density patterns also varied between the two groups in terms of body part preferences. While the densest areas, in terms of fixation patterns, for both groups were the face look zones, those most inclined to make comparisons targeted the legs next, followed, in order, by the arms, breasts, and legs. For those less inclined, the legs were the second densest area, followed by the breasts and then the arms. The least dense area for both groups was the thigh look zone.

CONCLUSION

The results of this study confirm our hypotheses that individuals with an inclination for making social comparisons visually seek out body parts typically associated with the assessment of body size and thinness—specifically the face, stomach, arms, and legs—when shown photographs and advertisements from women's beauty and fashion magazines. Importantly, our data confirm that unprompted social comparisons, and the related allocation of cognitive and sensory resources, can be observed empirically via eye-tracking technology.

Specifically, we believe our findings contribute to the ongoing examination of the media's role as a contributory factor in the rise in anorexia nervosa and bulimia nervosa among girls and women of all ages in two important ways. First, our findings corroborate previous research that suggests that social comparisons are an important factor in the etiology of body image disturbance and disordered eating. Second, and perhaps more importantly, our findings add to the body of knowledge by empirically demonstrating that the visual attention of those most inclined to make social comparisons is selectively and reflexively drawn to the ultra-thin images and ultra-thin body parts common in the photographs and illustrations found in women's beauty and fashion magazines, particularly when compared to individuals less inclined to make social comparisons. These findings suggest that ultra-thin images may be potentially harmful to an at-risk segment of the population, in part, because they appear to be more instinctively attracted to them. The correlational nature of the analysis does not make it possible to determine if the images contribute to the initiation and development of disordered cognitions and social comparison tendencies, but it does confirm that the two are clearly linked.

To test our hypotheses we focused on two important measures associated with viewing behavior—fixation density and total fixation duration (dwell time). As previously discussed, Liechty et al. (20) have proposed a two-phase viewing process that begins with a general scan of the image (global attention state) followed by more detailed and purposive viewing. They argue that the greatest level of selective visual attention occurs in the local attention state (the second phase) and produces a spatially dense fixation pattern. Our results are consistent with this theoretical model and confirm our belief that high social comparers would be more likely than those less inclined to make social comparisons to produce dense eye fixation patterns consistent with localized attention. Specifically, when comparing the high social comparers to those less inclined, we found that the high comparers fixated more frequently on faces, arms, stomachs, and legs and overall for longer periods of time on all ultra-thin body parts combined.

That the greatest fixation density for both groups overall occurred in the face looks zones should not be surprising. Past research has documented that both clinical and non-clinical populations exhibit a strong bias toward looking at faces when shown photographs that include people. This is particularly true for bulimic patients who may perceive attractive women as a sexual threat (28). Maner et al. (28) refer to this as the "female competition hypothesis," which they describe as "cognitive vigilance to perceived threats posed by other women" (p. 60). They argue that this effect is greatest among women who are insecure about their own physical appearance, a factor that often influences the need to make social comparisons and that contributes to body image disturbance. We believe our findings support this. As previously mentioned, our high SCS group also scored significantly higher than the low SCS group on measures of disordered-eating risk (i.e., the Mizes Anorectic Cognitions Scale, the Social Attitudes Toward Appearance Scale).

We also believe these findings address a number of the concerns raised by Wood (1) and others who have critiqued the methodological limitations of past social comparison studies and called for new research models. First, we feel that by observing fixation patterns and dwell times, we were able to pinpoint localized increases in cognitive activity and attentional bias associated with social comparisons and the process of thinking about social information. Second, we feel that our eye-tracking study was able to minimize potential distortion and constraints created when subjects are forced (or specifically instructed) to make social comparisons. Although our study was conducted in a laboratory setting, we attempted to minimize constraints and biases by a) allowing subjects to control the time an image was shown, b) not informing subjects of our primary research intent until after the eye-tracking sessions and data collection were complete, c) allowing a week to pass between the completion of the initial surveys and the eye-tracking so that any sensitivity from the survey questions might be reduced, and d) using distracter advertisements that did not include depictions of human bodies.

Finally, we believe our understanding of the differential viewing patterns based on potential eating disorder risk would be improved by future research that uses eye-tracking analysis to compare eating-disorder symptomatic and non-symptomatic populations. Although eye tracking is a time-consuming, labor-intensive process, future studies also would benefit from larger samples. Our decision to split our sample and compare upper and lower groups based on SCS scores, produced relatively small cells for comparison and thus may have limited our statistical power. Finally, future studies should consider examining the differential effects of motivations for making social comparisons, particularly among populations at risk for developing eating disorders, on eye-movement patterns and, in particular, pupillary response. We believe that these studies could contribute substantially to the growing theoretical understanding of social comparison and related cognitive processes.

REFERENCES

[1]   Wood JV. What is social comparison and how should we study it? Pers Soc Psychol B 1996;22(5):520-37.
[2]   Corning AF, Krumm AJ, Smithan, LA. Differential social comparison processes in women with and without eating disorder symptoms. J Couns Psychol 2006;53(3):338-49.
[3]   Festinger L. A theory of social comparison processes. Hum Relat 1954;7:117-40.
[4]   Martin MC, Kennedy PR. Advertising and social comparison: Consequences for female pre-adolescents and adolescents. Psychol Market 1993;10:513-30.
[5]   Richins ML. Social comparison and the idealized images of advertising. J Consum Res 1991;18:71-83.
[6]   Aspinwall LG, Taylor SE. Effects of social comparison direction, threat, and self-esteem on affect, self-evaluation, and expected success. J Pers Soc Psychol 1993;64(5):708-22.
[7]   Wheeler L, Miyake K. Social comparison in everyday life. J Pers Soc Psychol 1992;62(5):760-73.
[8]   Jansen A, Nederkoorn C, Mulkens S. Selective visual attention for ugly and beautiful body parts in eating disorders. Behav Res Ther 2005;43(1):183-96.
[9]   Schneider WX. An introduction to "Mechanisms of visual attention: A cognitive neuroscience perspective." In: Schneider WX, Maasen S. Mechanisms of visual attention: A neuroscience perspective. East Sussex, UK: Psychology Press, 1998:1-8.
[10]   Lynn R. Attention, arousal and the orientation reaction. Oxford: Pergamon Press, 1966.
[11]   Näätänen R. Attention and brain function. Hillsdale, NJ: Lawrence Erlbaum, 1992.
[12]   Rayner K. Eye movements in reading and information processing: 20 years of research. Psychol Bull 1998;124(3):372-422.
[13]   Andreassi JL. Psychophysiology: Human behavior and physiological response (5th ed.). Mahwah, NJ: Lawrence Erlbaum, 2007.
[14]   Just MA, Carpenter PA. A theory of reading: From eye fixations to comprehension. Psychol Rev 1980;87:329-54.

[15] Crespo A, Cabestrero R, Grzib G, Quirso P. Visual attention to health warnings in tobacco advertisements: An eye-tracking research between smokers and non-smokers. Stud Psychol 2007;49:39-50.

[16] Radach R, Lemmer S, Vorstius C, Heller D, Radach K. Eye movement in the processing of print advertisements. In: Hyönä J, Radach R, Deubel H. The mind's eye: Cognitive and applied aspects of eye movement research. Amsterdam: Elsevier, 2003:609-32.

[17] Lohse GL. Consumer eye movement patterns on Yellow Pages advertising. J Advertising 1997;25(1):61-73.

[18] Hayhoe M, Ballard D. Eye movements in natural behavior. Trends Cogn Sci 2005;9(4):188-94.

[19] Rayner K, Miller B, Rotello CM. Eye movements when looking at print advertisements: The goal of the view matters. Appl Cognitive Psychol 2008;22:697-707.

[20] Liechty J, Pieters R, Wedel M. Global and local covert visual attention: Evidence from a Bayesian hidden marker model. Psychometrika 2003;68(4):519-41.

[21] Freeman, R., Touyz, S., Sara, G., Rennie, C., Gordon, E., & Beumont, P. In the eye of the beholder: Processing body shape information in Anorexic and Bulimic patients. Int J Eat Disord 1991;10(6):709-14.

[22] Hewig J, Cooper S, Trippe RH, Hecht H, Straube T, Miltner WHR. Drive for thinness and attention toward specific body parts in a nonclinical sample. Psychosom Med 2008;70:729-36.

[23] Roefs A, Jansen A, Moresi S, Willems P, van Grootel S, van der Borgh A. Looking good. BMI, attractiveness bias and visual attention. Appetite 2008;51:552-5.

[24] Thompson JK, Heinberg LJ, Tantleff S. The Physical Appearance Comparison Scale (PACS). Behav Ther 1991;14:174.

[25] Tiggemann M, McGill B. The role of social comparison in the effect of magazine advertisements on women's mood and body dissatisfaction. J Soc Clin Psychol 2004;23(1):23-44.

[26] Mizes JS. Validity of the Mizes anorectic cognitions scale: A comparison between anorectics, bulimics, and psychiatric controls. Addict Behav 1992;17:283-9.

[27] Heinberg LJ, Thompson JK, Stormer S. Development and validation of the Sociocultural Attitudes Towards Appearance Questionnaire. Int J Eat Disord 1995;17:81-89.

[28] Maner JK, Holm-Denoma JM, Van Orden KA, Gailliot MT, Gordon KH, Joiner TE. Evidence for Attentional Bias in Women Exhibiting Bulimotypic Symptoms. Int J Eat Disord 2006;39(1):55-61.

In: Food, Nutrition and Eating Behavior
Editors: Joav Merrick and Sigal Israeli

ISBN: 978-1-62948-233-0
© 2014 Nova Science Publishers, Inc.

Chapter 16

RECOMMENDATIONS FOR FAMILY INTERVENTIONS FOR EATING DISORDERS

Uri Pinus, MSW*

Adolescent Psychiatric Day-Care Unit, Hadassah University Hospital,
Jerusalem, Israel

ABSTRACT

This chapter is a brief review of empirical support for family therapy of eating disorders. It highlights the most important recommendations that emerge from recent research. While key theoretical concepts in the field were developed in the 1970s, clinical trial-based practice guidelines for treating patients suffering from eating disorders have been developed in recent years. Inspired by traditional family therapy, nutrition-focused family therapy has proven effective, especially in treating younger non-chronic patients with eating disorders.

INTRODUCTION

In the past 30 years, important theoretical concepts linking families with eating disorders have been published, along with various models for family therapy. While the theoretical concepts drew largely on clinical experience, there was very little research backing to substantiate them (1, 2). Given the high morbidity and mortality rates, detecting effective family interventions for eating disorders is critical. The purpose of this paper is to summarize the main findings of recent literature on treatment and their contribution to effective family treatment for eating disorders.

For decades, researchers have agreed that the most likely cause of eating disorders is the family (3). This belief has deep historical roots. Physicians in the nineteenth century recommended that anorexic girls be separated from their families to ensure proper nutrition:

---

* Correspondence: Uri Pinus, MSW, Child Psychiatry Unit, Hadassah University Medical Center, POBox 1200, IL-91120 Ein Karem, Jerusalem, Israel. E-mail: uri.pinus@mail.huji.ac.il.

"The patients should be fed at regular intervals and surrounded by persons who would have moral control of them, relatives and friends being generally the worst attendants" (1, 4). Assumptions about the family as the source of eating disorders abounded, and these gave rise to models for family intervention (1).

Although the contribution of the family to the disorders is the focus of some research, we have yet to find definitive evidence for their causes. Interestingly, while recent research has tended to disclaim family background as the source, these same studies point to the importance of family involvement in advancing treatment (5).

The family approach that has been the subject of the most comprehensive research is based heavily on the systematic-structural model. Other models, such as the strategic-systemic and cognitive-behavioral, have also had their influence (6). The systematic-structural model, as its name suggests, focuses on family structure and relationship issues, such as hierarchies, problematic alliances and coalitions, communication disturbances, inappropriate emotional involvement, high levels of parental criticism of children, and conflicts that perpetuate symptoms. According to this model, the issue of control is central and becomes the focus for family intervention. In cases of eating disorders, the issue of control is addressed with regard to food, whether from the point of view of the patient's food intake or the family's helplessness in the face of the patient's illness (7). In utilizing systematic-structural family therapy, the therapist reinforces inter-generational limits by re-enacting family situations in the treatment room. In these situations, the therapist assists the re-organization of family interactions. The therapist blocks or encourages interaction patterns in keeping with the level of intimacy or privacy best suited to the developmental needs of the family members, thereby preventing them from reverting to their symptomatic behavior (7).

In 1978, Minuchin et al. (8) published the results of an uncontrolled follow-up study of systemic-structural family therapy employed in the cases of 53 adolescent girls suffering from anorexia for less than a year who had requested therapy for the first time. Some had been hospitalized for a short time, but most were treated as outpatients for six months on average. Results were measured at the completion of therapy and also at follow-ups at intervals of 18 months to seven years. Approximately 80% of the patients sampled were monitored for at least two years. The criteria for measuring the impact of the therapy were linked to the patients' physical condition and psycho-social functioning (within the family, in society and at school) (8). Surprisingly, family functioning was not measured. The reported rate of success using the systematic-structural approach was remarkably high: 86%. The 1978 study (8) was followed by additional uncontrolled research measuring the results of this therapy with non-chronic, anorexic adolescent girls, and the results indicated that the underlying therapeutic model was satisfactory (9, 10). There was some criticism of the methodology used in these follow-up studies, particularly the lack of control groups and the absence of other types of intervention for purposes of comparison (11).

In their research, Minuchin et al. (12) set out to measure the influence of therapy on what they described as a typical family structure for eating disorders – a "psycho-somatic family" characterized by enmeshment, over-protectiveness, rigidity, and an inability for conflict resolution. In this type of family, the ailing child plays a central role in the pattern of conflict avoidance, and communication takes place most often in the form of body language. The psycho-somatic (or "anorexogenic") family, conclude the researchers, not only fuels the disorder but creates it (12). Studies that followed did not find evidence of these characteristics in the families of anorexic or bulimic children (13-15). Many studies over the last two decades conducted on families in which one member suffers from an eating disorder describe family risk factors and characteristics. However, the correlation between these factors and instances of eating disorders is not necessarily causative, as the pioneers of the systemic-structural approach argued (3, 16).

The main limitation of the systemic-structural model was its focus on etiology rather than on an understanding how families organize themselves to deal with a life-threatening problem. However, once symptoms appear, the model can help the therapist understand how these symptoms are perpetuated by the family. Treatment providers, therefore, can implement family resources in order to advance healing and coping processes through development assignments appropriate to the patient's age (2, 17).

Today, family therapists who treat eating disorders are faced with questions that demand evidence-based responses:

- Of the various therapeutic approaches involving the family, which is the most effective for treating eating disorders?
- Which basic family therapy techniques have proven effective, specifically in relation to eating disorders?
- Which family members should be included in family therapy, and when is it advisable to alter the composition of family members participating in treatment?
- Which aspects of the eating disorder should be included in family intervention?
- What are the phases of family intervention for treatment of eating disorders?
- Are different types of intervention necessary for various types of eating disorders (anorexia, bulimia, binging, and ED-NOS), age groups (young girls, adolescents, adults), stages of the illness, and degree of severity (acute, chronic, fluctuating)?

It appears that evidence-based answers exist only for some of these questions.

EVIDENCE-BASED FAMILY THERAPY

Like other fields of health care, family therapy, and family therapy for eating disorders in particular, needs to employ treatment that is grounded in empirical evidence. This demand comes from those who finance mental health services and from those who provide the services – the therapists – both of whom seek proven methods of treatment for specific problems (18-20). Evidence-based therapy is administered according to systematically applied, written guidelines. This type of manual-based therapy is a relatively new approach and differs from clinical, experience-based treatment, which reflects the conventional opinions of therapists and those considered experts in the field, without the backing of research evidence (21).

Many clinicians have expressed their unease with treatment manuals and are suspicious of guidelines for family therapy. In recent years, however, research-based recommendations were published in the U.S. and Britain, where there were also attempts to formulate a handbook for family intervention that could be used universally to examine the degree of treatment effectiveness, compare results, and formulate recommendations for improving treatment methods (22, 23).

EVIDENCE-BASED FAMILY THERAPY FOR ANOREXIA NERVOSA

Family intervention trials for anorexia nervosa have employed various forms of family therapy. Two studies focused on adults, five exclusively on adolescents, and one on adults and adolescent patients together (24). Family interventions that have proved effective in treating anorexia are found to include the following components (6, 25):

- An effort to mobilize the adolescent and her parents for therapy, with the objective of building, strengthening, and maintaining motivation for treatment and eliminating the risk of drop-out. (Therapy drop-out rates are reported to reach 50%, a particularly worrisome figure given the life-threatening nature of the disorder).
- Psycho-educational intervention that addresses the characteristics of the disorder and its risks.
- Prioritization of weight rehabilitation and regular follow-up by a dietician.
- A shift in focus from nutrition to issues related to appropriate adolescent development (increased independence, greater distance from family members, etc.) with the objective of identifying factors that reinforce symptomatic behavior in the adolescent girl.
- An effort to prevent a relapse after improvement has been achieved.

Most of the family interventions found to be effective took place on an outpatient basis. They continued for a maximum of 15 months and 18 sessions.

The first controlled study of eating disorders, published in 1987, compared the results of treatment for anorexic and bulimic patients who, after inpatient weight restoration, were randomly referred to one of two methods of outpatient treatment. One group was treated through family therapy, while the other received what was defined as individual, supportive, "non-specific" intervention. While the family therapy relied to some extent on Minuchin's model, it parted company with this approach by encouraging parents to help in re-feeding their adolescent children until weight restoration was achieved. General adolescent and family issues were deferred until the eating disorder behavior was under control. The emphasis in the therapy was on the need for the parents to cooperate with and support each other and to remain firm and consistent in their responses to their child's symptoms.

A follow-up a year later found family therapy to be more effective than individual therapy for relatively young patients, under the age of 19, who had been ill for a relatively short period of less than three years. For older patients, individual treatment tended to be more effective with regard to weight rehabilitation, but for the majority of patients studied this improvement later ceased (26). A subsequent follow-up study five years later showed that therapeutic achievements were maintained and that family therapy had proven to achieve better results than supportive individual treatment for the defined population of non-chronic younger girls (27).

In another study, published in 1991, anorexic patients were randomly assigned to one of four types of treatment: hospitalization, outpatient family therapy, outpatient group therapy, or follow-up with no additional treatment. The family intervention worked to establish appropriate limits, block the tendency toward excess intervention and invasiveness by the family, and encourage problem-solving while taking into account the desire to avoid conflict in the family. A one-year follow-up showed that the family intervention was as effective as the other interventions with regard to weight and psychological, sexual, and socio-economic functioning. It was also more effective than follow-up with no additional treatment (28). A two-year follow-up study in 1994 indicated that the achievements of the family therapy were maintained over time (29).

Another study, in 1994, assessed treatment of adolescents suffering from anorexia nervosa. Two types of randomly assigned intervention were compared: one group received system-behavioral family therapy and the other ego-oriented individual therapy. The family therapy promoted communication skills, problem-solving skills, and cognitive change for distorted beliefs and conceptions within the family. It also addressed familial processes, such as inter-generational coalitions, that hamper communication. The family therapist encouraged the parents to work as a team and to take responsibility for instituting the menu they were given for their child. When the adolescent reached the target weight, control of nutrition was gradually returned to her. At this stage, the family therapy focused on reinforcing the adolescent's autonomy and improving communication patterns in the family.

In the second group, the adolescents underwent individual treatment that aimed to reinforce ego strengths and clarify the latent dynamic that hindered proper nutrition. The parents of the treated adolescents were seen periodically by the therapist, without their daughters.

The results indicated similar improvement for the two types of intervention with regard to nutrition, depression level, and family relationships. Family therapy proved more effective than individual treatment, both at the end of the treatment and at a one-year follow-up, with regard to weight rehabilitation and the date of resumption of the menstrual cycle, (30).

A decade later, a similarly designed study showed the same trend. The characteristics of the sample were only slightly different with regard to depression rates, duration of the disorder, and duration of the therapy (31).

In the year 2000, a study on treatment of anorexia nervosa compared two randomly assigned types of family intervention. The first was conducted through separate sessions with parents and the ailing adolescent (separated family therapy). The sessions with parents focused on mobilizing the resources needed to overcome their feeling of powerlessness and developing mechanisms for coping with the symptomatic behavior of their daughter. At the same time, the therapist conducted sessions with the adolescent alone. In the second form of intervention, the parents and the adolescent sat together (conjoint family therapy). The frequency and length of the sessions were similar in both interventions. The duration for both was about a year, and approximately 25 sessions were conducted.

A comparison of the results of both interventions after a year revealed no significant differences with regard to their shared therapeutic goals of achieving normal weight and preventing relapse and re-hospitalization. In cases where the adolescent and parents met the therapist separately, slightly more psychological improvement was recorded for the adolescent. In a follow-up study two years after the treatment ended, it was found that the family members who participated in the separated family therapy reported a higher level of satisfaction with their current relations (fewer power struggles, accusations and quarrels). Another important finding was that families characterized by a high level of parental criticism (especially on the part of the mother) toward the adolescent at the beginning of the therapy had a more favorable treatment outcome when the parents and adolescent were seen separately (32, 33).

Follow-up at the end of five years showed that the improvement achieved in both types of treatment sessions was maintained: for 75% of the patients significant improvement was observed, for 15% the improvement was moderate, and the remaining 10% showed poor results (32).

The results of the comparison between the two family therapy groups (separated and conjoint) are especially meaningful for family therapists, and it is therefore worth taking a closer look at some of the key features of these interventions (32):

- The therapist clarified to the parents at the start of treatment that the family is not the source of the disorder but the best resource for its effective treatment.
- The therapist provided detailed information to both the parents and the patient about physical and psychological consequences of malnourishment.
- The therapist explained to both the parents and the patient the compulsive nature of anorexic behaviors that tend to govern the lives of adolescents and their families.
- To the parents, the therapist stressed the need for parental involvement in nutritional rehabilitation, without resorting to criticism of the adolescent. Consistency, firmness, and determination in promoting nutritional rehabilitation, it was emphasized, should not be translated as insults and accusations.
- The therapist encouraged the parents to support their daughter to help her take back control as soon as possible.
- The therapist supported and encouraged the parents to maintain a positive marital relationship, in part to enable the adolescent to realize that her parents have lives together beyond the mutual care of their children.

In both the separate and conjoint sessions, the initial focus was on parental control of nutritional rehabilitation. At a later stage, as the patient's physical condition improved, the focus shifted gradually to family relationship and adolescent development issues. The guiding therapeutic principle was to help the family separate undesirable eating habits and patterns of interaction related to nutrition from psychological problems within the family.

These two forms of family therapy express concern about the dangers of malnutrition and urge the parents to act firmly to rehabilitate their daughter's eating habits while, on the other hand, they encourage the adolescent to claim her right to privacy, autonomy, and personal aspirations. Anorexia was described by the family therapist as an internal enemy that deludes the young girl into thinking that the condition is her real voice, when in fact the anorexia makes her insignificant and rules her through the psychology of hunger.

In the session with parents only, the therapist discussed strategies to achieve a change in eating habits without intervening directly in the parent-child interaction. The therapist took a supportive and empathic position toward the parents, while encouraging them to avoid criticizing their daughter. Issues surrounding the marital relationship were not raised unless doing so would reinforce the parental coalition as a means of facilitating the key objective of the nutritional rehabilitation.

During the first phase of treatment, nutrition at home should be the parents' responsibility, since they are charged with buying, preparing, and serving the food according to a predetermined menu. The parents, as opposed to the adolescent, are responsible for their own nutrition and that of the entire family. If the patient seeks autonomy, it should not be in the area of nutrition; she should be given other, age-appropriate ways of achieving it (34).

Meals should be planned in advance according to the instructions provided by the treatment staff, and they should end after a predetermined length of time. It appears that there is no benefit to preparing or ordering special foods for the adolescent (34). The individual sessions with the adolescent had a counseling-supportive style aimed to prepare her for discussions about further sensitive topics. One component of all sessions with adolescents was the influence of the anorexic symptoms on family relationships. The sessions with the younger adolescents were most effective when they focused on subjects directly connected to the eating problem. With older adolescents, the therapeutic discussions were effective when they widened to address how the girls themselves felt about their social life, family life and more.

To summarize, the purpose of the study was to compare two types of family therapy. The findings reinforce the conclusions of previous research showing that encouragement of direct parental intervention in regulating nutrition brought about symptomatic improvement and positive psychological change in their daughters (26, 28, 30, 32, 35). Moreover, it appears that parents are interested in taking on this role for the sake of their children. A study published in 2004, showed that 88% of the participating parents related positively to the role given to them in regulating their daughter's nutrition (36).

Treatments that encourage parents to play an active role in addressing their daughter's eating habits seem the most effective. Methods that instruct parents to refrain from attempting to influence their daughter's eating habits, at the same time encouraging her to understand her condition were found to be less effective (30). The absence of parental intervention in regulating nutrition was also found to delay recovery (26, 27).

The encouraging results for family therapy for adolescents were not duplicated for older patients (2, 26, 27, 37). While the parents of adolescents should be responsible for nutritional rehabilitation, the preferred method for adult patients is to distance the eating problem as quickly as possible from its dominant role in family relationships (38). There is little convincing data regarding the effectiveness of family interventions with adult patients (over age 19) who suffer from anorexia nervosa (11). In addition, family therapy has been found to be less effective than other methods for patients with chronic or late-onset eating disorders (37).

A controlled study published in 2001 compared family therapy with individual therapy for adult patients suffering from anorexia nervosa after hospitalization. In one-year and five-year follow-ups, it was found that, compared with a control group that did not undergo therapy, both family and individual intervention correlated with a greater improvement in weight. Although there was no significant difference between the types of treatment, there was a slight advantage to individual treatment with regard to psychological adaptation (37).

EVIDENCE-BASED FAMILY THERAPY FOR BULIMIA NERVOSA

While there is evidence of the effectiveness of family therapy for anorexia nervosa, systematic research on family therapy for bulimia nervosa is nearly non-existent (11-39). This gap may stem from the fact that bulimia was categorized diagnostically only in recent decades and therefore a useful body of knowledge about its therapeutic dynamics has yet to be accumulated.

Some researchers have suggested reassessing the diagnostic distinction between bulimia nervosa and anorexia nervosa. Both disorders may exhibit binging and vomiting, and it appears that the single outstanding difference between them is the severity of the weight loss. At any rate, it has been found that family intervention is effective for both restrictive anorexics and anorexics with bulimic symptoms (27).

In 1995, a controlled study that examined the application of family intervention for eight adolescent girls suffering from bulimia nervosa showed a significant lessening of bulimic symptoms, which was maintained in the follow-up a year after completion of treatment (40).

A recent randomized controlled trial conducted for adolescents with bulimia nervosa showed a clinical and statistical advantage for family-based treatment over supportive individual psychotherapy at post-treatment and at a six-month follow-up. Family therapy also appears to be a more efficient means for achieving early symptomatic relief. This form of treatment is impartial about the cause of the disorder but assumes that normal adolescent development is negatively affected by the condition. The model shares many characteristics with the previously existing family-based treatment model applied for anorexia (41). The usual treatment for bulimia proceeds through three phases: sessions are weekly in phase 1 (2-3 months), every second week in phase 2, and monthly in phase 3. In the first phase, the therapist tells the family about the physical and psychological risks of the disorder. Although this often arouses anxiety in the parents, the ultimate objective is to involve them in the course of the treatment, foster awareness of their daughter's condition and increase their motivation for treatment. At the same time, the therapist makes it explicitly clear to the parents that there is no place for blaming or criticizing the patient, and that there is no proof that any blame for the disorder lies with the family. The treatment aims at empowering parents to disrupt binge eating, purging, restrictive dieting, and any other pathological weight control behaviors. It also aims to separate the adolescent herself from her disordered behaviors in order to promote parental action and lessen adolescent resistance to their assistance. Once the adolescent's disordered eating habits and related behaviors begin to wane, phase 2 begins, and parents gradually pass control over eating issues back to the adolescent. Phase 3 focuses on the ways the family can help counter the effects bulimia on adolescent developmental processes (42).

Despite the use of this procedure, there is still some doubt as to whether the treatment model initially designed for anorexic patients is also suitable for bulimic patients, who sometimes exhibit different traits: greater independence, rebelliousness, higher risk for sexual promiscuity, and abuse of addictive substances (26).

In another recent study, 85 adolescents with bulimia nervosa or ED-NOS were randomly assigned to family therapy (at least 13 sessions, plus two individual sessions, over six months) or to therapist-supported, self-guided, manual-based, cognitive-behavioral therapy (15 sessions over six months). The findings suggest that while adolescents with bulimia nervosa can benefit from family therapy, their conditions improved more dramatically with cognitive-behavioral therapy (43).

PRACTICE GUIDELINES FOR THE TREATMENT OF PATIENTS WITH EATING DISORDERS

To date, three comprehensive guidelines for the treatment of eating disorders have been published. The first, "Practice guideline for the treatment of patients with eating disorders", was published in 1993 by the American Psychiatric Association and based on the most current research findings at the time (44). A third revised edition was published in 2006 (45). The chapter on family therapy for anorexia nervosa recommends that therapists mobilize family support for the benefit of the patient and her treatment. Family intervention has been found to be especially effective for adolescents under the age of 19 years, who are living at home with their families and whose disorder was diagnosed less than three years earlier. The publication recommends therapy when family problems perpetuate and reinforce eating disorder symptoms.

For bulimic patients, family therapy should be considered whenever possible, particularly for adolescent patients living with their families and adult patients with problematic family relationships. Similarly, adult patients are likely to benefit from intervention by their partners.

In 2004, a clinical guideline was published by the National Institute for Clinical Excellence (NICE) in England, in cooperation with the Association of Psychologists and Union of Psychiatrists (46). The document strongly promotes family intervention that directly addresses eating disorders, and it recommends their use for children and adolescents with anorexia nervosa. In a chapter specifically devoted to family intervention, therapists are advised to include a psycho-educational component in their work – basic information about the disorder that includes its cause(s), factors that perpetuate and reinforce it, proven ways of helping the patient, and the anticipated course of the disorder and results of the treatment. The chapter also recommends providing the patient and her family with information about the risks accompanying the disorder, warning signs of possible physical dangers, and concrete steps that can be taken to reduce risk.

The degree of family intervention recommended, according to the 2004 guideline, depends on a number of factors, including the age of the patient the relevant developmental issues, and the severity and risk level of the illness. In addition, it was recommended that the therapist update the families of minors about any unusual findings, worsening of the condition, or possible danger to the patient.

For minors suffering from anorexia nervosa, the guideline recommends guided family intervention at the onset of treatment. The immediate objective is to involve the family in the therapy. While anorexic patients often lack insight into their condition and their level of motivation for therapy is low, parents are sometimes skeptical about categorizing anorexia as an emotional disorder, and they are not certain of the need for any sort of psychological counseling. The therapist, therefore, must first try to build a good working relationship with the family.

For patients suffering from bulimia nervosa, the 2004 guideline recommends treatment that includes cognitive-behavioral therapy, anti-depressants, and family intervention, as appropriate. The guideline further suggests that parents and siblings of minors suffering from all types of eating disorders be routinely included in the treatment procedure. Intervention may consist of sharing information, counseling for behavioral management, and advice on facilitating communication. It is also recommended that parents be involved in meal planning for minors.

In 2004, a clinical practice guideline for the treatment of anorexia nervosa was published by the Royal Australian and New Zealand College of Psychiatrists. It notes that family therapy has been found to be a valuable component of treatment, particularly for children and adolescents. With regard to "schools" of family therapy, no specific family approach is superior to any other (47).

The 2001 "Treatment manual for anorexia nervosa" is the first published guideline for the family-based approach. Extending beyond traditional family therapy techniques, this model is geared specifically for intervention by families of patients suffering from anorexia nervosa (43). It was inspired by Minuchin and his colleagues and developed at Maudsley Hospital in London. The model has been widely adopted and implemented in treatment centers around the world.

The 2001 manual was designed to empower parents to disrupt the powerful behaviors maintaining their child's low weight. The model is impartial to the cause of the eating disorder and assumes that normal adolescent development is negatively affected by the disorder. The treatment aims to achieve behavioral change as soon as possible, again, without focusing on the reason for the occurrence of the disorder. It is conducted on an outpatient basis and includes 20-25 sessions of about one hour each, divided into three phases over the course of a year. Sessions are weekly in phase 1 (two-three months), every two weeks in phase 2 and monthly in phase 3.

At the beginning of the intervention, parents are given responsibility for their daughter's nutrition. With the support of the treatment staff, the parents give the girl the message that the food is a form of medication and that self-starvation is not an option. The parents are encouraged to find suitable ways of guiding their daughter toward a nutritional routine that will rehabilitate her physical condition. Though assisted by the staff, the parents must have a high degree of determination and persistence. The therapists free the parents from guilt over the appearance of the illness; it is portrayed as something that has taken over patient. This approach is reminiscent of what narrative family therapy calls "externalization," (48) which also helps parents refrain from blaming their child for the illness.

In the second phase, after attaining the desired weight, the adolescent gradually regains control of her nutrition. This is the time to deal with difficulties within the family.

In the third and final phase, the intervention focus shifts to problem-solving and critical adolescent development issues. It is best to discuss these issues only after the signs of anorexia recede, thereby opening the possibility of building family relationships without the intervening factor of the eating disorder and all it entails. Family therapy is contraindicated for families with a history of violence and exploitation.

CONCLUSION

Family Therapy in the treatment of eating disorders has come a long way in the last three decades. Current evidence shows that family therapy is especially effective for non-chronic adolescents below the age of 19 who live at home with their families. Controlled studies of this population, especially for anorexia, have shown that family therapy is more effective than any other therapeutic format.

The findings accumulated in recent years indicate that family therapy at the beginning of intervention on nutrition issues has proven its effectiveness in treating eating disorders, especially with adolescents. While the treatment of adult patients may include family members and spouses as needed, the most effective approach has proven to be cognitive individual intervention.

Despite the progress in the field, further research is needed to establish a useful, evidence-based body of knowledge for family therapists who treat eating disorders.

REFERENCES

[1]   Vanderlinden J, Vandereycken W. Overview of the family therapy Literature. In: Vandereycken W, Kog E, Vanderlinden J, eds. The family approach to eating disorders: Assessment and treatment of anorexia nervosa and bulimia, New York: PMA, 1989:189-225.

[2]   Dare C, Eisler I, Family therapy and eating disorders. In: Brownell K, Fairburn CG, eds. Eating disorders and obesity: A comprehensive handbook. New York: Guilford, 1995.

[3]   Polivy J, Herman C, Causes of eating disorders. Ann Rev Psychol 2002;53:187-213.

[4]   Gull W. Anorexia nervosa (apepsia hysterica, anorexia hysterica). Transactions Clin Soc London 1874;7:22-8. Reprinted in: Andersen A. Practical comprehensive treatment of anorexia nervosa and bulimia. Baltimore, MD: John Hopkins Univ Press, 1985:13-8.

[5]   Rosen D. Eating disorders in children and young adolescents: Etiology, classification, clinical features and treatment. Adolesc Med 2003;14:49-59.

[6]   Wilson T, Fairburn C. Treatments for eating disorders. In: Nathan P, Gorman J, eds. A guide to treatments that work. New York: Oxford Univ Press, 1998:501-30.

[7]   Cottrell D, Boston P. Practitioner review: The effectiveness of systemic family therapy for children and adolescents. J Child Psychol Psychiat 2002;43(5):573-86.

[8]   Minuchin S, Rosman B, Baker L. Psychosomatic families: anorexia nervosa in context. Cambridge, MA: Harvard Univ Press, 1978.

[9]   Herscovici C, Bay L. Favorable outcome for anorexia nervosa patients treated in Argentina with a family approach, Eat Disord 1996;4:59-66.

[10]   Martin F. The treatment and outcome of anorexia nervosa in adolescents: a prospective study and five year follow-up. J Pychiatr Res 1985;19:509-14.

[11]   Asen E. Outcome research in family therapy. APT 2002;8:230-8.

[12]   Minuchin S, Baker L, Rosman B, Liebman R, Milman L, Todd T. A conceptual model of psychosomatic illness in children. Arch Gen Psychiatry 1975;32:1031-8.

[13]   Stice E. Risk and maintenance factors for eating pathology: A metaanalytic review. Psychol Bull 2002;128:825-48.

[14]   Dare C, Le Grange D, Eisler I, Rutherford J. Redefining the psychosomatic family: family process of 26 eating disorder families. Int J Eat Disord. 1994;12:347-57.

[15]   Crisp A, Hsu L, Harding B, Hartshorn J. Clinical features of anorexia nervosa: A study of a consecutive series of 102 female patients. J Psychosom Res 1980;24:179-91.

[16]   Haworth-Hoeppner S. The critical shapes of body image: The role of culture and family in the production of eating disorders. J Marriage Fam 2000;62:212-27.

[17]   Yager J. Anorexia Nervosa and the family. In: Lansky MR, ed. Family therapy and major psychopathology. New York: Grune Stratton,1981:249-80.

[18]   Russell D, McArthur H. Meeting the needs of evidence-based practice in family therapy: developing the scientist-practitioner model. J Fam Ther 2002;24:113-24.

[19]   Carr A. Evidence-based practice in family therapy and systemic consultation I: Child-focused problems. J Fam Ther 2000;22:29-60.

[20]   Carr A. Evidence-based practice in family therapy and systemic consultation II: Adult-focused problems. J Fam Ther 2000;22:273–95.

[21]   Chambless D, Ollendick T. Empirically supported psychological interventions: controversies and evidence. Ann Rev Psychol 2001;52:685-716.

[22]   Pote H, Stratton P, Cottrell D, Shapiro D, Bostonb P. Systemic family therapy can be manualized: research process and findings. J Fam Ther 2003;25:236-62.

[23]   Lock J, Le Grange D. Can family-based treatment of anorexia be manualized? J Psychother Pract Res 2001;10:253-61.

[24]   Bulik C, Berkman N, Brownley K, Sedway J, Lohr K. Anorexia nervosa treatment: A systematic review of randomized controlled trials. Int J Eat Disord 2007;40(4):310-20.

[25]   Fairburn C, Harrison P. Eating disorders. Lancet 2003;361:407-16.

[26]   Russell G, Szmukler G, Dare C, Eisler I. An evaluation of family therapy in anorexia and bulimia nervosa. Arch Gen Psychiatry 1987; 44:1047-56.

[27]   Eisler I, Dare C, Russell G, Szmukler G, Le Grange D, Dodge E. A five-year follow-up of a controlled trial of family therapy in severe eating disorders: the results of controlled comparison of two family therapy interventions. Arch Gen Psychiatry 1997;54:1025-30.

[28]   Crisp A, Norton K, Gowers S, Halek C, Bowyer C, Yeldham D, Levett G, Bhat A. A controlled study to the effect of therapies aimed at adolescent and family psychopathology in anorexia nervosa. Br J Psychiatry 1991;159:325-33.

[29]   Gowers S, Norton K, Halek C, Crisp A. Outcome of outpatient psychotherapy in a random allocation treatment study of anorexia nervosa. Int J Eat Disord 1994;15:165-77.

[30]   Robin A, Siegel P, Koepke T, Moye A, Tice S. Family therapy versus individual therapy for adolescent females with anorexia nervosa. J Dev Behav Pediatr 1994;15:111-6.

[31]   Robin A, Siegel P, Moye A, Gilroy M, Baker-Dennis A, Sikard A. A controlled comparison of family versus individual therapy for adolescents with anorexia nervosa. J Am Acad Child Adolesc Psychiatry 1999;38:1482-9.

[32]   Eisler I, Dare C, Russell G, Hodes M, Russell G, Dodge E, Le Grange D. Family therapy for adolescent anorexia nervosa: The results of a controlled comparison of two family interventions. J Child Psychol Psychiatr 2000;41:727-36.

[33]   Haworth-Hoeppner S. The critical shapes of body image: The role of culture and family in the production of eating disorders. J Marriage Fam 2000;62:212-27.

[34]   Treasure J. Anorexia nervosa: A survival guide for families, friends and sufferers. East Sussex: Psychol Press, 1999.

[35]   Le Grange D, Eisler I, Dare C, Russell GFM. Evaluation of family treatments in adolescent anorexia nervosa: a pilot study. Int J Eat Disord 1992;12(4):347-57.

[36]   Krauttera T, Lock J. Is manualized family-based treatment for adolescent anorexia nervosa acceptable to patients? Patient satisfaction at the end of treatment. J Fam Therapy 2004;26:66-82.

[37]   Dare C, Eisler I, Russell G, et al. Psychological therapies for adults with anorexia nervosa: a randomized controlled trial of out-patient treatments. Br J Psychiatry 2001;178:216-21.

[38]   Dare C. The place of psychotherapy in the management of anorexia nervosa. In: Holmes J, ed. Psychotherapy in psychiatric practice. Edinburgh: Churchill Livingstone, 1991:395-418.

[39]   Le Grange D, Lock J, Dymek M. Family-based therapy for adolescents with bulimia nervosa. Am J Psychother 2003;57:237.

[40]   Dodge E, Hodes M, Eisler I, Dare C. Family therapy for bulimia nervosa in adolescents: An exploratory study. J Fam Therapy 1995;17:59-77.

[41]   Lock J, Le Grange D, Agras, S, Dare C. Treatment manual for anorexia nervosa: A family-based approach. New York: Guilford, 2001.

[42]   Le Grange D, Crosby R, Rathouz P, Levental B. A randomized controlled comparison of family-based treatment and supportive psychotherapy for adolescent bulimia nervosa. Arch Gen Psychiatry 2007;64(9):1049-56.

[43]   Schmidt U, Lee S, Beecham J, et al. A randomized controlled trial of family therapy and cognitive behavior therapy guided self-care for adolescents with bulimia nervosa and related disorders. Am J Psychiatry 2007;164:5918.

[44] American Psychiatric Association. Practice guidelines for eating disorders. Am J Psychiatry 1993;150(2):212-28.

[45] American Psychiatric Association. Treatment of patients with eating Disorders, third ed. Arlington, VA: APA, 2006.

[46] National Collaborating Centre for Mental Health. Core interventions in the treatment and management of anorexia nervosa, bulimia nervosa and related eating disorders. London: Gaskell, 2004.

[47] Beumont P, Hay P, Beumont D, et al., Australian and New Zealand clinical practice guidelines for the treatment of anorexia nervosa. Aust NZ J Psychiatry 2004;38(11-12):659-70.

[48] White M, Epston D. Narrative means to therapeutic ends. New York: Norton, 1990.

In: Food, Nutrition and Eating Behavior
Editors: Joav Merrick and Sigal Israeli

ISBN: 978-1-62948-233-0
© 2014 Nova Science Publishers, Inc.

Chapter 17

STUDENT FOOD DECISIONS

Jennifer L Zuercher, PhD, RD and Sibylle Kranz, PhD, RD*

Department of Foods and Nutrition, Purdue University, West Lafayette, Indiana, US

ABSTRACT

Though all age groups have been impacted, late adolescents, including college students, have experienced some of the largest increases in obesity. Poor eating habits contribute to excessive body weight and other health issues. Unfortunately, college students do not tend to eat well. Further, eating habits developed during the college years often persist beyond graduation. Although dietary recommendations, gender, and place of residence are among the most frequently researched influences on college students' food selections and diet quality, awareness of how these factors moderate students' food choices is necessary to facilitate the development of more effective educational and environmental interventions, and to better prepare students to move beyond college with a better understanding about how to make healthier food choices and keep themselves well. The objective of this review was to elucidate and describe the factors that influence college students' food choices.

INTRODUCTION

Overweight and obesity continue to be at the forefront of health concerns in the United States. Some of the largest increases in overweight and obesity have been observed among late adolescents and young adults. Between 1991 and 2001, obesity among 18-29 year olds doubled from 7.1% to 14% (1, 2). More recently, Behavioral Risk Factor Surveillance System (BRFSS) 2009 data indicate that among 18 to 24 year olds, 25.3% and 17.8% are overweight and obese, respectively (3). Similarly, of those college students who completed the National College Health Assessment in 2010, 21.9% were overweight and 11.6% were obese (4).

* Correspondency: Sibylle Kranz, PhD, RD, Associate Professor, Department of Nutrition Science, Purdue University, 700 W State Street, West Lafayette, IN 47907 United States. E-mail: kranz@purdue.edu.

The period of life from the late teens to the mid-20s is characterized by much "change and exploration". Leaving home for college demands taking greater responsibility for one's own day-to-day activities. Unfortunately, college students frequently engage in risky health behaviors, including poor eating habits, that worsen throughout their college careers (5, 6), putting them at risk for serious diet-related health problems in the short term as well as in the future. Improving these behaviors and health during this malleable life-stage for the over 11 million 18-24 year olds enrolled in college in the United States (7) is a substantial challenge. The objective of this review is to discuss the factors that contribute to the food intake decisions made by college students.

KNOWLEDGE

Though knowledge of healthy eating practices is not necessarily associated with putting that information into practice, students who have a better knowledge of and familiarity with the Dietary Guidelines (8) do tend to have better eating habits (9). Additionally, students who perceive themselves as "healthy eaters" likely consume a "healthy diet" more often than those who don't perceive themselves as healthy (10). Unfortunately, research suggests that college students generally have a low level of familiarity with particular topics related to nutritional guidelines, including healthful eating (11), and find incorporating variety into their diets challenging (12). College students are often not meeting MyPyramid food group recommendations (13, 14), with fruits and vegetables, as well as fiber (15, 16), cited most frequently as areas for concern. According to the most recent National College Health Assessment (4), 64% of college students are consuming two or fewer servings of fruits and vegetables per day (roughly one cup total) compared to the 2.0 cups of fruit and 2.5 to 3.0 cups of vegetables per day recommended for this age group (14). Further, highly-processed convenience-type foods (i.e., fried potatoes, whole grain bread/rolls, and Mexican mixtures) are frequently cited as main fiber sources (17), resulting in mean fiber intakes well below the DRI recommendation of 14 g/1000 kcal (18-20). This reliance on convenience foods that are easily accessible, low in cost, and require a short preparation time, adds to the complexity of promoting healthy food choices among college students (21).

One method of providing nutrition information to the consumer, Point-of-Purchase (POP) labeling, is intended to facilitate informed food choices. A review of studies assessing the impact of labeling revealed mostly positive, though weak, associations with healthier food choices (22). Studies specifically focused on providing POP nutritional information in on-campus food establishments, including campus convenience stores and dining facilities, indicate that POP labels providing nutrient information (23, 24) and promotional messages (25,26) are effective in encouraging students to choose healthier food items and increasing purchases of labeled items. The effectiveness of POP labels among college students is encouraging and warrants additional efforts to assess the circumstances and individual characteristics associated with their use.

Gender

Gender plays a significant role in food decision-making among college students. For instance, females are more mindful about food-related decisions (27) and nutrition trends (28) than males. This is likely a consequence of inherent gender differences related to health in that men tend to have less healthy lifestyles than women (29). Further, females are more likely than males to use POP information to make more informed choices in the dining hall (30,31) and at fast food restaurants (32).

Among those living on their own, males have been found to have a low level of participation in food preparation in spite of similar self-reported adequacy of cooking skills between genders (33). Increasing participation in food preparation for both males and females can increase the likelihood that the student will have a dietary intake that meets the Healthy People 2010 recommendations (33).

RESIDENCE

Place of residence (i.e., campus dormitories, off-campus apartments, living at home) influences dietary choice as well. Regardless of residence, college students generally do not meet food group recommendations, though those living on campus generally have healthier intakes than those living off campus or with their parents (34). Consistent trends over the last 30 years suggest that students living on campus tend to eat more fruits and vegetables than those living off campus (35, 36), and those living off campus have less variety in their intake of fruits, vegetables, and dairy products (37).

There is some evidence that students living off campus are more likely to be overweight or obese than those living on campus or with their parents (37). A contributing factor may be the greater variety of foods as well as the increased consumption (13) of nutrient dense foods (i.e., fruits and vegetables) by those living on-campus compared to those living off campus. While students living off campus engage in food purchasing and preparation activities more frequently than those living on campus, the majority of young adults are not engaging in these activities, with more than one-third of participants in one study reporting that they did not have enough time for food preparation (33).

Parental influence on food decisions generally decreases when children gain more independence and again when they move away to college. In spite of this, parents' contributions to foods in the dorm room, including among students enrolled in a university/college meal plan, demonstrate continued parental influence (38). Unfortunately, as researchers discovered, the foods purchased by parents may in fact be less healthy than the foods purchased by the students. Additional exploration into the intricacies of familial influence on college students' dietary intake is needed.

CONCLUSION

Students living both on- and off-campus face challenges in making healthy food choices. Their desire for convenience combined with the lack of concern for their health complicate the transition to a healthy, yet independent lifestyle. Feasible methods for positively influencing the food choices of male and female college students living both on- and off-campus that are inexpensive and unobtrusive need to be identified and examined further. Additional research and behavioral studies are needed to help facilitate healthy eating practices among college students.

ACKNOWLEDGEMENTS

Special thanks to Mary Brauchla for her research assistance and Onikia Esters for her thoughtful advice on this project.

REFERENCES

[1]   Mokdad AH, Ford ES, Bowman BA, Dietz WH, Vinicor F, Bales VS, et al. Prevalence of obesity, diabetes, and obesity-related health risk factors, 2001. JAMA 2003(289):76-69.
[2]   Mokdad A, Serdula M, Dietz W, Bowman B, Marks J, Koplan J. The spread of the obesity epidemic in the United States, 1991-1998. JAMA 1999;282:1519-22.
[3]   Centers for Disease Control and Prevention (CDC). Behavioral Risk Factor Surveillance System Survey Data. Atlanta, GA: US Department of Health and Human Services, Centers for Disease Control and Prevention; 2009.
[4]   American College Health Association. American College Health Association National College Health Assessment II: Reference Group Executive Summary Spring 2010. Linthicum, MD: American College Health Association, 2010.
[5]   Storer J, Cychosz C, Anderson D. Wellness behaviors, social identities and health promotion. Am J Health Behav 1997;21:260-8.
[6]   Berman W, Sperling M. Parental attachment and emotional distress in the transition to college. J Youth Adolesc 1991;20:427-40.
[7]   US Department of Education, National Center for Education Statistics. Digest of Education Statistics, 2008 (NCES 2009-020), Chapter 3. 2009. Accessed 2011 Feb 22. URL: http://nces.ed.gov/ fastfacts/display.asp?id=98.
[8]   US Department of Agriculture, US Department of Health and Human Services. Dietary Guidelines for Americans, 2010. 7th Edition. Washington, DC: US Government Printing Office, 2010.
[9]   Kolodinsky J, Harvey-Berino J, Berlin L, Johnson R, Reynolds T. Knowledge of current Dietary Guidelines and food choice by college students: better eaters have higher knowledge of dietary guidance. J Am Diet Assoc 2007;107(8):1409-13.
[10] Kendzierski D, Costello M. Healthy eating self-schema and nutrition behavior. J Applied Soc Psych 2004;34(12):2437-51.
[11] McArthur L, Grady F, Rosenberg R, Howard A. Knowledge of college students regarding three themes related to dietary recommendations. Am J Health Studies 2000;16(4):171-8.
[12] Anding JD, Suminski RR, Boss L. Dietary intake, body mass index, exercise, and alcohol: are college women following the Dietary Guidelines for Americans? J Am Coll Health 2001;49:167-71.
[13] Brown LB, Dresen RK, Eggett DL. College students can benefit by participating in a prepaid meal plan. J Am Diet Assoc 2005;105(3):445-8.
[14] US Department of Agriculture, Center for Nutrition Policy and Promotion. MyPyramid Food Guidance System. Washington, DC: Center for Nutrition Policy and Promotion; 2005. Accessed 2011 Feb 22. URL: http://www.mypyramid.gov/index.html.
[15] Huang T, Harris K, Lee R, Nazir N, Born W, Kaur H. Assessing overweight, obesity, diet, and physical activity in college students. J Am Coll Health 2003;52(2):83-6.

[16]   Center for Disease Control and Prevention. Behavioral Risk Factor Surveillance System WEAT: Web Enabled Analysis Tool. Atlanta, GA 2005. Accessed 2011 Feb 22. URL: http://apps.nccd.cdc.gov/s_broker/WEATSQL.exe/weat/freq_Year.hsql.

[17]   Byrd-Williams CE, Strother ML, Kelly LA, Huang TTK. Dietary fiber and associations with adiposity and fasting insulin among college students with plausible dietary reports. Nutrition 2009;25(9):896-904.

[18]   Bryd-Bredbenner C, Finckenor M. The dietary fiber and fat intake, dietary fat avoidance patterns, and diet-disease knowledge of college women. Int Electronic J of Hlth Educ 2001;4:105-10.

[19]   Institute of Medicine of the National Academy of Sciences. Dietary Reference Intakes for Energy, Carbohydrate, Fiber, Fat, Fatty Acids, Cholesterol, Protein, and Amino Acids (Macronutrients). Washington, DC: National Academy Press, 2002.

[20]   Rose N, Hosig K, Davy B, Serrano E, Davis L. Whole-grain intake is associated with Body Mass Index in college students. J Nutr Educ Behav 2007;39(2):90-4.

[21]   Betts N, Amos R, Keim K, Peters P, Stewart B. Ways young adults view foods. J Nutr Educ 1997;29(2):73-9.

[22]   Harnack LJ, French SA. Effect of point-of-purchase calorie labeling on restaurant and cafeteria food choices: A review of the literature. Int J Behav Nutr Phys Act [serial on the Internet] 2008;5(51).

[23]   Chu YH, Frongillo EA, Jones SJ, Kaye GL. Improving patrons' meal selections through the use of point-of-selection nutrition labels. Am J Public Health 2009;99(11):2001-5.

[24]   Freedman M, Connors R. Point-of-purchase nutrition information influences food-purchasing behaviors of college students: A pilot study. J Am Diet Assoc 2010;110(8):1222-6.

[25]   Buscher LA, Martin KA, Crocker S. Point-of-purchase messages framed in terms of cost, convenience, taste, and energy improve healthful snack selection in a college foodservice setting. J Am Diet Assoc 2001;101:909-13.

[26]   Peterson S, Duncan D, Null D, Roth S, Gill L. Positive changes in perceptions and selections of healthful foods by college students after a short-term point-of-selection intervention at a dining hall. J Am Coll Health 2010;58(5):425-31.

[27]   Levi A, Chan KK, Pence D. Real men do not read labels: The effects of masculinity and involvement on college students' food decisions. J Am Coll Health 2006;55(2):91-8.

[28]   Glanz K, Basil M, Maibach E, Goldberg J, Snyder D. Why Americans eat what they do: taste, nutrition, cost, convenience, and weight control concerns as influences on food consumption. J Am Diet Assoc 1998;98:1118-26.

[29]   Courtenay WH. Engendering health: A social constructionist examination of men's health beliefs and behaviors. Psychol Men Masculinity 2000;1(1):4-15.

[30]   Driskell JA, Schake MC, Detter HA. Using nutrition labeling as a potential tool for changing eating habits of university dining hall patrons. J Am Diet Assoc 2008;108(12):2071-6.

[31]   Conklin M, Cranage D, Lambert C. College students' use of point of selection nutrition information. Top Clin Nutr 2005;20(2):97-108.

[32]   Gerend MA. Does calorie information promote lower calorie fast food choices among college students? J Adolesc Health 2009;44(1):84-6.

[33]   Larson N, Perry C, Story M, Neumark-Sztainer D. Food preparation by young adults is associated with better diet quality. J Am Diet Assoc 2006;106(12):2001-7.

[34]   Laska M, Larson N, Neumark-Sztainer D, Story M. Dietary patterns and home food availability during emerging adulthood: do they differ by living situation? Public Health Nutr 2010;13(2):222-8.

[35]   Beerman K, Jennings G, Crawford S. The effect of student residence on food choice. J Am Coll Health 1990;38:215-20.

[36]   Melby C, Femea P, Sciacca J. Reported dietary and exercise behaviors, beliefs and knowledge among university undergraduates. Nutr Res 1986;6:799-808.

[37]   Brunt A, Rhee Y. Obesity and lifestyle in U.S. college students related to living arrangements. Appetite 2008;51:615-21.

[38]   Nelson M, Story M. Food environments in university dorms: 20,000 calories per dorm room and counting. Am J Prev Med 2009;36(6):523-6.

In: Food, Nutrition and Eating Behavior
Editors: Joav Merrick and Sigal Israeli

ISBN: 978-1-62948-233-0
© 2014 Nova Science Publishers, Inc.

Chapter 18

SNACK CONSUMPTION AND ADOLESCENT URBAN SCHOOL GIRLS

Alphonsus N Onyiriuka[1], Eruke E Egbagbe[2] and Eucharia PA Onyiriuka[3]

[1]Department of Child Health, [2]Department of Medicine, University of Benin Teaching Hospital and [3]Department of Health Education and Human Kinetics, Faculty of Education, University of Benin, Benin City, Nigeria

ABSTRACT

The worldwide dramatic increase in the prevalence of obesity in childhood and adolescence has led to a greater public health concerns relating to the dietary and snacking behaviours among the paediatric age group. Objective: To describe the pattern of snack consumption among adolescent Nigerian urban secondary schoolgirls. Methods: In this school-based-cross-sectional study, we assessed the snack consumption pattern of 2,304 adolescent girls (aged 12-19 years) in two urban public girls' only secondary schools selected by balloting. Data was obtained using an anonymous-structured-self-administered questionnaire. All the students were invited to participate. Results: Among the 2,304 participants, 1693(73.5%) admitted consuming snacks in the last two weeks preceding the survey. The contexts in which adolescent girls most frequently snacked were after school but before dinner (74.8%) and during their leisure time while watching television or hanging out with friends (78.3%). The majority (76.4%) of the adolescent girls consumed energy-dense snacks such as meat pie and egg buns along with soft drinks with only 9.4% of them consuming fruits 4-6 days in a week. Taste was the leading factor (88.2%) influencing the choice of type of snack. Among the 1,693 adolescent girls who snacked, 31.6% did so after dinner. Conclusion: The unhealthy snacking behaviours exhibited by adolescent schoolgirls in the present study included low consumption of fruits, consumption of energy-dense snacks along with soft drinks, snacking during leisure time as well as after dinner. Health education for promotion of healthy snacking behaviours should be given more attention in Nigerian school health programmes.

INTRODUCTION

A snack is a light food eaten in between the main meals; breakfast, lunch and dinner. Snacking is a key characteristic of the diet of majority of adolescents and it has been estimated to provide one-fourth to one-third of their daily energy intake (1). The choice of snacks in adolescents is based mainly on taste rather than nutrition, resulting in the tendency to choose salty, high-sugar or high-fat foods as snacks instead of healthier alternatives (2). Soft drinks are one of the most common snack choices among adolescent schoolgirls (3). Among adolescents, fruits and vegetables are chosen less frequently as snacks (2). The dramatic rise in the prevalence of obesity in the paediatric age group in the past three decades has led to concerns about the dietary pattern of children and adolescents (4, 5). In addition, habits acquired during adolescence tend to persist into adulthood. In this context, dietary behaviour developed in adolescence may have a major effect on the risk of chronic disease later in life. It has been emphasized that health-care providers should not only be alert toward unhealthy eating habits and nutrition-related issues among adolescents, but also, provide adequate and timely counselling (6). Health education and promotion in the schools cannot succeed in the absence of a carefully conceived school health programme based on data on snacking pattern. Yet these data are neither well known nor documented (7).

The prevalence of snacking among adolescents varies widely. The report of one study indicated that 80-90% of adolescent females consumed at least one snack per day, with a range of one to seven snacks daily (1). Different snacking rates have been reported from various countries. For instance, 87-88% in USA (2, 8), 62.1% in India (9) and 54.1% in Malaysia (10). A rising trend in the prevalence of snacking among adolescents has been reported (8). Generally speaking, adolescents as a group, are highly receptive to new food products and snack-type meals.

Some undesirable health outcomes that have been linked to snacking include obesity, skipping of meals, unhealthy food choices and poor nutrient intake (11-14). Despite the recognized undesirable health outcome of snacking among adolescents, published studies reporting pattern of snack consumption among Nigerian adolescents is very scarce. A search of the literature indicated that information on the specific contexts in which adolescent Nigerians snack is grossly lacking. The aim of the present study was to describe the pattern of snack consumption among adolescent Nigerian secondary schoolgirls. The knowledge derived from this study will assist those involved in health education and promotion of healthy eating habits among adolescents.

OUR STUDY

This descriptive-cross-sectional study was conducted in two public secondary schools located in Oredo Local Government Area (OLGA), Edo State, Nigeria. The two schools were for girls only. According to Edo State Ministry of Education Statistics, there are nine public secondary schools in the LGA comprising 4 females-only, 3 co-educational and 2 males-only (15). Consent for the study was obtained from the school authorities. The teachers distributed parental consent forms to parents via the students asking for permission for the child to participate in the study. Of the four girls' secondary schools, two were randomly selected by ballot. The total population of students in the two schools selected were school A 1,605 and school B 772, giving a grand total of 2,377 which was the target study population. The survey was designed to include all the students in the two schools. As a consequence, no sampling was performed. The principal of each of the two schools introduced the authors during the morning assembly. Subsequently, we addressed the students in their classrooms on the objectives of the study as well as on how to accurately fill the questionnaire. We also emphasized to the students that the questionnaires were anonymous and that their participation was voluntary.

Data was collected between October and November, 2011, using a structured-anonymous- self-administered questionnaire. The questionnaire was pre-tested on 30 school girls of similar age and class in another girls' only secondary school in the same LGA. The questionnaire was divided into two parts: the first part sought information on socio-demographic data, such as age of participants, the number of people in the household, educational status of father and mother, occupation of father and mother, religion and state of origin. The socio-economic status of the parents was determined using the classification suggested by Ogunlesi et al. (16). This was analyzed via combining the highest educational attainment, occupation and income of the parents (based on the mean income of each educational qualification and occupation). In this Social Classification System, classes I and II represent high social class, class III represents middle social class while classes IV and V represent low social class. In this way, the adolescent girls were categorized into high, middle and low socio-economic groups. The second part consisted of questions relating to pattern of consumption of snacks. The questions included frequency of consumption of snacks in the preceding two weeks, type of snacks, context of consumption of snacks, whether or not soft drinks accompanied the snacks, and various factors influencing choice of snacks. In the present study, the recall day was defined as from when the respondent gets up one day until the respondent gets up the next day (17). A snack is defined as a light food and/or a drink that is consumed outside the main meals. Main meals refer to breakfast, lunch and dinner.

The data were entered into excel spread sheet directly from the pre-coded questionnaire. Computer printouts of the data were reviewed for any information that was out of range. The statistical analysis was performed using the SPSS software package version 12.0. Descriptive statistics such as frequencies, means, ratios, standard deviations, confidence intervals, percentages were used to describe all the variables.

FINDINGS

At the time of this survey, a total of 2,377 female students (1,605 in school A and 772 in school B) were attending the two public, non-boarding girls' secondary schools in the LGA (randomly selected by ballot). Eleven students (8 from school A and 3 from school B) declined to participate. The response rates were 99.5% in school A and 99.6% in school B. The overall response rate was 99.5%. The questionnaires of 62 students were excluded from the final analysis because they were incompletely filled, thereby leaving a total of 2,304 questionnaires (respondents) for data analysis. Students in both schools had similar socio-demographic characteristics, thus further analysis of data was carried out for the combined group of students.

Among the 2,304 participants, 81.5%, 15.8% and 2.7% were from Christian, Muslim and Traditional religion families respectively. Based on the state of origin and the religion, the snacking pattern did not differ. Among the 2,304 participants, 1693 (73.5%) admitted consuming snacks at least once in the last two weeks preceding the day of the interview. The socio-demographic characteristics of the participants are depicted in table 1. More than half of the participants (53.8%) belong to the age group of 14-16 years. The majority of the participants (84.7%) lived with family members and over two-thirds (70.3%) in households with five to seven members. More than half of the participants were from families in the middle socio-economic status. The family SES did not appear to influence the frequency of snacking among adolescent schoolgirls. The snacking pattern of the participants is displayed in table 2 with ready-to-eat energy-dense snack items (meat pie, egg buns, ice cream and soft drinks) being the most frequently consumed. Among adolescent schoolgirls in this study, fruits were not popular as snacks as less than one in ten of the participants consumed fruits 4-6 days in a week. Over three-quarter (76.4%) of the participants consumed the snacks along with soft drinks. As depicted in table 3, snacking after school but before dinner was the most common context for snacking. Majority of the participants who snacked during school recess time admitted skipping breakfast and they purchased meat pie, egg buns and soft drinks from shops near their schools during recess because they were hungry. Comparing the frequency of snacking during the weekend and during the weekdays, it was 73.2% versus 41.5% OR = 1.8. The three leading factors that influenced choice of type of snack consumed were taste, cost and convenience (table 4).

Table 1. Socio-demographic characteristics of participants

Socio-demographic parameter	No(%)	Mean ± SD (95% CI)
Age groups		
Below 14 years	560(24.3)	
14-16 years	1281(55.6)	
17-19 years	463(20.1)	
Total	2304(100.0)	14.5 ±2.0 years (14.4-14.6)
Household members		
2-4 persons	286(12.4)	
5-7 persons	1682(73.0)	
8 or more persons	336(14.6)	
Total	2304(100.0)	4.6 ±1.5 (4.5-4.7)
Socio-economic status (SES) of parents		
High SES	302(13.1)	
Middle SES	1260(54.7)	
Low SES	742(32.2)	
Total	2304(100.0)	
Living arrangement		
Living with parents	1890(82.0)	
Living with guardian	414(18.0)	
Total	2304(100.0)	

Table 2. Snack consumption pattern among 1,693 adolescent school girls
Types of snacks Frequency of consumption per week

	1-3 times/wk	4-6 times/wk
	No*(%)	No*(%)
Soft drinks	1344(79.4)	867(51.2)
Meat pie	1239(73.2)	720(42.5)
Egg buns	1173(69.3)	571(33.7)
Ice cream	1056(62.4)	538(31.8)
Doughnut	1046(61.8)	503(29.7)
Cake	904(53.4)	466(27.5)
Biscuits (sweetened)	848(50.1)	430(25.4)
Plantain chips	633(37.4)	371(21.9)
Fruits	191(11.3)	154(9.1)

* Some respondents cited more than one type of snack.

Table 3. Mean snacking per week among 1,693 adolescent school girls according to seven snacking contexts

Snacking contexts	No* (%)	Mean ±SD	95%
		snacking	Confidence
		per week	Interval (CI)
During school recess time	254(15.0)	0.4±1.8	0.18 -0.62
After school but before dinner	1266(74.8)	4.2±2.0	4.09-4.31
Leisure time (watching TV and hanging out with friends	1325(78.3)	5.0±1.7	4.91-5.09
On the way to or from school	778(46.0)	1.2±1.5	1.09-1.31
Any time	705(41.7)	1.0±2.0	0.85-1.15
While doing homework or working	579(34.2)	1.0±1.9	0.83-1.17
Snacks after dinner	325(19.2)	0.7±1.1	0.58-0.82

SD= Standard Deviation.

* Some respondents cited more than one snacking contexts.

Table 4. Factors influencing choice of type of snack among 1,693 adolescent school girls

Factors	Respondents (adolescent school girls)	
	Number *	Percentage
Taste of snack	1493	88.2
Convenience	1092	64.5
Cost of snack	953	56.3
Conformity with peers	764	45.1
Nutritive value of snack	637	37.6

*Some respondents cited more than one factor.

DISCUSSION

Data from the present study showed that almost three-quarter of adolescent schoolgirls consumed snacks at least once fortnightly. A similar high prevalence of snacking has been reported among adolescent schoolgirls in Syria, Malaysia and India (9, 10, 17). This is not surprising as consumption of snacks is a recognized aspect of adolescent eating behaviour (18, 19). Although more than half of the participants were from families in the middle socio-economic status (SES), this socio-demographic factor did not appear to influence the frequency of snacking. This finding may be explained by the report of previous studies which proposed that social class gradient may fail to reflect because of the homogenizing effects of school experiences, youth culture and peer-group influence among adolescents (20, 21). Consistent with other studies (9, 10), the highest frequency of consuming various types of snacks was once to thrice a week.

The major snack items consumed by adolescent girls in this study were meat pie, egg buns, ice cream and soft drinks. This is generally consistent with the reports of previous studies (10). In contrast to the reports of some previous studies (10, 22), fruits were not popular as snacks as less than one in ten of the participants consumed fruits 4-6 days in a week in the present study. Indeed, those that consumed fruits in the present study did not regard it as snacks. The finding of low fruit consumption frequency is consistent with the report of previous studies (23-25). The practice of low fruit consumption is worrisome as some studies have reported an inverse association between overweight and fruit consumption (26, 28). Given that snacking is a common dietary behavior among adolescent girls, promotion of consumption of nutritious snacks (fruits inclusive) is needed. Soft drinks are known to have a high glycaemic index and are energy dense, consequently are obesity promoting. For instance, in a cluster randomized controlled trial in south west England, a reduction in consumption of soft drinks resulted in a decrease in the number of overweight and obese children over a period of 12 months (29).

In consonance with previous studies (2, 30), the present study revealed that the contexts in which adolescent schoolgirls most frequently snacked include after school but before dinner and during their leisure time. The finding that snacking occurs most frequently after school suggests that girls snack most frequently in the afternoon. This in keeping with the finding in other studies (2, 30). The high frequency of snacking after school may be related to the fact that in the Nigerian school system snacking is not permitted during class time, therefore the first opportunity students have to snack is after school. Another noteworthy snacking context in this study was snacking after dinner. The practice of snacking after dinner represents a major threat to both the present and future health of these adolescent girls because it corresponds to the time of the day when physical activity level is at its lowest. A review of the literature revealed that obesity is due to a chronic imbalance between energy intake and energy expenditure which is exemplified by consumption of energy-dense snacks in the face of low physical activity level after dinner (31). Data from the present study revealed a high prevalence of snacking during leisure time among adolescent girls. This eating behaviour is unhealthy. Given that most of the adolescents spend their leisure time watching television (TV) and home videos, consumption of high-calorie snacks during this sedentary activity will, overtime, results in an imbalance between energy intake and energy expenditure, predisposing to overweight and obesity. This finding linking TV viewing with snacking is not surprising as a previous report has revealed a positive association between TV viewing and snacking (32). In a previous study it was reported that snacking while watching TV is associated with increased overall caloric intake and calories from fat (33). Reports of previous studies indicated that overweight and obesity among school children were directly related to amount of time spent watching TV (34, 35).

In the present study, the leading factors in the adolescent girls' environment that influenced her choice of type of snack included taste, cost and convenience. This finding is consistent the report of previous studies (36). Given that establishment of identity is a key characteristics of the adolescent age group, food (snacks inclusive) choices may convey strong messages about the individual to her family and friends. A pattern of snacking may be adopted as a way of exploring new lifestyles and asserting one's independence. However, the adopted pattern of snacking may affect health adversely. One limitation of the present study is that it involved only girls, therefore the results cannot be generalized to include boys.

In conclusion, areas of unhealthy snacking practices among adolescent schoolgirls in the present study included low consumption of fruits, consumption of energy-dense snacks along with soft drinks and snacking after dinner.

REFERENCES

[1]   Bigler-Doughten S, Jenkins RM. Adolescent snacks: nutrient density and nutritional contribution to total intake. J Am Diet Assoc 1987; 87(12):1678-9.

[2]   Cross AT, Babicz D, Cushman LF. Snacking patterns among 1800 adults and children. J Am Diet Assoc 1994;94(12):1398-1403.

[3]   Ludwig DS, Peterson KE, Gortmaker SL. Relation between consumption of sugar-sweetened drinks and childhood obesity: a prospective, observational analysis. Lancet 2001;357:505-8.

[4]   Lobstein T, Baur L, Uauy R. Obesity in children and young people: a crisis in public health. Obes Rev 2004;5:4-104.

[5]   Nicklas TA, Baranwosski T, Cullen KW, Berenson G. Eating patterns, dietary quality and obesity. J Am Coll Nutr 2001;20:599-608.

[6]   Mascarenhas MR, Zemel BS, Tershakovec AM, Stallings VA. Adolescence. In: Bowman BA, Rusell RM eds. Present knowledge in nutrition, 8th ed. Washington DC: International Life Institutes Press, 2001:426-38.

[7]   Dukes G, Helsing E. Food and drugs: the peril of plenty. World Health Forum 1992;13:218-21.

[8]   Jahns L, Siega-Riz AM, Popkin BM. The increasing prevalence of snacking among US children from 1977 to 1996. J Pediatr 2001; 138:493-8.

[9]   Shrivastav M, Thomas S. Snack consumption among underprivileged adolescent girls. Indian Pediatr 2010;47:888-90.

[10]   Chin YS, Mohd Nasir MT. Eating behaviours among female adolescents in Kuantan District, Pahang, Malaysia. Pak J Nutr 2009;8(4):425-32.

[11]   Nicklas TA, Yang SJ, Baranowski T, Zakari I, Berenson G. Eating patterns and obesity in children: The Bogalusa Heart Study. Am J Prev Med 2003;25:9-16.

[12]   Cusatis DC, Shannon BM. Influences on adolescent eating behavior. J Adolesc Health 1996;18:27-34.

[13]   Haapalahti M, Mykkanen H, Tikkanen S, Kokkonen J. Meal patterns and food use in 10-to-11-year-old Finnish children. Public Health Nutr 2003;6:365-70.

[14]   Sjorberg A, Hallberg L, Hoglund D, Huithen L. Meal pattern, food, choice, nutrient intake and life style factors in The Goteborg Adolescent Study. Eur J Clin Nutr 2003;57:1569-78.

[15]   Ministry of Education. Directory of pre-primary, primary, junior and senior secondary institutions in Edo State. Benin City: Department Planning Research Statistics, 2006.

[16]   Ogunlesi TA, Dedeke IOF, Kuponiyi OT. Socio-economic classification of children attending specialist paediatric centres in Ogun State, Nigeria. Nig Med Pract 2008;54(1):21-5.

[17]   Lock K, Pomerleau J, Causer L, Altmann DR, Mckee M. The global burden of disease attributable to low consumption of fruit and vegetables: implication for the global strategy on diet. Bull World Health Organ 2005;83:100-8.

[18]   Qotba H, Al-Isa AN. Anthropometric measurements and dietary habits of school children in Qatar. Int J Food Sci Nutr 2007;58:1-5.

[19]   Bin Zaal AA, Musaiger AO, D'Souza R. Dietary habits associated with obesity among adolescent in Dubai, United Arab Emirates. Nutr Hosp 2009;24:437-44.

[20]   Starfield B, Robertson J, Riley AW. Social class gradients and health in childhood. Ambul Pediatr 2002;2(4):238-46.

[21]   Johansen A, Rasmussen S, Madsen M. Health behaviour among adolescents in Denmark:influence of social class and individual risk factors. Scand J Public Health 2006;34(1):32-40.

[22]   Liu Y, Zhai F, Popkin BM. Trends in eating behaviours among Chinese children (1991-1997). Asia Pac J Clin Nutr 2006;15:72-80.

[23]   Montazerifar F, Karajibani M, Dashipour AR. Evaluation of dietary intake and food patterns of adolescent girls in Sistan and Baluchistan Province, Iran. Functional Foods Health Dis 2012;2(3):62-71.

[24]   Washi SA, Ageib MB. Poor diet quality and food habits are related to impaired nutritional status in 13-to-18-year-old adolescents in Jeddah. Nutr Res 2010;30(8):527-34.

[25]   Paulus D, Saint-Remy A, Jeanjean M. Dietary habits during adolescence: results of the Belgian Adolux Study. Eur J Clin Nutr 2001; 55(2):130-6.

[26]   Hilsen M, Eikemo TA, Bere E. Healthy and unhealthy eating at lower secondary school in Norway. Scand J Public Health 2010;38:7-12.

[27]   Bernard L, Lavallee C, GrayDonald K, Dellsle H. Overweight in Cree schoolchildren and adolescents associated with diet, low physical activity and high television viewing. J Am Diet Assoc 1995; 95:800-2.

[28]   Kelishadi R, Ardalan G, Gheiratmand R, Gouya MM, Razaghi EM, Deavari A, et al. Association of physical activity and dietary behaviours in relation to the body mass index in a national sample or Iranian children and adolescents: CASPIAN Study. Bull World Health Organ 2007;85(1):19-26.

[29]   James J, Thomas P, Cavan D, Kerr D. Preventing childhood obesity by reducing consumption of carbonated drinks: cluster randomised controlled trial. BMJ 2004;328:1237-9.

[30]   Anderson AS, Macintyre S, West P. Adolescent meal patterns: grazing habits in the west of Scotland. Health Bull 1993;51:158-65.

[31]   Galuska DA, Khan LK. Obesity: A public health perspective. In: Bowman BA, Rusell RM, eds. Present knowledge in nutrition, 8th ed. Washington DC: International Life Sciences Institute Press, 2001:531-41.

[32]   Van den Bulck J, Van Mierlo J.Energy intake associated with television viewing in adolescents, a cross-sectional study. Appetite 2004;43:181-4.

[33]   Gore SA, Foster JA, DiLillo VG, Kirk K, Smith West D. Television viewing and snacking. Eating Behav 2003;4:399-405.

[34]   Ramic E, Kapidzic-Durakovic S, Karic E, Batic-Mujanoric O, Alibasic E, Zildzic M. Influence of lifestyle on overweight and obesity in school-age children. Med Arh 2009;63:280-3.

[35]   Robinson TN. Television viewing and childhood obesity. Pediatr Clin North Am 2001;48(4):1017-25.

[36]   Shannon C, Story M, Fulkerson JA, French SA. Factors in the school cafeteria influencing food choices by high school students. J Sch Health 2002;72(6):229-34.

SECTION 5: OBESITY

In: Food, Nutrition and Eating Behavior
Editors: Joav Merrick and Sigal Israeli

ISBN: 978-1-62948-233-0
© 2014 Nova Science Publishers, Inc.

Chapter 19

ALTERNATIVE WAY OF MEASURING FATNESS AMONG RURAL CHILDREN OF BENGALEE ETHNICITY

Gopal Chandra Mandal, PhD and Kaushik Bose, PhD*

Department of Anthropology,Bangabasi College, Kolkata, West Bengal, India
And Department of Anthropology, Vidyasagar University, Paschim Midnapore,
West Bengal, India

The prevalence of childhood obesity has been increasing during the last three decades. Obesity in children is a cause for concern and a new index Body Mass Abdominal Index (BMAI) has been derived by combining two separate indices – weight for height and waist circumference for height ratios. The aim was to measure the common indicators of abdominal adiposity – waist circumference (WC), waist-hip ratio (WHR), waist-height ratio (WHTR), conicity index (CI) and newly proposed body mass abdominal index (BMAI) and study relationship with BMI. Our cross sectional study was undertaken at 20 Integrated Child Development Service (ICDS) centers in Bali Gram Panchayet, Arambag, Hooghly District of West Bengal, India. A total of 1,012 children (boys = 498; girls = 514; all Hindu by religion) aged 2-6 years were included in the present study. The measurements (in centimeters) were taken following Lohman et al. Weight was measured in kg. and mathematically, the BMAI was calculated by multiplying BMI with waist circumference. Pearson's correlation coefficients (r) of the adiposity measures with BMI were calculated. Results showed that no significant correlations were observed for all adiposity measures except BMAI. Moreover, the magnitude of correlations of BMAI were very high ($p < 0.001$) with BMI (boys: $r = 0.907$, girls: $r = 0.881$, sex-combined: $r = 0.894$). Our results provided clear evidence that the new index BMAI had a distinct advantage in that it relates much strongly with overall adiposity (BMI) than the other commonly used indicators of adiposity. Its use may be advantageous in studies dealing with the evaluation of nutritional status of rural preschool children.

* Correspondence: Gopal Chandra Mandal, PhD, Associate Professor, Department of Anthropology, Bangabasi College, Kolkata, India. E-mail: golmal_anth@rediffmail.com.

INTRODUCTION

Obesity is the most rapidly growing form of malnutrition in developed as well as developing countries experiencing an economic transition (1, 2). Obese children are those who are 20 percent above the normal weight for age and they are more prone to become overweight adults as the tendency of obesity in such children persists throughout the life (3). The risk of obesity is two or three times greater for an individual with a family history of obesity and increases further with severe obesity (3). The most significant long-term consequence of obesity is the tracking of obesity from childhood to adulthood and its contribution to adult obesity-related morbidity and mortality (4, 5). The prevalence of childhood obesity has been increasing during the last three decades (6). Obesity has emerged as an epidemic in developed and developing countries during the last quarter of the 20th century affecting high and middle income people (7). The epidemic of childhood obesity is a major public health problem in US, where in 2003-04, 26.2% of children aged 2-5years, 37.2% of children aged 6-11 years and 34.3% of adolescents 12-19 yrs were at risk for overweight (8). Furthermore, the risk of excess body mass and adiposity in young First Nation's children is particularly relevant given their potentially increased risk for type 2 diabetes (9, 10). The economic cost of obesity and associated co-morbidities is skyrocketing which is beyond the capacity of the best health care system in the world (11, 12). Childhood obesity has emerged only recently in India, unlike the West where it existed since long. Obesity in children as young as two years onwards have been reported from Indian populations (13). The study of Wang and Hoy (14, 15) was able to describe both overall and central fat patterning through BMI, waist circumference and multiple skinfold measures, in recognition that overall obesity without excessive central obesity can also be predictive of adverse health outcomes.

Furthermore, obesity in children is a cause for concern because it may predict adult obesity and increased risk of coronary heart disease in adult life (16). Obesity is the result of a caloric imbalance (too few calories expended for the amount of calories consumed) and is mediated by genetic, behavioral, and environmental factors (17).The adiposity in preschool children is measured by using weight for length, waist-to-height index and body mass index (BMI) (18). While BMI is the recommended method for population based screening of children for obesity it was a poor predictor of body fat for individual children (19). Currently increase in weight gain and obesity in preschool children are measured independently either by weight for length index (20), waist − to - hip ratio (21), or BMI for age (20). Another index, waist-to-height ratio relates to abdominal obesity, but recent investigations stated that this ratio should also be adjusted with optimal power of height (22). Cole (23) has already shown that weight for height should be adjusted for age (weight / height) by determining appropriate power of height (p). The optimal value of 'p' is 2, 3, and 2 preschool, at 11 years of age and puberty respectively. Therefore 'p' is variable throughout the infancy and childhood. There is another index, Conicity Index, which is a function of weight, height and waist circumference, but it has been shown in one of the studies that BMI is better than conicity index in predicting coronary artery disease (24). Therefore all these ratios have mathematical complexity, advantages and limitations.

To counter obesity in a population, it is important to know its incidence, trend and differentials. The nutritional status of an individual or of a population can be assessed with clinical, biochemical and anthropometric measurements. Of these anthropometry has the advantage because it is easy to perform and requires simple apparatus (25). Some agents have an affect on obesity, low physical activity, high TV watching and computer usage, high caloric diet and high income (26, 27).

A Canadian Community Health Survey, completed in 2004, reported that Aboriginal children had an obesity prevalence of 20%, which was two and one-half times national average for children (28). In a study, Ng and others (26) found that, there is a high prevalence of overweight and obesity among this sample of Aboriginal children living in northern Quebec. Of particular concern is the level of central adiposity, as demonstrated by high waist circumferences and truncal skinfold thicknesses that are associated with the development of metabolic and cardiovascular diseases. This risk profile is intensified by the accompanying low physical fitness and inadequate activity levels. Further research is necessary to investigate the extent of the impact of excess body mass and unfavorable body fat distribution on disease risk and health outcomes, in conjunction with its relationships with physical fitness and activity levels in Canadian First Nations children.

Only limited data are available from Indian subcontinent about the changes in the prevalence of obesity (29). Recent evidence indicates a disturbing trend of increasing adiposity in developed and developing countries including India (30-32). The earliest age of documentation of this trend appears to be in primary school children and preschoolers in developed countries (33, 34). It would be of interest to determine if a similar trend is observable at an earlier age and that too from a developing country like India, which is currently undergoing a nutritional transition (35).

A hypothetical index for better measuring adiposity – "Body Mass Abdominal Index" (BMAI) was proposed in a recent article (18). The new index has been derived from by combining two separate indices – weight for height and waist for height ratios. The BMAI is mostly influenced by waist circumference which will mostly include fat component. This signifies that the measurement of adiposity is better reflected in BMAI rather than BMI or Waist/Height ratio alone (18). The author (18) stated that, BMAI is a very simple index to use and all the three main body measurements – weight, height, minimum waist circumference are included. The measurement of adiposity is included in BMAI in the form of waist-to-height ratio, therefore BMAI will be an important tool in assessing cardiovascular risk factors in preschool children.

Keeping these in mind, the aim of the present study was to measure the indicators of abdominal adiposity – waist circumference (WC), waist-hip ratio (WHR), waist-height ratio (WHTR), conicity index (CI) and the newly proposed body mass abdominal index (BMAI) and study their relationship with overall adiposity as measured by BMI among the rural Bengalee preschool children from Arambag, Hooghly District, West Bengal, India.

OUR STUDY

The present cross sectional study was undertaken during the period November 2005 to December 2006, at 20 Integrated Child Development Services (ICDS) centers in Bali Gram Panchayet, Arambagh, Hooghly District of West Bengal, India. The study area consists of remote villages located approximately 100 km. from Kolkata, the capital of West Bengal.

Figure 1 shows the area of study. All children (aged 2-6 years old) living in these areas are enrolled at these centers.

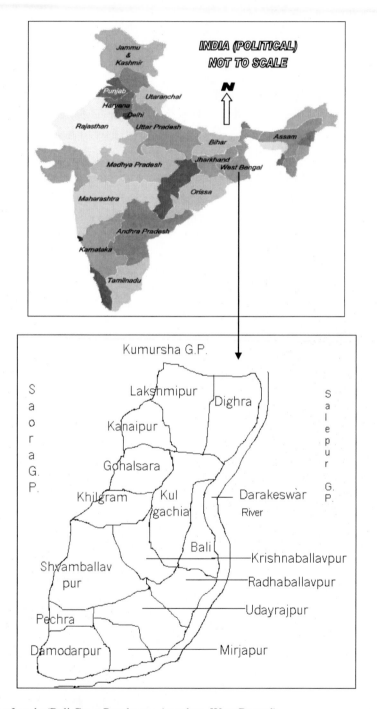

Figure 1. Area of study (Bali Gram Panchayat, Arambag, West Bengal).

The population

A total of 1012 rural Bengalee preschool children comprising of both boys (498) and girls (514) aged 2-6 years old, enrolled in these centers were studied. All children of aged 2 years enrolled their names at these (ICDS) centers and their names get eliminated when they cross the age of 6 years. Information on a number of non-anthropometric variables such as age, sex, were collected using a pre-structured interview schedule. All the children were Hindu by religion. The age and sex distribution of the subjects is given in Table 1. All children were given a daily food supplementation, in the form of porridge, consisting of approximately 60 grams of rice and 20 grams of lentils per day. They were also fed an egg per week.

Table 1. Age and sex distribution of the subjects

Age (years)	Boys	Girls	Total
2	91	92	183
3	125	106	231
4	110	131	241
5	115	124	239
6	57	61	118
Total	498	514	1012

Anthropometric measurements

All the measurements i.e., height, weight, minimum waist circumference, maximum hip circumference were taken following standard method (36) by the first author.

Indices

Body Mass Index (BMI) – a popular indicator of generalized adiposity was calculated following the formula of World Health Organization (37).

BMI = Weight in kg/(Height)^2 in m.

Conicity index (CI) and waist – hip ratio (WHR) – two typical measures of central adiposity were derived using the standard formula.

CI = Minimum waist circumference (cm)/[(0.109 x $\sqrt{}$ { weight (kg) / height (m)}].

WHR = Minimum waist circumference (cm) / Maximum hip circumference (cm).

Another measure of central adiposity, waist – height ratio (WHTR) was calculated also following standard equation.

WHTR = Minimum waist circumference (cm)/height (m).

The new hypothetical index - BMAI (17) was calculated in the following way:

BMAI = Weight / Height X minimum waist circumference / Height

= Weight / (Height)^2 X minimum waist circumference

= BMI X minimum waist circumference

where Weight is in Kg. and Minimum waist circumference and height are in meters.

The BMI includes lean mass and fat components of the body and it is mostly influenced by waist circumference which will mostly include fat component. This signifies that the measurement of adiposity is better reflected in BMAI rather than BMI or Waist / height ratio alone (18).

FINDINGS

Table 2 presents the means and standard deviations of the five important conventional and one new measures of adiposity among the studied preschool children of Bali Gram panchayat, Arambag, Hooghly district, West Bengal, India. Among boys, the mean (sd) values of BMI, WC, WHR, WHTR, CI and BMAI were 13.12 kg/m2 (1.7), 45.3 cm (2.8), 0.97 (0.05), 0.47 (0.04), 1.17 (0.07) and 5.94 kg/m (0.87), respectively. Whereas, in case of girls, the corresponding values were 13.14 kg/m2 (1.5), 44.8 cm (2.8), 0.96 (0.05), 0.47 (0.04), 1.17 (0.07) and 5.88 kg/m (0.78), respectively. The sex combined overall values were 13.13 kg/m^2 (1.6), 45.03cm (2.8), 0.97 (0.05), 0.47 (0.04), 1.17 (0.07) and 5.91 kg/m (0.82) respectively.

**Table 2. Mean values (sd) of the six measures of adiposity
among the studied children**

Measures of adiposity	Boys (n = 498)	Girls (n = 514)	Sex combined (N = 1012)
BMI	13.12 (1.7)	13.14 (1.5)	13.13 (1.6)
WC	45.30 (2.8)	44.80 (2.8)	45.03 (2.8)
WHR	0.97 (0.05)	0.95 (0.05)	0.97 (0.05)
WHTR	0.47 (0.04)	0.47 (0.04)	0.47 (0.04)
CI	1.17 (0.07)	1.17 (0.07)	1.17 (0.07)
BMAI	5.94 (0.87)	5.88 (0.78)	5.91 (0.82)

Standard deviations are presented in parentheses.

Table 3 shows the correlation coefficient (r) of age with adiposity measures among the studied children. Overall (sex combined) waist circumference (r = 0.402) and BMAI (r = 0.166) had positively correlations with age significantly at 0.01 level (p < 0.01). Sex specific results also showed the same trend. However, WHR and WHTR had significant correlation with age but in a negative way. No significant correlations were found in case of CI and BMI. This has been graphically presented in figure 2.

Table 3. Pearson Correlation Coefficient (r) of age with adiposity measures among the children

Measures of adiposity	Boys (N= 498)	Girls (N= 514)	Sex combined (N= 1012)
WC	0.386**	0.427**	0.402**
WHR	-0.297**	-0.320**	-0.310**
WHTR	-0.660**	-0.680**	-0.670**
CI	-0.002	-0.035	-0.035
BMAI	0.152**	0.183**	0.166**
BMI	-0.012	-0.021	-0.015

** = p < 0.01

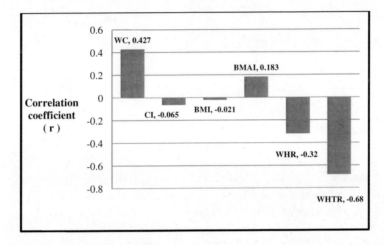

Figure 2. Correlation of age with adiposity measures.

The correlation coefficients (r) of the adiposity measures with BMI are presented in table 4. From the table, it can be seen that no significant correlations were observed for all adiposity measures except BMAI. Among girls, the correlations of WC and CI with BMI were negative. Moreover, the magnitude of correlations of BMAI were very high (p < 0.001) with BMI (boys: r = 0.907, girls: r = 0.881, sex-combined: r = 0.894). The correlation of BMAI with BMI in case of the boys was slightly higher than the girls. This has been graphically presented in figure **3**.

Table 4. Pearson Correlation Coefficients (r) of WC, WHR, WHTR, CI and BMAI with BMI among the studied children

Measures of adiposity	Boys (N= 498)	Girls (N= 514)	Sex combined (N= 1012)
WC	0.005	-0.009	0.023
WHR	0.049	0.010	0.029
WHTR	0.084	0.023	0.054
CI	0.007	-0.017	0.005
BMAI	0.907**	0.881**	0.894**

** = p < 0. 001.

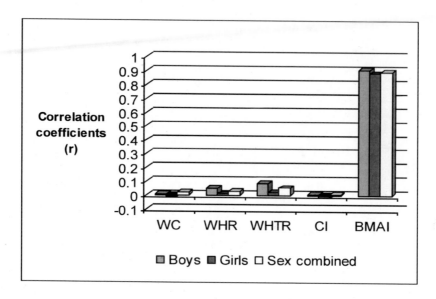

Figure 3. Correlation of BMI with WC, WHR, WHTR, CI and BMAI.

DISCUSSION

Ideally, any acceptable and good adiposity measure must have a strong positive relationship with BMI which is an indicator of overall adiposity. This should be equally true for both sexes. Conversely, an adiposity measure at any particular site which does not have a strong relationship with BMI may accurately reflect regional adiposity, but it fails to relate adequately with overall adiposity (BMI). Hence, it may be of limited use in epidemiological studies, particularly those dealing with the anthropometric evaluation of nutritional status. WHTR is better than WC and BMI at predicting adiposity in children and adolescents. It can be a useful surrogate of body adiposity when skinfold measurements are not available (38).

In conclusion, our results provided clear evidence that the new index BMAI had a distinct advantage in that it relates much strongly with overall adiposity (BMI) than the other commonly used indicators of adiposity. Its use may be advantageous in studies dealing with the evaluation of nutritional status of rural preschool children. A study on 2,016 rural preschool children aged 3-5 years from randomly selected 66 Integrated Child Development Services (ICDS) centres in the Nadia District of West Bengal,India, revealed the strongest correlation ($p < 0.01$) with BMAI (boys: $r = 0.856$, girls: $r = 0.868$, sex-combined: $r = 0.863$). Results of linear regression of adiposity measures with BMI revealed that BMAI had the strongest significant impact ($t = 76.73$) on BMI (39). Thus, there is a valid justification in preferring the use of BMAI over other measures of central adiposity. Our results clearly vindicate the theoretical hypothesis propounded by Kumar (18) regarding the utility and efficacy of BMAI.

However, it is well established that there exits significant ethnic differences in the relationship between regional adiposity and overall adiposity. Thus, we suggest that similar studies, utilizing this new index, be undertaken among other ethnic groups. These would provide us with valuable results as to whether the findings obtained by us holds true across ethnic groups. This is particularly important for country like India which is ethnically heterogeneous. Lastly, it would be of much interest to investigate whether this utility of BMAI holds its validity among individuals of higher age groups also.

ACKNOWLEDGMENTS

All subjects who participated in the study are gratefully acknowledged. Special thanks are due to the ICDS authorities of these centers. Gopal Chandra Mandal received financial assistance in the form of a Minor Research Project from the University Grants Commission, Government of India [PSW-046/03 – 04 (ERO), Dt. 12.03.2004]. Conflict of interest: None

REFERENCES

[1]   Chopra M, Galbirth G, Darnton-Hill. A global response to a global problem; The epidemic of over-nutrition. Bull World Health Organization 2005;80:925-58.

[2]   Madanat HN, Trontman KP and Al-Madi B. The nutrition transition in Jordon: the political, economic and food consumption contexts. Promot Educ 2008;15:6-10.

[3]   Kaur Sangha J, Kaur Pandhar A, Kochhar A. Anthropometric profile and adiposity in the obese Punjabi children and their parents. J Hum Ecol 2006;19(3):159-62.

[4]   Kotani K, Nishida AM, Yamashita S, Funahashi T, Fujioka S, Tokunga K, et al. Two decades of annual medical examination in Japanese obese children: Do obese children grow into obese adults? Int J Obes 1997;21:912-21.

[5]   Whitaker RC, Wright JA, Pepe MS, Seidel KD, Dietz WH. Predicting obesity in young adulthood from childhood and parental obesity. N Engl J Med 1997;337:869-73.

[6]   Golan M, Weizman A, Apter A, Fainaru M. Parents as the exclusive agents of childhood obesity. Am J Clin Nutr 1998;67: 1130-5.

[7]   Popkin BM, Doak CM. The obesity epidemic is a world wide phenomenon. Nutr Rev 1998;56:106-14.

[8]   Ogden CL, Carroll MD, Curtin LR, McDowell MA, Tabak CJ, Flegal KM. Prevalence of overweight and obesity in the US, 1999-2004. JAMA 2006;295:1549-55.

[9]   Young TK, Dean HJ, Flett B and Wood-Steiman P. Childhood obesity in a population at high risk for type 2 diabetes. J Pediatr 2000, 2000;136:365-9.

[10] Dean H. Type 2 diabetes in youth: a new epidemic. Adv Exp Med Biol 2001;498;1-5.

[11] Viad I. Obesity counts UK economy L 2bn a year. BMJ 2003;327: 1308.

[12] Bontayeb A, Bontayeb S. The burden of non-communicable diseases in developing countries. Int J Equity Health 2005;4:2.

[13] Sharma M. Roly poly children make unfit adults. Tribune (Spectrum) 2002 Mar 03.

[14] Wang Z, Hoy WE. Body size measurements as predictors of type 2 diabetes in Aboriginal people. Int J Obes Relat Metab Disord 2004; 28:1580-4.

[15] Wang Z, Hoy WE. Waist circumference, BMI, hip circumference and waist to hip ratio as predictors of cardiovascular diseases in Aboriginal people. Eur J Clin Nutr 2004;58:888-93.

[16] Must A, Strauss RS. Risks and consequences of childhood and adolescent obesity. Int J Obes Relat Metab Disord 1999;23:S 2-11.

[17] Daniels SR, Arnett DK, Eckel RH, et al. Overweight in children and adolescents: Pathophysiology, consequences, prevention, and treatment. Circulation 2005;111:1999-2002

[18] Kumar P. A hypothetical index for adiposity "Body mass abdominal index" – will predict cardiovascular disease risk factors in children. Int J Pediatr Neonat 2009;11:1.

[19] Ellis KJ, Abrams SA, Wong WW. Monitoring childhood obesity: assessment of the weight / height index. Am J Epidemiol 1999;150: 939-46.

[20] Taveras EM, Rifas-Shiman SL, Belfort MB, Kleinman KP, Oken E, Gillman MW. Weight status in the first 6 months of life and obesity at 3 years of age. Pediatrics 2009;123:1173-83.

[21] Li C, Ford ES, Mokdad AH, Cook S. Recent studies in waist circumference and waist – height ratio among US children and adolescents. Pediatrics 2006;118:e1390-8.

[22] Tybor DJ, Lichtenstein AH, Dallal GE, Must A. Waist-to-height ratio is corrected with height in US children and adolescents aged 2-18 years. Int J Pediatr Obes 2008;3(3):148-51.

[23] Cole TJ. Weight/height compared to weight / height 2 for assessing adiposity in childhood: influence of age and bone age on p during puberty. Ann Hum Biol 1986;13(5):433-51.

[24] Kim KS, Owen WL, William D, Sdams-Campbell LL. A comparison between BMI and Conicity index on predicting coronary heart diseases: The Framingham heart study. Ann Epidemiol 2000;10:424-31.

[25] Gholamreza V, Mohsen S. The comparative study of Body Mass Index distribution among preschool children in a 7 years period in North Iran. J Appl Scs 2007;7(18):2681-5.

[26] Ng C, Marshal D, Willows ND. Obesity, adiposity, physical fitness and activity levels in Cree children. Int J Circumpolar Health 2006;65:4.

[27] Kang HT, Ju YS, Park KH, Kwon YJ, Im HJ, Paek DM, Lee HJ. Study on the relationship between childhood obesity and various determinants, including socioeconomic factors, in an urban area. J Prev Med Publ Health 2006;39:371-8.

[28] Shields M. Measured obesity, Overweight Canadian children and adolescents. Statistics Canada. Ottawa: Catalogue no. 82-620- MVVE 2005001, 2005.

[29] Sidhu S, Kaur N and Kaur R. Overweight and obesity in affluent school children of Punjab. Ann Hum Biol 2006;33(2):255-9.

[30] Nunez-Rivers HP, Monge-Rojas R, Leon H, Rosello M. Prevalence of overweight and obesity among Costa Rican elementary school children. Rev Panam Salud Publica 2003;13:24-32.

[31] Livingstone MB. Childhood obesity in Europe: a growing concern. Public Health Nutr 2001;4:109-16.

[32] Kapil U, Sing P, Dwivedi SN, Bhasin S. Prevalence of obesity amongst affluent adolescent school children in Delhi. Indian Pediatr 2002,39:449-52.

[33] Chinn S, Rona RJ. Secular trends in weight, weight-for-height and triceps skinfold thickness in relative weight and adiposity among children over two decades: the Bogalusa Heart Study. Pediatrics 1987;99:420-6.

[34] Chinn S, Rona RJ. Trends in weight-for-height and triceps skinfold thickness for English and Scottish children, 1972-1982 and 1982-1990. Pediatr Perinat Epidemiol 1994;8:90-106.

[35] Sachdev HPS. Recent transitions in anthropometric profile of Indian children: Clinical and public health implications. NFI Bull 2003;24: 6-8.

[36] Lohmann TG, Roche AF, Martorell R. Anthropometric standardization reference manual. Chicago: Human Kinetics Books, 1988.

[37] World Health Organization. Physical status: The use and interpretation of anthropometry: Technical Report Series no. 854. Geneva: World Health Organization, 1995.

[38] Brambilla P, Bedogni G, Heo M, Pietrobelli A. Waist circumference-to-height ratio predicts adiposity better than body mass index in children and adolescents. Int J Obesity 2013;37:943-6.

[39] Biswas S, Bose K. The utility of a new index for adiposity among Pre-school Children. Mal J Nutr 2010;16(3):121-4.

In: Food, Nutrition and Eating Behavior
Editors: Joav Merrick and Sigal Israeli

ISBN: 978-1-62948-233-0
© 2014 Nova Science Publishers, Inc.

Chapter 20

INSULIN SENSITIVITY AND SURROGATES FOR ADIPOSITY IN YOUTH

Robert G McMurray[*], *PhD*[1], *Shrikant I Bangdiwala, PhD*[2,3], *Diane J Catellier, PhD*[2,3] *and Joanne S Harrell, PhD*[4]

[1]Department of Exercise and Sport Science,
[2]Department of Biostatistics,
[3]Collaborative Studies Coordinating Center,
[4]School of Nursing, University of North Carolina at Chapel Hill,
Chapel Hill, North Carolina, US

ABSTRACT

In this chapter we identify which surrogate of adiposity best identifies the risk of insulin resistance (HOMA-IR) in youth and could be used for all ages, both sexes, and both Caucasians and African Americans. The participants were 1,511 youth; 8-17 yrs old, 37.5% African American and 55.4% Caucasians. Cross sectional analyses (ROC & regression) of HOMA-IR and several obesity surrogates. Measurements included fasting insulin and glucose, body mass, height, waist circumference, and triceps & subscapular skinfolds. These were used to determine BMI, BMI percentile (& z-score), waist percentiles, waist to height ratio (WHtR) and the HOMA-IR. The WHtR cut-point derived from the ROC was the same for both sexes; whereas all other surrogates had sex-specific cut-points. Logistic regression to determine the odds ratios for insulin resistance found that the cut-points for all adiposity surrogates were highly associated with HOMA-IR; OR > 6.5. BMI percentiles had the highest OR for the girls, while waist circumference had the highest OR for the boys. WHtR and sum of skinfolds were most consistent for both sexes. The results indicate that all the surrogates for adiposity are useful for assessing the risk of insulin resistance. Although sum of skinfolds may be least influenced by age, sex and race of all the adiposity surrogates, waist-height ratio provides a good alternative for both sexes.

INTRODUCTION

The significance of the relationship between obesity and health risk is clear (1, 2). In addition, childhood obesity appears to be predictive of later development of these maladies (3). Thus, there is ample support for measuring weight status (obesity) as part of clinical screening and epidemiologic study for both children and adults. Body fat can be directly measured by many means; dual energy x-ray absorptiometry (DEXA), underwater weighing, bioelectrical impedance analysis (BIA) or air displacement plethsmography; however, these techniques are not suitable in clinical practice or for large-scale epidemiologic research. Skinfolds can be measured to estimate body fat, but The American Academy of Pediatrics Expert Committee has recommended against their clinical use for defining obesity because of measurement problems (4). Thus, other indirect estimates, or surrogates of body fat have been used, such as body mass index (BMI: body mass/height^2), BMI percentile, BMI z-scores, waist circumference, waist/hip ratio, or waist/height ratio.

Although these indirect measures correlate fairly well with direct measures of body fat, they do have limits of applicability (5). In children, BMI may inadequately reflects body fat and appears to have less predictive value for cardiovascular disease risk than either waist or waist/height ratio (6). Also, in children, the use of BMI percentiles requires age and sex-specific norm tables. Waist circumference may be a better indicator of central adiposity than BMI, but has limitations with children, because waist naturally increases as children grow (6-9). The American Academy of Pediatrics Expert Committee noted that waist circumference may be a good indicator of insulin resistance, but does not recommend its use for determination of obesity, because of the lack of clinical guidelines (4). To counter this argument, Fernandez et al. (10) have proposed to use waist circumference percentiles; but these require the use of race, age, and sex-specific tables to properly interpret the results. Several investigators suggested the use of waist/height ratio (WHtR), especially for children (1, 11, 12). Thus, clinicians and epidemiologists have several choices at their disposal, some quite simple and others requiring age, sex, and race specific tables. From the perspective of the clinician, the optimal surrogate for body fat would be predictive of health risk regardless of age, sex, pubertal stage, and race. Although all of these surrogates for adiposity relate to health risk, the relative predictive capability of each surrogate in children is not clear. While studies have compared some of these surrogates to insulin resistance, to our knowledge no one has compared the strength of the association between all of these surrogates and insulin resistance measured in a large sample of children and adolescents (1, 11).

Therefore, the purpose of this report is to examine the relationship between insulin resistance and surrogates of adiposity in a wide age-group of ethnically mixed children and determine which surrogate is most strongly associated with, and which best identifies the risk for insulin resistance while being least influenced by age, sex and ethnicity.

OUR STUDY

The participants in the study were 1,511 children and adolescents from the Cardiovascular Health in Children Study (CHIC II & III; J.S. Harrell, P.I.). The sample consisted of volunteers obtained from ten schools in eastern North Carolina. They ranged in age from eight to 17 years and were mostly Caucasians (55.4%) and African American (37.5%), with small proportions of Hispanics, Asians, and those who self defined as "other". Before participation in the study consent was obtained from a parent and assent was obtained from the child, using University IRB approved forms.

Procedures

All measurements were obtained at the schools. Age, sex, and ethnicity were self-reported and verified with school records. Pubertal status was estimated using the Pubertal Development Scale (PDS), which is a self-administered questionnaire with 5-item subscales, one for each gender (13). Height was measured to the nearest 0.1 cm using a stadiometer (Perspective Enterprises, Kalamazoo, MI, USA). Body mass was measured to the nearest 0.1 kg using either a balance beam scale (Detecto Scale, Model 439) or an electronic scale (Scaletronix, White Plains, NY, USA). BMI (kg/m^2) was computed from these measures and BMI percentiles were extracted from sex and age specific growth chart data using the SAS program from the CDC website. Waist circumference was measured in the horizontal plane at a site just above the iliac crest as recommended by the NHANES III (14). Waist measurements were done on bare skin with subjects standing erect, on both feet, after a normal minimal inspiration. Waist percentiles were derived from Fernandez et al. (10). Triceps and subscapular skinfolds were measured using a Lange skinfold caliper. Each measurement was made in triplicate following NHANES III procedures and the average of the three measures used for analysis (14). All research assistants were trained to measure each adiposity surrogate and met strict certification criteria to insure quality control.

Venous blood samples were obtained from 7 to 9 am, after an overnight fast. The fast was verified and youth not fasting were excluded. The blood samples were immediately processed and placed on dry ice for shipment back to the chemistry laboratory, where they were stored at −80°C. The serum glucose levels were measured using a Johnson and Johnson 950 automated chemistry system (UNC Hospital Core Chemistry Lab; certified by the College of American Pathologists). Insulin was measured from fasting plasma specimens by Penn Laboratory (MedStar Research Institute, Washington, DC, USA) using radio-immunoassay technique (RIA). Any hemolyzed samples were not analyzed. To estimate insulin resistance (IR) HOMA-IR values were computed from glucose and insulin measures (15): (glucose [mmol/L] x insulin [μU/L])/22.5.

Analytical methods

Means and standard deviations were computed for all variables of interest by sex. Pearson correlations were computed between all the surrogates of adiposity, as well as between the surrogates and the markers of glucose status (glucose, insulin and HOMA-IR). Although no standard definition of insulin resistance exists, for the purposes of developing the receiver operating characteristic (ROC) curves, the presence of insulin resistance was defined by a HOMA-IR = 4.0 as suggested by Bonora et al. (16) and Reinehr et al. (17). ROC curves were constructed by plotting the sensitivity and specificity for all possible values of each surrogate against a HOMA-IR of = 4.0 (18). The area under the ROC curve (AUC) represents the probability of correctly distinguishing between the presence and absence of insulin resistance. A surrogate that correctly classified insulin resistant individuals 100% of the time and never misclassifies individuals as insulin resistant would result in an ROC curve that has an AUC = 1, while an AUC = 0.5 suggests a predictive capability that is no better than chance. Our overall intent was to determine which surrogate most strongly identified the risk of insulin resistance for all youth, regardless of age, sex, and ethnicity. However, we did analyze the data (ROC curves) by sex to determine if one surrogate better identified insulin resistance for each sex.

The critical or cut-point value for each adiposity surrogate was defined as the value that minimized overall misclassification (i.e., least false positive and false negative results) and was determined from the ROC curves. Differences in the accuracy of detection of insulin resistance across surrogates were assessed by pair-wise comparisons of AUC statistics using the method described by Hanley and McNeil (18). Curves for BMI z-scores were not presented, since their rank ordering was identical to the BMI percentile (overlapping ROC curves). Then, each of the surrogate variables were dichotomized using the critical or cut point value and the odds ratio of insulin resistance (HOMA-IR = 4.0) was estimated using logistic regression, first overall and then by sex. Data were analyzed using SAS v.9.1 (SAS Institute, Cary, NC) and MedCalc v.9.1 (source www.medcalc.be) statistical software packages.

Finally, multiple regression models were run to determine which of the surrogates for obesity was least influenced by age, sex and ethnicity; thus, would be most generally useful to identify potential insulin resistance in a clinical or screening setting. The presence or absence of insulin resistance (HOMA-IR = or < 4.0; coded 0 or 1) was the dependent variable, while the independent variables were one of the adiposity surrogates dichotomized by the cut point risk level (coded 0 or 1), age, sex and ethnicity.

FINDINGS

The 1,511 children and adolescents ranged in age from 8 to 17 years of age, with about half girls and boys. Fifty five percent of the children were Caucasian, with about 37% African American, 2% Hispanic/Latino and 5% other. Their characteristics are presented by their insulin resistance (IR) status in table 1. Three hundred ninety four, or 26%, were found to have HOMA-IR values above 4.0, suggestive of insulin resistance. This IR group consisted of 252 girls and 142 boys (χ^2; p= 0.0001) and was 67% Caucasian and 25% African American (χ^2; P = 0.0001). The IR group was similar in age to the non-IR youth, but differed from the non-IR group in all other variables listed in Table 1 (P < 0.05). Sex differences were compared within the two groups. In those youth with normal insulin status (HOMA-IR < 4.0), there were no significant sex-differences in height, body mass, waist, waist percentile, or waist height ratio (P > 0.05), but there were differences by sex in other variables. Compare to the girls, the boys were slightly older, had higher BMI percentiles (or BMI z-scores), and blood glucose concentrations (P < 0.005), but had significantly lower skinfolds, BMIs, circulating insulin concentrations, and HOMA-IR (P < 0.001). In the insulin resistant group, the boys were slightly taller than the girls and had a lower sum of skinfolds (P < 0.008); no other sex-related differences existed.

Table 1. Characteristics of the participants, presented by insulin resistance status[a] and gender (mean±SD)

Characteristic	Normal		Insulin Resistant[a]	
	Females	Males	Females	Males
	(n = 500)	(n=617)	(n=252)	(n=142)
Age (y)	11.5±3.0	11.0±2.7[*]	11.4±2.6	11.8±2.7
Height (cm)	147±13	148±16	152±10	155±15[*]
Body Mass (kg)	44.4±15.3	45.3±16.6	62.7±21.1	65.5±24.0
BMI (kg/m^2)	20.3±4.3	20.1±4.1	26.9±6.9	26.4±6.4
BMI percentile	64.7±26.6	69.4±26.7[*]	90.6±15.1	89.7±18.2
BMI z-score	0.49±1.00	0.67±1.05[*]	1.71±0.84	1.70±0.90
Waist (cm)	67.1±11.0	67.9±11.6	82.2±15.5	85.3±17.2
Waist Percentile	48.4±27.9	51.7±29.9	80.1±19.4	79.5±23.2
WHtR	0.46±0.06	0.46±0.06	0.54±0.09	0.55±0.10
SSF (mm)	24.5±11.8	20.3±11.1[*]	42.8±17.2	35.9±16.6[*]
Glucose (mmol/L)	4.80±0.60	4.96±0.42[*]	5.14±0.58	5.25±0.59
Insulin (mmol/L)	84±28	76±31[*]	197±88	194±85
HOMA-IR	2.47±0.80	2.30±0.80[*]	6.23±2.81	6.28±3.02

[a] Insulin resistance: HOMA-IR> 4.0.

[*] p< 0.01; females vs. males.

Note: The insulin resistant group was significantly different from the normal group in all variables except age.

The values from the ROC curves, summarizing the ability of the adiposity surrogates to predict the presence of insulin resistance are presented in table 2. Overall and sex-specific curves were fairly similar, with the AUC ranging from 76 to 84%; all had fairly narrow confidence limits. The overall AUC for body mass was found to be significantly less than for the other measures (P < 0.05). All other methods were fairly similar in the ability to correctly classify insulin resistant participants. The critical or cut-points values were derived from the ROC curves and represented the value at which there were the fewest misclassifications. Body mass produced the overall most misclassifications and a very large proportion of false negative predictions. Except for body mass, the cut-points for the other six adiposity surrogates resulted in more false positive (False +) predictions of IR than false negative (False -) predictions.

The sex-specific ROC analyses are also presented in table 2. The critical, or cut-point, values for WHtR were the same for the boys and girls and there was only a one 1 mm difference in skinfolds between the sexes. The cut-point values differed somewhat by sex, as the BMI, waist circumference and waist percentile cut-points were lower for the girls than the boys. In contrast, the cut-point values for BMI percentiles and body mass were higher for the girls than the boys and resulted in more false positive than false negative misclassifications especially for the boys. The use of BMI percentile resulted in fewer misclassifications for the girls than the boys (23% vs. 37.7%, respectively); whereas waist circumference resulted in fewer misclassifications for the boys than the girls (19.4% vs.25.5%, respectively).

Table 2. Area under the ROC curve (AUC)[a] and critical or cut-point value[b] for the relationship between the adiposity surrogates[c] and the HOMA-IR. Also presented are the percentage of false positive (+) and false negative (-) classification based on the critical value

	BMI	BMI	ΣSF	Waist	Waist	WHtR	Mass
	kg/m^2	%tile	mm	cm	%tile	cm/cm	kg
Overall							
AUC	0.812	0.812	0.818	0.796	0.799	0.791	0.766
95% C.I.	.79-.83	.79-.83	.80-.84	.78-.82	.78-.82	.77-.81	.74-.79
Value	23.5	89th	27.3	73.9	75th	0.49	40.2
False +	13.5%	19.9%	18.6%	19.3%	12.6%	16.3%	2.5%
False -	9.0%	6.3%	6.3%	7.9%	9.7%	7.8%	37.8%
Girls							
AUC	0.817	0.839	0.821	0.802	0.819	0.801	0.772
95% C.I.	.79-.84	.81-.86	.79-.85	.77-.83	.79-.85	.77-.83	.74-.80
Value	23.1	89th	27.3	74.5	50th	0.49	49.7
False +	12.5%	15.3%	19.6%	14.1%	21.7%	13.4%	9.6%
False -	11.0%	7.7%	6.4%	11.4%	5.9%	10.1%	21.5%
Boys							
AUC	0.804	0.790	0.791	0.800	0.785	0.781	0.764
95% C.I.	.77-.83	.76-.82	.76-.82	.77-.83	.75-.81	.75-.81	.73-.79
Value	23.5	83rd	28.3	79.5	75th	0.49	44.5
False +	15.7%	34.3%	16.2%	12.5%	15.9%	19.1%	3.7%
False -	6.3%	3.4%	6.5%	6.9%	6.7%	5.5%	32.0%

[a] AUC: 1=100% or perfect agreement and 0.5 = 50% or purely chance.
[b] Critical value is the cut-point for the surrogate that minimized misclassification, derived from the ROC analysis.
[c] Since the results for BMI z-score were the same as for BMI percentile only the percentile is presented..

Logistic regression analyses to determine the odds ratios, with 95% confidence limits, for the presence of insulin resistance based on the critical or cut-points values for each of the adiposity surrogates are presented overall and for each sex in table 3. Overall, the cut-points were highly predictive of insulin resistance, with all odds ratios being above 6.25. Sum of skinfolds had the highest OR (9.35), while waist circumference had the lowest OR (6.58). Odds ratios for BMI, BMI %tile, waist %tile, WHtr and body mass were similar (8.13-8.93). With regard to the sex-specific logistic regression analyses (table 3), the least predictive for the girls was the waist circumference (OR = 6.57), while the most predictive was BMI percentile or BMI z-score (OR = 10.52). For the boys the least predictive was body mass (OR = 6.25) or BMI percentile (OR = 6.41) and the most predictive was waist circumference (OR = 9.52).

Table 3. Summary of logistic regression results presenting the odds ratios and 95% confidence interval for predicting insulin resistance (HOMA-IR > 4.0) overall and for each gender with respect to the ROC derived cut-point value (Table 2) for each adiposity surrogate[a]

Surrogate	Sex	Value	O.R.	Lower	Upper
BMI (kg/m^2)	All	23.5	8.48	6.58	10.99
	F	23.1	8.00	5.87	11.49
	M	23.5	8.26	5.56	12.34
BMI %tile	All	89	8.85	6.76	11.49
	F	89	10.52	7.40	14.92
	M	83	6.41	4.09	10.10
SSF (mm)	All	27	9.35	7.14	12.20
	F	27.3	9.35	6.49	13.51
	M	28.3	7.69	5.18	11.49
Waist (cm)	All	73.9	6.58	5.12	8.48
	F	74.5	6.57	4.69	9.17
	M	79.5	9.52	6.32	14.28
Waist %tile	All	75	8.13	6.29	10.53
	F	50	9.80	6.71	14.28
	M	75	7.30	4.92	10.86
WHtR	All	0.49	8.26	6.41	10.75
(cm/cm)	F	0.49	9.17	6.45	12.99
	M	0.49	7.58	5.05	11.36
WHtR	All	0.54	8.85	6.71	11.63
	F	0.54	8.93	13.15	6.06
	M	0.54	9.62	14.49	6.37
Body Mass	All	40.2	8.93	6.29	12.82
(kg)	F	49.7	9.25	5.78	14.92
	M	44.5	6.25	4.01	9.80

[a] Since the results for BMI z-score were the same as for BMI percentile only the percentile is presented.

The results of the multiple regression models examining the influence of age, sex and ethnicity on the relationship between insulin resistance and the adiposity surrogates are presented in table 4. In each of the nine models, sex had an R^2 of approximately 2% for all except skinfolds, in which the R^2 for sex was less than 1%. The R^2 for age was greater than 0.01 for only waist circumference and body mass, but was least for skinfolds and the WHtR ratios. Ethnicity had an R^2 of approximately 0.01 for all waist measures, as well as body mass. The least R^2 was for BMI and SSF. The three characteristics combined accounted for approximately 6.2% of the variance when body mass was used in the model and only 1.5% of the variance when using SSF. The same three demographic characteristics accounted for 3.1-4.9% of the variance for all other surrogate models. Therefore, of the six obesity surrogates examined, the cut-point for sum of skinfolds appears to be least influenced by age, sex and ethnicity.

Table 4. Total and partial R^2 for the multiple regression models for the relationship of insulin resistance (HOMA-IR) with each of the adiposity surrogates focusing on the variance accounted for by age, gender, and race

Variable	Adiposity	Age	Gender	Ethnicity	Total
BMI	.2025	.0043	.0208[*]	.0057[*]	.2332
BMI%tile	.1929	.0031	.0244[*]	.0084[*]	.2287
BMIz	.1921	.0029	.0254[*]	.0091[*]	.2294
Skinfolds	.2098	<.0001	.0085[*]	.0067[*]	.2250
Waist	.1567	.0112[*]	.0274[*]	.0120[*]	.2073
Wst %tile	.1946	.0028	.0251[*]	.0113[*]	.2338
WHtR (0.49)	.1966	.0012	.0218[*]	.0137[*]	.2333
WHtR (0.54)	.1907	.0013	.0229[*]	.0104[*]	.2254
Body Mass	.1252	.0330[*]	.0188[*]	.0101[*]	.1871

All models significant at p=0.0009.
[*] p<0.001 significant contribution to model.

DISCUSSION

The results of the study suggest that all the surrogates for adiposity have the capacity to be used as a means for screening for insulin resistance. Sum of skinfolds resulted in the highest AUC, OR and R^2, while having the least influence of age, sex, and ethnicity; but there was still a 24.9% misclassification; mostly false positive classifications. Using the sex, age- and ethnic-specific 75th waist percentiles cut-point values resulted in a slightly lower misclassification than skinfolds, but the AUC, OR and R^2 analyses were somewhat lower and the influence of the three characteristics was higher (R^2>3%). Using the ROC curve derived cut-point values and the proportion of misclassifications suggest that for girls, BMI percentile or BMI z-score appear to be best choice, while waist circumference appears to be the best for boys. Although in general the adiposity surrogates appear somewhat comparable in their abilities to predict insulin resistance, there are advantages and disadvantages for each, which could potentially limit their use in specific situations or specific populations.

Presently, BMI and BMI percentiles (or BMI-z scores) are used commonly in clinical situations to screen for insulin resistance; BMI is used in adults and BMI percentiles in children. A positive relationship exists between age and BMI or HOMA (i.e., both increase with age); whereas the BMI percentile is adjusted for age. When we reviewed the data for IR based on absolute BMI, we noted that the majority of false negative misclassifications for IR were for younger boys (8-10 yrs). Thus, the BMI results may only suggest that older youth may be more at risk for IR than younger boys. In adolescents using a BMI cut-point of 23.1, or 23.4, may appear to provide an adequate screening method for IR, but may not be appropriate for young children, suggesting absolute BMI is not the optimal method.

BMI percentile is widely used in children and adolescents as a screening tool for both IR and CVD risk (13, 19). Although the ROC curves and logistic regression analyses suggest that BMI percentile, or BMI z-score, are salient IR screening methods in girls, our results, however, suggest that BMI percentiles may not be as good a predictor of IR as waist circumference or WHtR for boys. Interestingly, BMI percentiles are age and sex-specific by design; yet in our regression model sex was a small, but significant confounder; suggesting that the relationship between these estimates of adiposity and IR supersedes the percentile (z-score) alone. Although BMI is easily obtained and our cut-point of the 89th and 83rd percentile appears logical, the concern is that the clinician must have the age and sex-specific tables available to interpret the results. However, in the US these BMI percentile tables are commonly used by pediatricians.

Several investigators have suggested that waist circumference is the most appropriate adiposity surrogate for screening for diabetes or the metabolic syndrome (6-9). Our logistic regression and misclassification results suggest that waist circumference is the best of the surrogates for predicting IR in boys but not for girls. The regression model for waist circumference (table 4) also showed that 4.9% of the 20.7% total variance was accounted for by age, sex, and race. Thus, for waist to be useful for a pediatric population, the sex-, age- and race-specific tables developed by Fernandez and associates (10) need to be more available to the clinician. The results of the logistic regression suggest that use of these waist percentiles improved the ability to screen for insulin resistance over waist circumference, especially for the girls (table 3); however, there was still a high number of misclassifications (false positive), especially for the girls. Since waist percentiles appears to have a similar relationship to IR as other surrogates and the requirement for multiple tables, then waist circumference percentiles may be less than optimal for a clinical setting or a community screening program. Also, in our experience with over 8,000 waist measures, waist circumference is surprisingly difficult to accurately assess.

If body fat is the component directly related to insulin resistance, then a measure of fat should produce the best results. Our estimate of body fat was the sum of the triceps and subscapular skinfolds. The ROC derived critical values differed only by one millimeter between the sexes and the differences between sexes in predictability was one of the lowest. Sum of skinfolds had one of the largest AUC of the ROC curves and had one of the higher amounts of variance accounted for in explaining the variability of the HOMA-IR. Also, the multiple regression analysis suggested the relationship between skinfolds and HOMA-IR was minimally influenced by age, sex or ethnicity, making it an acceptable measure for all children, with no special tables needed for interpretation of the results. The small sex-difference in critical/cut-points for sum of skinfolds was not expected, since one might suspect that the girls would have had a higher value than the boy. Typically, girls have more body fat than boys at a given sum of skinfold. If the prediction equation of Slaughter et al. (20) is applied to our cut-point of 27 mm, the computed body fat is approximately 29% for the girls and only 23% for the boys. Thus, the use of a single sum of skinfold value does adjust for sex-differences in body fat content. This result also suggests that boys have a tendency for insulin resistance at a lower percent body fat than girls, in agreement with Rommich et al. (21). Although skinfolds appear to be the best fit, there were still a considerable number of misclassifications (22-25%). In addition, accurate measurement of skinfolds is difficult and takes practice. Furthermore, studies in youth suggest that the measurement of skinfolds adds little to the ability to assess adiposity when using BMI percentiles (22, 22). In contrast, the findings of the Amsterdam Growth and Health Longitudinal Study suggest that skinfolds are more useful than BMI to predict adult fatness (24). Thus, with some training skinfolds could be used in a clinical setting, but may be of limited value in a community screening setting, when trained individuals are not readily available. Hence, the American Academy of Pediatrics does not recommend skinfolds to determine obesity (4).

Waist-height ratio appears to be a simple measure that can be obtained in clinical and community settings. Ashwell and Hseih (12) suggested that, for children, this ratio is more sensitive to health changes than BMI, is easier to interpret than BMI or waist alone, and may have the same values for children and adults. After the age of four years, waist and height appear to simultaneously increase during childhood and adolescence (11). Therefore, in theory, WHtR should account for growth and could provide a practical estimate of adiposity that could be consistently applied for all age groups. Indeed, age appeared to have little influence on the predictability of WHtR for IR (Age R^2 ~ 0.001; table 4); however, sex and ethnicity did account for an additional 3% of the variance. Overall, a WHtR of 0.49 provided an adequate cut-point for both sexes, similar to the findings of Kahn et al. (11); however, the ratio of 0.49 appeared more predictive of IR in girls than boys (OR 9.17 vs. 7.58, respectively). Kahn et al. (11) and Savva et al. (6) have suggested that although the WHtR of 0.49 may be adequate, although a slight higher value of ~ .51-.54 may be optimal. Therefore, we also examined a WHtR cut-point value of 0.54 and found that the overall odds ratios were somewhat improved over the 0.49 cut-point (overall OR: 8.85 vs.8.26). Intriguingly, as noted in table 3, when using the WHtR of 0.54, the difference in odds ratios between the sexes was slightly smaller when using the 0.49 WHtR (ΔOR: 0.69 vs. 1.61, respectively). In addition, the misclassification rate was the lowest of any method overall (20.5%) and especially for the boys (17.7%); while the misclassification rate for the girls (23.5%) was similar to the other methods. These results suggest that a WHtR of 0.54 may be a better cut-point than the ROC produced ratio of 0.49. One concern with WHtR is that waist circumference is more difficult to measure than body mass and some practice is required to accurately assess waist on the varying body sizes of youth and adolescents. The real advantage of WHtR is that it is easy to calculate and because it has a single cut-point value for all ages and both sexes; it does not require complicated tables to interpret the results.

Clearly, pubertal status could have influenced the results (25). However, we attempted to determine the most relevant screening method for all youth regardless of developmental stage and we were looking for a method that could be used without other sophisticated measures. Once again, aposteriori, we examined our data with regard to pubertal status and found the pre-pubertal girls had lower HOMA-IR than their counterparts in stages 2-5 (P = 0.0001), while there were no significant differences in the HOMA-IR with respect to pubertal stage in the boys (P > 0.05). Also, when we added pubertal status to our regression analyses, its contributions were ≤ 1% of the variance; thus, we feel the obesity surrogates could be used without consideration for pubertal status. A possible criticism of the study was the use of the HOMA-IR to indicate insulin resistance. However, the HOMA-IR has been evaluated for decades and appears to provide an adequate estimate for insulin resistance (15-17). The strength of the study is the size and heterogeneity of the age, sex, and to some extent, ethnicity, included in the sample. Thus, we feel confident in our findings.

In summary, all the surrogates for adiposity were able to assess the risk of insulin resistance. Sum of skinfolds (triceps plus subscapular), which is the hardest of all the surrogates to accurately assess, may be the best predictor of insulin resistance. The absolute cut-point of ~27 mm provides an appropriate marker with the least influence of age, sex and race of all the adiposity surrogates. BMI percentiles above the 89th and BMI z-scores above

1.27 appear to be adequate cut-points for screening, particularly for girls. Absolute measures of BMI or waist circumference, although related to insulin resistance, tend to produce false negative results in younger children; therefore, their interpretation is somewhat dependent upon the age, sex and race of the youth. Furthermore, waist circumference appears to have the lowest odds ratio to predict IR of all the surrogates for girls, but appears to be a better predictor for boys. Waist-height ratio of 0.54 may provide a good alternative to BMI, BMI percentile or waist measures to identify those youth with IR. Once a clinician or researcher learns to accurately measure waist circumference, the WHtR is comparatively easy to measure and does not require extensive computation or sex, race, and age specific tables to understand the results.

ACKNOWLEDGEMENTS

This study was supported by grant #NR01837 from the National Institute of Nursing Research of the National Institutes of Health

REFERENCES

[1]   Bosy-Westphal A, Geisler C, Onur S, et al. Value of body fat mass vs anthropometrics obesity indices in the assessment of metabolic risk factors. Int J Obes (Lond) 2006;30(3):475-83.

[2]   Must A, Spadano J, Coakley EH, Field AE, Colditz G, Dietz WH. The disease burden associated with overweight and obesity. JAMA 1999; 282:1523-9.

[3]   Kemper HC, Post GB, Twisk JW, van Mechelen W. Lifestyle and obesity in adolescence and young adulthood: results from the Amsterdam Growth and Health Longitudinal Study (AGAHLS). Int J Obes 1999;23(Suppl 3): S34-40.

[4]   American Academy of Pediatrics. Expert Committee recommendations on the assessment, preventions, and treatment of child and adolescent overweight and obesity. Accessed 2013 Aug 01. URL: www.ama-assoc.org/ama/pub/category/11759.html.

[5]   Lindsay RS, Hanson RL, Roumain J, Ravussin E, Knowler WC, Tataranni PA. Body mass index as a measure of adiposity in children and adolescents: Relationship to adiposity by dual exergy X-ray absorptiometry and to cardiovascular risk factors. J Clin Endocrin Metab 2001;86:4061-7.

[6]   Savva SC, Tornaritis M, Savva ME, et al. Waist circumference and waist-to-height ratio are better predictors of cardiovascular disease risk factors in children than body mass index. Int J Obes 2000;24: 1453-8.

[7]   Han TS, van Leer EM, Seidell JC, Lean ME. Waist circumference action levels in the identification of cardiovascular risk factors: prevalence study in a random sample. BMJ 1995;311:1401-5.

[8]   Janssen I, Katzmarzyk PT, Ross R. Waist circumference and not body mass index explains obesity-related risk. Am J Clin Nutr 2004;79:379-84.

[9]   Taylor RW, Jones IE, Williams SM, Goulding A. Evaluation of waist circumference, waist-to-hip ratio, and the conicity index as a screening tool for high trunk fat mass, as measured by dual-energy X-ray absorptiometry, in children aged 3-19 y. Am J Clin Nutr 2000; 72:490-5.

[10]   Fernandez JR, Redden DT, Pietrobelli A, Allison DB. Waist circumference percentiles in nationally representative sample of African-American, European-American and Mexican-American children and adolescents. J Pediatr 2004;145:439-44.

[11]   Kahn HS, Imperatore G, Cheng YJ. A population-based comparison of BMI percentiles and waist-to-height ratio for identifying cardiovascular risk in youth. J Pediatr 2005;146:482-8.

[12] Ashwell M, Hsieh SD. Six reasons why the waist-to-height ratio is a rapid and effective global indicator for health risk of obesity and how its use could simplify the international public health message on obesity. Int J Food Sci Nutr 2005;56:303-7.

[13] Petersen AC, TobinRichards M, Boxer A. Puberty: Its measurement and its meaning. J Early Adolesc 1983;3:47-62.

[14] US Department of Health and Human Services, PHS. NHANES III Anthropometric Procedures Video. #017-022-01335-5. Washington, DC: US GPO, Public Health Service, 1996.

[15] Matthews DR, Hosker JP, Rudenski AS, Naylor BA, Treacher DF, Turner RC. Homeostasis Model Assessment: Insulin resistance and ?-cell function from fasting plasma glucose and insulin concentrations in man. Diabetologica 1985;28:412-9.

[16] Bonora E, Targher G, Alberiche M, et al. Homeostasis model assessment closely mirrors the glucose clamp technique in the assessment of insulin sensitivity. Diabetes Care 2000;23:57-63.

[17] Reinher T, Andler W. Changes in the atherogenic risk factor profile according to degree of weight loss. Arch Dis Child 2004;89:419-22.

[18] Hanley JA, McNeil BJ. A method of comparing the areas under the receiver operating characteristic curves defined from same cases. Radiology 1983;148:839-43.

[19] Thompson DR, Obarzanek E, Franko DL, et al. Childhood overweight and cardiovascular disease risk factors: The National Heart, Lung and Blood Institute Growth and Health Study. J Pediatr 2007;150:18-25.

[20] Slaughter MH, Lohman TG, Boileau RA, et al. Skinfold equations for estimation of body fatness in children and youth. Hum Biol 1988;60:709-23.

[21] Roemmich JN, Clark PA, Lusk M, et al. Pubertal alterations in growth and body composition. VI. Pubertal insulin resistance: relation to adiposity, body aft distribution and hormone release. Int J Obes 2002;26:701-9

[22] Mei Z, Grummer-Strawn LM, Wang J, et al. Do skinfold measurements provide additional information to body mass index in the assessment of body fatness among children and adolescents? Pediatr 2007;119:1306-13.

[23] Watts K, Naylor LH, Davis EA, et al. Do skinfolds accurately assess changes in body fat in obese children and adolescents? Med Sci Sports Exerc 2006;38:439-44.

[24] Nooyens ACJ, Koopes LLJ, Visscher TLS, et al. Adolescent skinfold thickness is a better predictor of high body fatness in adults than is body mass index: the Amsterdam Growth and Health Longitudinal Study. Am J Clin Nutr 2007;85:1533-9.

[25] Goran MI, Gower BA. Longitudinal study on pubertal insulin resistance. Diabetes 2001;50:2444-50.

In: Food, Nutrition and Eating Behavior
Editors: Joav Merrick and Sigal Israeli

ISBN: 978-1-62948-233-0
© 2014 Nova Science Publishers, Inc.

Chapter 21

OBESITY AND QUALITY OF LIFE

Eveline J Wouters, MD and Rinie Geenen, PhD*

Fontys University of Applied Sciences, Eindhoven Department of Clinical and Health
Psychology, Utrecht University, the Netherlands

ABSTRACT

Obesity, especially morbid obesity, is a major health problem with considerable impact
on physical, mental and social quality of life. Assessment of quality of life is considered
crucial to understand and evaluate the consequences of obesity. However, the
heterogeneity of the quality of life concept makes it difficult to compare and value studies
on quality of life. Both generic -applying to any disease- and obesity specific quality of
life instruments can be used for assessment in obesity. Obesity has major consequences
for quality of life, as a result of co-morbidities of obesity, weight stigmatization, and
other less frequently ventilated problems. Bariatric surgery has been proven to lead to
significant weight loss and improvement of quality of life. Instruments differ in the
suitability to asess quality of life after surgery and weight loss, and they differ in the
domains of quality of life that are tapped by the instruments. Besides obesity, also
personal and psychosocial variables influence quality of life and affect the outcome of
surgery. Obesity, even after substantial weight loss by gastric bypass surgery, is a chronic
disease requiring life long consideration, in order to attain long standing quality of life
improvement.

INTRODUCTION

Obesity, especially morbid obesity, is a major health problem with considerable impact on
physical, mental and social quality of life. Morbidly obese persons report problems with their
mobility and activity level, vitality, social relations, eating behavior, and sexual life (1). A
higher body weight is associated with proportionally reversed quality of life (2, 3). Of all
obese groups, women seeking bariatric surgery report the lowest quality of life and surgery is

---

* Correspondence: Eveline JM Wouters, MD, Fontys University of Applied Sciences, Postbox 347, 5600 AH
Eindhoven, the Netherlands. E-mail: e.wouters@fontys.nl.

often the last resort for patients after many attempts to lose weight with dietary therapy (4,5). Patients mention several reasons to apply for surgery; many of them are related to co-morbidity and experienced restrictions in several domains of quality of life (6,7). Thus, quality of life is an important issue for obese people who seek surgical treatment. Divergent quality of life domains have been widely accepted as health outcomes after bariatric surgery, next to co-morbidity and weight loss.

Quality of life often improves considerably after bypass procedures (8,9) and most patients are satisfied with the results several years after surgery. Some specific problems, such as binge eating and skin abundance after treatment, might negatively impact on quality of life and need attention in order to improve the results.

HISTORY

In 1948, the World Health Organization gave a strong impetus to the quality of life concept by stating that "health is a state of complete physical, mental and social well-being and not merely the absence of disease or infirmity" (10). The statement induced discussions on the best way to measure health in practice. By defining health not merely as the absence of disease, but in a more positive manner, the focus of health shifted to the subjective perception of health. This implies that conventional health measurement instruments that assess presence or absence of disease and disease signs no longer suffice. Another consequence is that to get a full picture of someone's health, not only disease, but also the person's response to the disease is important. Here illness rather than disease is a more appropriate word to be used. Illness also includes the perceived part of health. Both mental and social determinants and consequences play a role in the new health concept (11).

Along with the implementation of the new health concept in clinical practice, the International Classification of Diseases (ICD) was complemented with the International Classification of Impairments, Disabilities and Handicaps (ICIDH, developed in the eighties) and the more recently and more positively formulated International Classification of Functioning, disability and health (ICF, 2001) (12).

Quality of life as an outcome measure in medical literature has been gaining more popularity due to several reasons, among others to oblige to the desire to incorporate the perspective of the patient in therapies such as chemotherapy, which put a high load on patients. This eagerness brought about the construction of numerous so called quality of life measurement instruments. These instruments mostly are not based on a uniformly and clearly defined concept of quality of life. This problem can be partly attributed to the simultaneous occurrence of two separate lines of development which have influenced the concept. First, form a medical line of history, the concept of quality of life was derived from the functional health status concept. A patient's daily behavior and activities was added to the strictly biological assessment of the patient (13). A list of impairments, disabilities and handicaps was developed, resulting in the ICIDH. Second, from a psychosocial science point of view, quality of life was related to psychological and environmental factors. Public life determinants, such as education, employment, security, and neighborhood were appraised as indicators of quality of life in this perspective (14).

These separate lines of development are to date still reflected in the absence of a uniform definition of quality of life (15). In literature, depending on the scope of the researcher or clinician, the full range of 'health status' and 'happiness' up till multifaceted domain models, can be encountered as definitions of quality of life. This makes it difficult to compare the studies. Some definitions are too parsimonious to do justice to the threat to quality of life that is experienced by the patient. Other definitions include as many domains as physical health, mental health, extent of independency, social relationships, and sometimes also the environmental and spiritual domains (16, 17). Some stress that the perspective of the patient, i.e., the extent to which the patient values a specific position in life regarding the context and everything that is considered important, is core to the evaluation of quality of life (16, 17). A brief straightforward definition of quality of life then is that it is a personal perception, indicating how a person feels about his or her health status including nonmedical aspects of life (18).

In conclusion, the heterogeneity in quality of life concepts may lead to confusion of tongues. For understanding and rightly valuing research on quality of life with respect to obesity, the heterogeneity of definitions has to be born in mind. However, it is impossible to think about interventions nowadays without considering quality of life. The last four decennia have shown a shift from the biomedical into the biopsychosocial model of health and disease (11). A great number of assessment instruments have been developed, many generic, and some especially designed for obesity. Taking the shortcomings into account, the introduction of these measurement instruments has added to the understanding of patients' position and perspectives in medicine.

ASSSESSMENT OF QUALITY OF LIFE

Assessing quality of life is important from both a clinical and a scientific point of view. It is important from a clinical perspective, because of the increasing prevalence of chronic diseases due to aging, and because diseases that used to be fatal such as myocardial infarction, cancer and HIV, have better treatment options. To improve the match between the care that is given and the care that is needed, quality of life aspects can be guiding. Also in research, not only the biomedical outcome, but also quality of life and improvement of quality of life, have become established as outcome measures.

Quality of life measurement instruments can be roughly divided into generic and disease-specific instruments. Sometimes domain-specific questionnaires are used, for instance instruments that predominantly apply to the physical domain. Generic instruments are multi-dimensional and can be used in different patient groups, with different health problems, different interventions, and demographics (19). By using generic instruments, comparisons of the relative burden of disease can be made between diseases and interventions. These instruments may lack the sensitivity to demonstrate characteristic aspects of certain diseases. An example of such a generic quality of life questionnaire is the World Health Organization Quality Of Life assessment instrument (WHOQOL-100) (20). Another widely used instrument, the Medical Outcomes Study (MOS) Short Form (SF-36) (21) is also often categorized within this group, although it has been argued that this questionnaire actually measures health status (22). This instrument asks about health themes, but does not explicitly ask the patient how they personally value these adverse consequences of health for quality of life.

Disease specific instruments are developed to measure quality of life in specific patient groups. They focus on problems that are common or specific for certain diseases. The disease specific and the generic instruments can, as a result of their different focus, give different results in the same patients. The disease specific measurements are, compared to generic instruments, better able to evaluate subtle changes due to alterations in the course of the disease, they tend to react more promptly when successful interventions are given, and are able to discriminate within subgroups of a population with a specific disease, e.g., between obesity groups that differ in body weight or clinical versus general population groups of obese persons. A drawback of the use of disease specific instruments is that comparison with other disease groups is impossible and the instruments may fail to assess valuable aspects of quality of life in the lives of individual patients.

In the evaluation of quality of life in obesity, the diversity of measurement instruments used in different studies should be considered (23). For instance, when using generic instruments, most studies find an association between body weight and physical health, but not between body weight and mental health (24, 25). Weight related measurements on the other hand, are also able to discriminate on the emotional and social domains, as well as on physical functioning between groups with different body weight (3, 26, 27).

Because generic and disease specific scales are complementary, it is useful to use both types of instruments, in order to be able to make comparisons across different populations and at the same time to discriminate within the disease population of interest (28).

In studies of obesity, a large variety of measurement instruments have been used to assess the relationship between obesity and quality of life. Some of the commonly applied generic and weight-related instruments will be presented.

Generic instruments

The generic instrument most often used in obesity studies, is the SF-36 questionnaire (21). This instrument, with 36 questions, consists of eight scales. These are: physical functioning, role limitations as a result of physical health, role limitations due to emotional health, bodily pain, general health, vitality, social functioning, and mental health. The scores on each scale are transformed to scores from 0 till 100, and to two summary scores, a physical component summary score and as a mental component summary score. The SF-36 is widely used, which is mainly because the access is easy and for free, and the questionnaire has been translated and validated in many languages and for several diseases (29, 30). In table 1 example questions and answering categories from each scale of the SF-36 are presented. An abbreviated version of the SF-36, the SF-12, also captures the eight domains and both the mental and physical summary scores of the SF-36. In obesity, this easily applicable instrument has proven to be reliable, and even better able to measure differences in quality life as related to body weight compared to the SF-36 (31).

Table 1. Example questions with answering categories from each scale of the SF-36

Scale	Example question	Range and number of answering categories (n)
Physical functioning	Climbing several flights of stairs?*	Yes, limited a lot – No, not limited at all (3)
Role limitations due to physical health	Cut down the amount of time you spent on work or other activities?**	Yes – No (2)
Role limitations due to emotional problems	Didn't do work or other activities as carefully as usual?**	Yes – No (2)
Bodily pain	Did pain interfere with your normal work?**	Not at all – Extremely (5)
General health	I am as healthy as anybody I know	Definitely true – Definitely false (5)
Vitality	Did you have a lot of energy?**	All of the time – None of the time (6)
Social functioning	How much of the time has your physical health or emotional problems interfered with your social activities?**	All of the time – None of the time (6)
Mental health	Have you felt so down in the dumps that nothing could cheer you up?**	All of the time – None of the time (6)

* perceived limitation during a typical day.
** perceived problems or limitations during the past four weeks.

Table 2. Example questions with answering categories from each domain of the WHOQOL

Domain	Example question	Range of answering categories
Physical domain	How much do you worry about your pain or discomfort?	Not at all – An extreme amount
Psychological domain	How much do you enjoy life?	Not at all – An extreme amount
Level of independence	How much do any difficulties in mobility bother you?	Not at all – To an extreme amount
Social relations	How satisfied are with your personal relationships?	Very dissatisfied – Very satisfied
Environment	How available to you is the information you need in your daily life?	Not at all - Completely
Spiritual domain	To what extent do you feel your life to be meaningful?	Not at all - Extremely

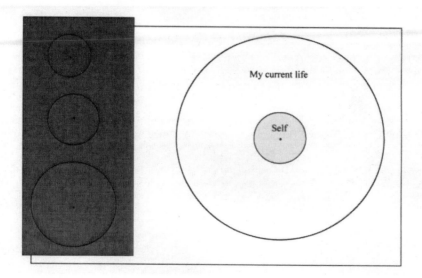

Figure 1. The Pictorial Representation of Illness and Self measure (PRISM); The outer circle represents one's current life, the yellow circle represents one's self, the red circles represent possible representations of the medical problem.

Another instrument, designed for measurement of generic quality of life, is the WHOQOL-100, which measures six domains of quality of life, i.e., physical health, psychological health, independency, social relations, environment, and spirituality/religion or personal beliefs. The WHOQOL-100 has good psychometric properties (20). Example questions with the range of the answering categories are shown in table 2. All questions have five answering categories. Because of its length a short form version has been developed, the WHOQOL-BREF, a 26-item questionnaire covering four domains: physical, psychological, social relations, and environment. The WHOQOL-BREF is reliable and valid across cultures and in clinical samples (32). The WHOQOL questionnaires, compared to e.g., the SF-36, explicitly include the patient perspective in the questions by asking how satisfied the respondent is with certain aspects of health.

The EQ-5D is an instrument less frequently used, and is rating health in the dimensions mobility, self-care, usual activities, pain and discomfort, and anxiety and depression (33, 34). The domains that are assessed by this instrument are closely related to health status.

Another instrument that might be considered a to assess quality of life, is the Pictorial Representation of Illness and Self measure (PRISM) (35-37). The instrument measures the burden imposed by disease and can be used for several health problems, including obesity. The instrument consists of a white rectangular sheet of firm paper, on which a circle is depicted, representing the patient's current life. In the centre of this is a yellow circle, representing one's 'self' (figure 1).

The patients imagine themselves as the yellow circle and are asked (with a standard oral or written instruction) to stick one of three different sized red (adhesive) disks, representing their illness (e.g., obesity), somewhere on the white sheet of paper. Also, they are asked to communicate why they chose for a particular size and position, thus eliciting qualitative information on the problem. A greater distance between the yellow circle and the illness-disk is hypothesized to represent less suffering, and a higher size of the illness-disk to indicate a greater perceived severity of the illness (38). There is preliminary support for the feasibility and validity of the variables assessed by PRISM in measuring aspects of suffering (38). The strength of this instrument is that is assesses overall suffering and that the instrument offers the possibility to start a conversation with patients on relevant aspects of their illness. Further evaluation for the use in bariatric surgery patients is necessary.

Weight specific quality of life instruments

Several weight specific quality of life instruments have been developed in different settings. A selection will be presented. The Impact of Weight on Quality Of Life (39), short version (IWQOL-lite) (40) includes 31 items and five scales on physical function, self-esteem, sexual life, public distress and work. In table 3 example statements with corresponding answering categories are presented. All questions have five possible answer categories. The IWQOL-lite is a reliable and valid instrument in both clinical and community samples (40, 41) and can discriminate between obesity subgroups (40-42). Translations in several languages are available (43) as well as a validated version for adolescents between 11 and 19 years of age (27). The IWQOL-lite is often used together with generic instruments, such as the SF-36 (44).

Table 3. Example statements with answering categories from each domain of the IWQOL-lite

Scale	Example question	Range of answering categories
Physical function	Because of my weight I have trouble using stairs	Always true – never true
Self esteem	Because of my weight I don't like myself	Always true – never true
Sexual life	Because of my weight I do not enjoy sexual activity	Always true – never true
Public distress	Because of my weight I experience discrimination by others	Always true – never true
Work	Because of my weight I am less productive than I could be	Always true – never true

The Obesity-Related Problem Scale (OP) was developed for the Swedish Obese Subjects (SOS) study (45). The aim of the instrument is to assess effects of obesity and long term effects of weight loss on psychosocial functioning in everyday life. The scale has eight items, asking about how much patients are bothered by certain everyday activities, such as swimming in public places and trying and buying clothes. The OP is psychometrically valid and responsive to weight change in several interventions, including surgery (46-48). Strong points of the instrument are the user friendliness, and the explicit focus on the patient's evaluation of obesity specific situations. Weaknesses are the narrow focus on social situations, and that the scale has not been widely used outside the SOS study (49).

The Obesity Specific Quality of Life (OSQOL) scale is specifically developed for the French population (26). This is an 11-item scale with four dimensions: physical state, vitality, relations with others and psychological state. The psychometric properties of this instrument were found to be satisfactory (26). The instrument has not been thoroughly tested on its responsiveness and little information is available as on interpretation of the scores (50).

For bariatric surgery patients, a specific instrument has been developed: the Bariatric Analysis and Reporting Outcomes System (BAROS) (51, 52). This instrument evaluates the result of obesity treatment on quality of life (using the Moorehead-Ardelt questionnaire (53)), but also on percentage of weight loss and co-morbidities. The instrument also reports on surgery complications and re-operations (52). The quality of life assessment instrument consists of six questions, with a 10-point Likert scale scoring key (52).

Although there are several other obesity specific quality of life instruments available, most of these have not been extensively evaluated in bariatric surgery patients. An overview of instruments has been given (50).

QUALITY OF LIFE IN PERSONS WITH OBESITY

The body of evidence in literature indicates that obesity is related to a lower (health related) quality of life. It has been frequently shown that obesity is associated with decreased vitality and physical, sexual, social and occupational functioning as measured with frequently used assessment instruments such as the SF-36 or the IWQOL-lite (39). There are several potential mechanisms linking obesity to poor quality of life. The risks and symptoms associated with co-morbidities such as diabetes, osteoarthritis and hypertension, partly explains such an association (54). When controlled for co-morbidity, obesity still has an independent impact on quality of life, as a consequence of physical limitations and of the stigma of being obese that affects mental and social domains of quality of life (55, 56). Body dissatisfaction and low self esteem are common in obesity (4, 39) and are considered to mediate the association between stigmatization and weight status (57).

Apart from co-morbidities and stigmatization, several other problems may influence quality of life (58). Not all obese persons suffer from an equally hampered quality of life. Quality of life will also depend on individual characteristics of persons that are part of personality or are related to experiences in the past.

In this paragraph the stigma of being overweight and minor, not often ventilated ailments influencing quality of life will be described, as well as moderating factors that influence the association between obesity and quality of life.

STIGMA OF BEING OBESE

Obese persons may daily experience the adverse consequences from the physical and psychological load of their overweight. Discrimination and stigmatization are pervasive phenomena, even now that the prevalence of overweight and obesity is high and obesity is relatively common. Many perceive that obese persons cause their own overweight and that overweight can and should be controlled (59). Negative stereotypes, such as obese people being lazy, unmotivated, incompetent, lacking of self-discipline, are common (60). Discrimination in work, educational possibilities, and in family relationships is not unusual (61, 62). There is no law against discrimination at work due to obesity, as there is a law that prohibits such discrimination based on gender, race, nationality or religion. The obese persons themselves also associate obesity with negative characteristics (63), and even in professionals in health care and research settings, who are dealing with the obesity problem and obese patients daily, a prejudice against obesity is not uncommon (60, 64). These stereotypes about obesity, when not addressed properly, will influence the quality of life of obese persons (60). Gaining consciousness is therefore important, among others in the context of bariatric surgery.

OTHER CO-MORBIDITIES

Apart from the well known co-morbidities of obesity that obviously influence aspects of quality of life such as cardiovascular disease, diabetes and osteoarthritis, some problems are less often diagnosed when a patient applies for gastric bypass surgery.

A problem of obese persons, which will obviously influence body satisfaction, self esteem and social quality of life, is the existence of excessive perspiration and the general inability to clean oneself properly (58).

A common, often under-diagnosed problem in morbid obesity is obstructive sleep apnea (65, 66). Sleep apnea causes sleep deprivation, both for the patient and for the bed partner. A person with sleep apnea will often not feel refreshed after awakening and is excessively fatigued during daytime, with consequences for mental and social life (66, 67). Also hypertension may occur as a consequence of sleep apnea (68). Furthermore, sleep apnea is related to sexual dysfunction and depression (69). Whether the sleep apnea causes depression or vice versa, is not exactly clear, but the treatment of sleep apnea can also alleviate depressive symptoms (70).

Independent of obstructive sleep apnea, sexual problems can arise as a result of obesity. Sexual life in most patients with obesity is associated with lack of enjoyment of sexual activity, lack of sexual desire, difficulties with sexual performance, and avoidance of sexual encounters (1). Especially women suffer in this respect (1, 71). Also, as a result of hormonal changes, both in men and women, sexual dysfunction is relatively common in obesity (72). Sexual and hormonal disturbances decrease fertility both in men and women: in women because of increased androgen function causing anovulation (73), in men amongst others as a consequence of lower testosterone levels (74).

Obesity is, next to pregnancy and childbirth, an important factor causing strain on the pelvic floor in women, which may result in pelvic organ prolapse and stress incontinence (75, 76). Stress incontinence can cause social and hygienic problems. Weight loss can improve the level of pelvic floor insufficiency and these associated clinical problems (77). Finally, uterine prolapse can, apart from the direct consequences of obesity, aggravate sexual dysfunction (78).

MODERATING FACTORS

Most of the quality of life studies in obesity have a cross sectional design. A limitation of this design is the difficulty of disentangling possible causal relationships and crucial intervening variables –mediators- that explain the association between a determinant and an outcome variable. For instance, a behavior such as lack of exercise can be one of the causal factors of obesity that subsequently causes a reduced quality of life, but it can also be a common cause of both obesity and a low perceived quality of life. Also, quality of life seems to be unequally influenced by differences between obese people. Individually different variables that interact with other determinants to produce a specific effect are called moderator variables. Some of the factors known to moderate the relationship between obesity and quality of life will be discussed here.

Gender is a major moderator influencing the extent to which a person's quality of life is decreased by obesity (79). In the general population, women report a more severely reduced quality of life in most domains than men (3, 80). In women seeking bariatric surgery, especially self-esteem, sexual life, and physical functioning are more severely affected compared to men, which may explain –among other variables- why more women than men apply for bariatric surgery (39, 81). This reduced quality of life in women may be partly explained by the fact that receiving weight stigma is more a problem for women than for men in romantic relationships (71). Men, more than women, judge women on their appearances and regard overweight women as less suitable partners (71, 82).

Race is also moderating the relationship between quality of life and obesity. In comparison to whites, black adults seem to experience less impact of obesity on quality of life (3, 80). In adolescents, these observations are only partly confirmed (83, 84). It seems that quality of life in both black and white adolescents is related to weight related teasing, and that, whereas in whites this most often results from peers, in blacks there is more often teasing within the family (85).

The impact of obesity on quality of life in different age groups also tends to be dissimilar. As can be expected, physical function, sexual life, and work related quality of life tend to decrease with age in obese persons (86). On the other hand, self-esteem and problems in public related to their obesity tend to improve with age (87).

QUALITY OF LIFE AFTER BARIATRIC SURGERY

Whether or not quality of life assessments are part of the outcome evaluation after bariatric surgery, an important goal of bariatric surgery is to improve health and quality of life by means of losing weight.

Gains from surgery

The large effects of gastric bypass surgery on weight loss are beyond discussion. Surgery also positively influences quality of life. The outcome for quality of life is more subtle and complex compared to the weight loss and depends on several concomitant factors.

Significant weight loss and improvement in weight-related co-morbidities, such as diabetes, hypertension, gastro-esophageal reflux, and medication use, which appear within a few months after surgery, immediately improve the health status of the patient (88-90). Self-perceived quality of life is also better: most patients report improved vitality, physical functioning, self-esteem, and satisfaction with their physical appearance (90, 91). Many every day life activities change after surgery and weight loss: patients experience less difficulty when moving around and are better able to perform daily tasks such as cleaning the home, cleaning themselves, and doing the shopping. With respect to body satisfaction after surgery, the extent of weight loss is not the most important factor. Also in people who lose less weight after surgery, the body satisfaction is high and in some even better compared to those who have experienced very rapid weight loss after surgery, resulting in excess skin (92, 93). Scale scores on quality of life instruments, which deviated significantly from norm values at baseline, reach norm values or are sometimes even higher than norm values years after surgery (88, 93). Even in patients experiencing complications during or after surgery, in super-obese patients and in patients with less than 50 percent excess weight loss, the quality of life after the operation is higher than it was before the operation (90, 93, 94). A drawback of the measurement scales needs to be considered. Disease specific questionnaires relate weight to aspects of quality of life. This hampers the quality of the postoperative assessment. In the IWQOL-lite, all questions start with "because of my weight…". Because some patients will have returned to normal weight after surgery, these questions are not entirely suitable even if some adverse consequences of the previous state of obesity, like low self esteem, would still exist.

Psychosocial determinants of success

In pre-surgical screening, few personality traits and psychosocial determinants have been found to influence the postsurgical weight outcome, but many psychological determinants do predict postsurgical mental and physical well being, which are two essential domains of quality of life (95, 96). Preoperative depressive mood has been shown to be a significant predictor of postoperative quality of life, even if weight loss is substantial (97). Therefore, although pre-surgical psychosocial functioning is not predictive for subsequent weight loss, it is important to identify those patients needing extra pre- or postsurgical interventions, resulting in better long term quality of life (98).

A specific problem, often considered to be a risk factor for insufficient weight loss after surgery, is the pre-existence of Binge Eating Disorder (BED), the consumption of an objectively large amount of food within a brief period of time (less than two hours), with the patient experiencing a loss of control and significant emotional stress. This behavior, which is not followed by vomiting, is present for at least six months, and at least two times a week (4). In normal weight persons, BED is present in about two percent, whereas in obesity, it is present in 15 to 30 percent of the patients (4). BED has been a major concern related to surgery failure and some research indicated poorer outcome with respect to weight loss and quality of life after surgery, when patients showed BED prior to surgery (99). In contrast, binge eating in many patients is reported to improve or totally disappear after surgery (91, 94, 100, 101). Some patients on the other hand, after an improvement in the first months, experience recurrence of BED and concomitant weight gain (102, 103). It is therefore important to evaluate postoperative, rather than only pre-operative behavior, for sustained weight loss success and for improvement of quality of life (104).

Sexual abuse is related both to depression and to obesity (105). Mechanisms thought to relate abuse to obesity are manifold, e.g., by inducing actual physical changes, psychological consequences (e.g., low self-esteem, sense of powerlessness), or behavioral problems (105). A history of sexual abuse has been related to adult obesity and the failure of conservative obesity treatment, as a result of non-compliance and lack of self-efficacy (106). In surgery, results are somewhat different. For weight loss success, patients with and without a history of abuse had the same results but the group with a history of childhood sexual abuse showed a higher level of depression (107). As a consequence, sexual abuse is not considered to be a contra-indication for surgery, but these patients need additional psychological treatment for their mental health problems (107).

It can be concluded that pre- and postsurgical evaluation and treatment of psychosocial problems are of great importance for targeting patients at risk for poor psychological outcomes, in order to improve the long term success of surgery with respect to weight loss as well as with respect to quality of life.

Long term quality of life outcomes after surgery: Special issues

Although the majority of patients benefit from bariatric surgery and experience enhanced quality of life, in most if not all domains, some problems can threat the outcome. Issues reported by patients most often, will be described briefly.

An important issue is surplus skin, situated most commonly on the abdomen, the upper arms, the inside of the thighs, and also on the back, the cheek and over the knees. As a result fungal infections, itching and hampered physical activity are experienced, which together may cause severe psychosocial problems (108). Many of these problems can be approached with reconstructive surgery after weight loss, and most patients feel more self-confident and attractive after such a procedure (109). With the increased application of bariatric surgery in morbid obesity, it would be advisable to address the problem of skin abundance, and the possibility of plastic surgical interventions, in the evaluation of patients.

Neither frequently mentioned by patients nor frequently described in literature, is the occurrence of diarrhea and malodorous flatulence (110). Also vomiting and "plugging", a feeling that food is not going down in the gastro intestinal tract, is a phenomenon reported by gastric bypass patients after surgery (111). These problems can reduce quality of life and are only partly if at all mirrored in most routine quality of life assessments. To assess these factors that threat quality of life the Gastrointestinal Quality of Life Index could be used (112, 113). Because this instrument has been developed for chronic gastrointestinal disease in general, it is not specific for all the post surgery problems of bariatric patients.

Another physical consequence related to malnutrition post-surgery, is the development of bone loss and skeletal fragility because of weight loss and altered nutrient metabolism. Long term evaluation and treatment of bone deficiencies, especially in post-menopausal women with a substantially reduced weight, may be necessary to prevent an increase of fractures in this group (114).

Perhaps most relevant for the valuation of quality of life, are the possibilities of patients to deal with their new body after surgery. Patients perceive their post surgical life as a rebirth or transformation (115), which poses them for specific changes and adaptations. Examples of such changes are increased feelings of vulnerability, changes in the social environment, such as marital dynamics or friendships (116), and the need of new skills such as implementing non-dietary means of coping with emotions (115). The extent to which patients are able to adjust to their new life, highly impacts on their perceived quality of life. These important topics are not covered by routine quality of life measurement scales that focus on adjustment outcomes instead of adjustment processes that improve the outcome.

CONCLUSION

Gastric bypass surgery is highly effective in attaining weight loss and improving quality of life. Patients experience an immense transformation in physical, mental, and social well-being and functioning. Bariatric weight loss surgery is a large undertaking for patients. Obesity is a chronic disease, just like diabetes, chronic obstructive pulmonary disease, or alcohol addiction. Even if much of the excess weight is lost as a result of surgery, the disease requires a lifelong commitment of both the people that were once obese and the people in their social environment, as well as a of a (multidisciplinary) treatment team. Both pre- and post surgical support, and a support that is unbiased by stigmatization, are mandatory in order to achieve a satisfying quality of life for patients (117, 118).

For the assessment of quality of life in bariatric patients, most disease specific instruments are not fully applicable after surgery when patients have lost large amounts of weight. However, also the use of generic quality of life instruments can be of limited value, because patients after surgery, even if they report a relatively good generic quality of life, can perceive specific problems not included in these instruments. There is a need for the development of quality of life instruments addressing these specific themes. Another possibility would be the evaluation of generic instruments like the Pictorial Representation of Illness and Self measure. With such instruments both the short and the long-term quality of life of the individual bariatric patient, or a group of patients in a research setting, can be evaluated.

Another issue that needs consideration is the large group of morbidly obese people, especially men, that does not apply for surgery. Both the health and the quality of life of this group may be less severely reduced than for the group that does apply for surgery. However, in the long term, reduction of overweight is also very important for this group. It is possible that the quality of life outcome studies after bariatric surgery will be become a little bit less spectacular when also this morbidly obese group with a relatively high quality of life will be operated.

Even after successful surgery, patients have a life-long chronic disease which, like any other chronic disease, requires sufficient health care support and permanent consideration and life style adjustment from the patient, in order to result in long term good quality of life. A multi-disciplinary, person centered approach, and the evaluation of such an approach, in different (e.g., gender and age specific) groups, is the most relevant future challenge.

REFERENCES

[1] Kolotkin RL, Binks M, Crosby RD, Ostbye T, Gress RE, Adams TD. Obesity and sexual quality of life. Obesity (Silver Spring) 2006;14(3):472-9.

[2] Chang CY, Hung CK, Chang YY, Tai CM, Lin JT, Wang JD. Health-related quality of life in adult patients with morbid obesity coming for bariatric surgery. Obes Surg 2008;20(8):1121-7.

[3]   Kolotkin RL, Crosby RD, Williams GR. Health-related quality of life varies among obese subgroups. Obes Res 2002;10(8):748-56.

[4]   Wadden TA, Stunkard AJ, eds. Handbook of obesity treatment. New York: Guilford, 2004.

[5]   Hsu LK, Benotti PN, Dwyer J, Roberts SB, Saltzman E, Shikora S, et al. Nonsurgical factors that influence the outcome of bariatric surgery: a review. Psychosom Med 1998;60(3):338-46.

[6]   Duval K, Marceau P, Lescelleur O, Hould FS, Marceau S, Biron S, et al. Health-related quality of life in morbid obesity. Obes Surg 2006;16(5):574-9.

[7]   Munoz DJ, Lal M, Chen EY, Mansour M, Fischer S, Roehrig M, et al. Why patients seek bariatric surgery: a qualitative and quantitative analysis of patient motivation. Obes Surg 2007;17(11):1487-91.

[8]   Van Hout GC, Fortuin FA, Pelle AJ, Blokland-Koomen ME, van Heck GL. Health-related quality of life following vertical banded gastroplasty. Surg Endosc 2009;23(3):550-6.

[9]   Muller MK, Wenger C, Schiesser M, Clavien PA, Weber M. Quality of life after bariatric surgery--a comparative study of laparoscopic banding vs. bypass. Obes Surg 2008;18(12):1551-7.

[10]   WHO. WHO definition of Health 2003 [updated 2003; cited 2009 May 22nd]; Available from: http://www.who.int/about/definition/en/print.html.

[11]   Engel GL. The need for a new medical model: a challenge for biomedicine. Science 1977;196(4286):129-36.

[12]   Bornman J. The World Health Organisation's terminology and classification: application to severe disability. Disabil Rehabil 2004;26(3):182-8.

[13]   McDowell I, Newell C. Measuring health: a guide to rating scales and questionnaires. New York: Oxford Univ Press, 1996.

[14]   Campbell A. Subjective measurements of well-being. American Psychologist 1976:117-24.

[15]   Hunt SM. The problem of quality of life. Qual Life Res 1997;6(3):205-12.

[16]   Felce D, Perry J. Quality of life: its definition and measurement. Res Dev Disabil 1995;16(1):51-74.

[17]   Group W. The World Health Organiszation quality of life assessment instrument (WHOQOL): position paper for the World Health Organization. Geneva: WHO, 1995.

[18]   Gill TM, Feinstein AR. A critical appraisal of the quality of quality-of-life measurements. JAMA 1994;272(8):619-26.

[19]   de Vries J. Assessment in behavioral medicine. Hove UK: Brunner-Rouledge, 2002.

[20]   Bonomi AE, Patrick DL, Bushnell DM, Martin M. Validation of the United States' version of the World Health Organization Quality of Life (WHOQOL) instrument. J Clin Epidemiol 2000;53(1):1-12.

[21]   Ware JE, Jr., Sherbourne CD. The MOS 36-item short-form health survey (SF-36). I. Conceptual framework and item selection. Med Care 1992;30(6):473-83.

[22]   Van Heck GL. Confusion concerning Quality of Life: a fault confessed is half redressed. Psychol Gezondheid 2008;36(2):72-8.

[23]   Jones GL, Sutton A. Quality of life in obese postmenopausal women. Menopause Int 2008;14(1):26-32.

[24]   Fontaine KR, Bartlett SJ, Barofsky I. Health-related quality of life among obese persons seeking and not currently seeking treatment. Int J Eat Disord 2000;27(1):101-5.

[25]   von Lengerke T, Janssen C, John J. Sense of coherence, health locus of control, and quality of life in obese adults: physical limitations and psychological normalcies. Int J Public Health 2007;52(1):16-26.

[26]   Le Pen C, Levy E, Loos F, Banzet MN, Basdevant A. "Specific" scale compared with "generic" scale: a double measurement of the quality of life in a French community sample of obese subjects. J Epidemiol Community Health 1998;52(7):445-50.

[27]   Kolotkin RL, Zeller M, Modi AC, Samsa GP, Quinlan NP, Yanovski JA, et al. Assessing weight-related quality of life in adolescents. Obesity (Silver Spring) 2006;14(3):448-57.

[28]   Maly M, Vondra V. Generic versus disease-specific instruments in quality-of-life assessment of chronic obstructive pulmonary disease. Methods Inf Med 2006;45(2):211-5.

[29]   Syddall HE, Martin HJ, Harwood RH, Cooper C, Aihie Sayer A. The SF-36: a simple, effective measure of mobility-disability for epidemiological studies. J Nutr Health Aging 2009;13(1):57-62.

[30]   Lim LL, Seubsman SA, Sleigh A. Thai SF-36 health survey: tests of data quality, scaling assumptions, reliability and validity in healthy men and women. Health Qual Life Outcomes 2008;6:52.

[31]   Wee CC, Davis RB, Hamel MB. Comparing the SF-12 and SF-36 health status questionnaires in patients with and without obesity. Health Qual Life Outcomes 2008;6:11.

[32]   Skevington SM, Lotfy M, O'Connell KA. The World Health Organization's WHOQOL-BREF quality of life assessment: psychometric properties and results of the international field trial. A report from the WHOQOL group. Qual Life Res 2004;13(2):299-310.

[33]   Sach TH, Barton GR, Doherty M, Muir KR, Jenkinson C, Avery AJ. The relationship between body mass index and health-related quality of life: comparing the EQ-5D, EuroQol VAS and SF-6D. Int J Obes (Lond) 2007;31(1):189-96.

[34]   Rabin R, de Charro F. EQ-5D: a measure of health status from the EuroQol Group. Ann Med 2001;33(5):337-43.

[35]   Buchi S, Buddeberg C, Klaghofer R, Russi EW, Brandli O, Schlosser C, et al. Preliminary validation of PRISM (Pictorial Representation of Illness and Self Measure) - a brief method to assess suffering. Psychother Psychosom 2002;71(6):333-41.

[36]   Buchi S, Sensky T, Sharpe L, Timberlake N. Graphic representation of illness: a novel method of measuring patients' perceptions of the impact of illness. Psychother Psychosom 1998;67(4-5):222-5.

[37]   Buchi S, Villiger P, Kauer Y, Klaghofer R, Sensky T, Stoll T. PRISM (Pictorial Representation of Illness and Self Measure)- a novel visual method to assess the global burden of illness in patients with systemic lupus erythematosus. Lupus 2000;9(5):368-73.

[38]   Wouters EJ, Reimus JL, van Nunen AM, Blokhorst MG, Vingerhoets AJ. Suffering quantified? Feasibility and psychometric characteristics of 2 revised versions of the Pictorial Representation of Illness and Self Measure (PRISM). Behav Med 2008;34(2):65-78.

[39]   Van Nunen AM, Wouters EJ, Vingerhoets AJ, Hox JJ, Geenen R. The health-related quality of life of obese persons seeking or not seeking surgical or non-surgical treatment: a meta-analysis. Obes Surg 2007;17(10):1357-66.

[40]   Kolotkin RL, Crosby RD, Kosloski KD, Williams GR. Development of a brief measure to assess quality of life in obesity. Obes Res 2001;9(2):102-11.

[41]   Kolotkin RL, Crosby RD. Psychometric evaluation of the impact of weight on quality of life-lite questionnaire (IWQOL-Lite) in a community sample. Qual Life Res 2002;11(2):157-71.

[42]   Kolotkin RL, Crosby RD, Williams GR, Hartley GG, Nicol S. The relationship between health-related quality of life and weight loss. Obes Res 2001;9(9):564-71.

[43]   Hamilton MA, Kolotkin RL. ProQolid. 2008 [updated 2008; cited 2009 May 24th]; Available from: http://www.proqolid.org/instruments/impact_of_weight_on_quality_of_life_lite_iwqol_lite.

[44]   Kolotkin RL, Norquist JM, Crosby RD, Suryawanshi S, Teixeira PJ, Heymsfield SB, et al. One-year health-related quality of life outcomes in weight loss trial participants: comparison of three measures. Health Qual Life Outcomes 2009;7:53.

[45]   Karlsson J, Sjostrom L, Sullivan M. Swedish obese subjects (SOS)--an intervention study of obesity. Two-year follow-up of health-related quality of life (HRQL) and eating behavior after gastric surgery for severe obesity. Int J Obes Relat Metab Disord 1998;22(2):113-26.

[46]   Ryden A, Karlsson J, Persson LO, Sjostrom L, Taft C, Sullivan M. Obesity-related coping and distress and relationship to treatment preference. Br J Clin Psychol 2001;40(Pt 2):177-88.

[47]   Sullivan M, Karlsson J, Sjostrom L, Backman L, Bengtsson C, Bouchard C, et al. Swedish obese subjects (SOS)--an intervention study of obesity. Baseline evaluation of health and psychosocial functioning in the first 1743 subjects examined. Int J Obes Relat Metab Disord 1993;17(9):503-12.

[48]   Karlsson J, Taft C, Sjostrom L, Torgerson JS, Sullivan M. Psychosocial functioning in the obese before and after weight reduction: construct validity and responsiveness of the Obesity-related Problems scale. Int J Obes Relat Metab Disord 2003;27(5):617-30.

[49]   Wadden TA, Phelan S. Assessment of quality of life in obese individuals. Obes Res 2002;10 Suppl 1:50S-7S.

[50]   Duval K, Marceau P, Perusse L, Lacasse Y. An overview of obesity-specific quality of life questionnaires. Obes Rev 2006;7(4):347-60.

[51]   Oria HE, Moorehead MK. Bariatric analysis and reporting outcome system (BAROS). Obes Surg 1998;8(5):487-99.

[52]   Oria HE, Moorehead MK. Updated Bariatric Analysis and Reporting Outcome System (BAROS). Surg Obes Relat Dis 2009;5(1):60-6.

[53]   Moorehead MK, Ardelt-Gattinger E, Lechner H, Oria HE. The validation of the Moorehead-Ardelt Quality of Life Questionnaire II. Obes Surg 2003;13(5):684-92.

[54]   Banegas JR, Lopez-Garcia E, Graciani A, Guallar-Castillon P, Gutierrez-Fisac JL, Alonso J, et al. Relationship between obesity, hypertension and diabetes, and health-related quality of life among the elderly. Eur J Cardiovasc Prev Rehabil 2007;14(3):456-62.

[55]   Rogge MM, Greenwald M, Golden A. Obesity, stigma, and civilized oppression. ANS Adv Nurs Sci 2004;27(4):301-15.

[56]   Friedman KE, Ashmore JA, Applegate KL. Recent experiences of weight-based stigmatization in a weight loss surgery population: psychological and behavioral correlates. Obesity (Silver Spring) 2008;16(Suppl 2):S69-74.

[57]   Fox CL, Farrow CV. Global and physical self-esteem and body dissatisfaction as mediators of the relationship between weight status and being a victim of bullying. J Adolesc 2009;32(5):1287-301.

[58]   Kral JG, Sjostrom LV, Sullivan MB. Assessment of quality of life before and after surgery for severe obesity. Am J Clin Nutr 1992;55(2 Suppl):611S-4S.

[59]   Wadden TA, Stunkard AJ. Social and psychological consequences of obesity. Ann Intern Med 1985;103(6):1062-7.

[60]   Puhl RM, Heuer CA. The stigma of obesity: a review and update. Obesity (Silver Spring) 2009;17(5):941-64.

[61]   Puhl RM, Brownell KD. Confronting and coping with weight stigma: an investigation of overweight and obese adults. Obesity (Silver Spring) 2006;14(10):1802-15.

[62]   Puhl RM, Moss-Racusin CA, Schwartz MB, Brownell KD. Weight stigmatization and bias reduction: perspectives of overweight and obese adults. Health Educ Res 2008;23(2):347-58.

[63]   Schwartz MB, Vartanian LR, Nosek BA, Brownell KD. The influence of one's own body weight on implicit and explicit anti-fat bias. Obesity (Silver Spring) 2006;14(3):440-7.

[64]   Schwartz MB, Chambliss HO, Brownell KD, Blair SN, Billington C. Weight bias among health professionals specializing in obesity. Obes Res 2003;11(9):1033-9.

[65]   Foster GD, Sanders MH, Millman R, Zammit G, Borradaile KE, Newman AB, et al. Obstructive sleep apnea among obese patients with type 2 diabetes. Diabetes Care 2009;32(6):1017-9.

[66]   Flemons WW. Measuring quality of life in patients with sleep apnoea: whose life is it anyway? Thorax 2004;59(6):457-8.

[67]   Flemons WW. Clinical practice. Obstructive sleep apnea. N Engl J Med 2002;347(7):498-504.

[68]   Hirshkowitz M. The clinical consequences of obstructive sleep apnea and associated excessive sleepiness. J Fam Pract 2008;57(8 Suppl):S9-16.

[69]   Schroder CM, O'Hara R. Depression and Obstructive Sleep Apnea (OSA). Ann Gen Psychiatry 2005;4:13.

[70]   Rakel RE. Clinical and societal consequences of obstructive sleep apnea and excessive daytime sleepiness. Postgrad Med 2009;121(1):86-95.

[71]   Chen EY, Brown M. Obesity stigma in sexual relationships. Obes Res 2005;13(8):1393-7.

[72]   Trischitta V. Relationship between obesity-related metabolic abnormalities and sexual function. J Endocrinol Invest 2003;26(3 Suppl):62-4.

[73]   Nelson SM, Fleming R. Obesity and reproduction: impact and interventions. Curr Opin Obstet Gynecol 2007;19(4):384-9.

[74]   Jarow JP, Kirkland J, Koritnik DR, Cefalu WT. Effect of obesity and fertility status on sex steroid levels in men. Urology 1993;42(2):171-4.

[75]   Whitcomb EL, Lukacz ES, Lawrence JM, Nager CW, Luber KM. Prevalence and degree of bother from pelvic floor disorders in obese women. Int Urogynecol J Pelvic Floor Dysfunct 2009;20(3):289-94.

[76]   Miedel A, Tegerstedt G, Maehle-Schmidt M, Nyren O, Hammarstrom M. Nonobstetric risk factors for symptomatic pelvic organ prolapse. Obstet Gynecol 2009;113(5):1089-97.

[77]   Aye C, Price N, Jackson SR. Urinary incontinence: Can weight loss treat urinary incontinence in obese women? Nat Rev Urol 2009;6(5):247-8.

[78] Handa VL, Cundiff G, Chang HH, Helzlsouer KJ. Female sexual function and pelvic floor disorders. Obstet Gynecol 2008;111(5):1045-52.

[79] Muennig P, Lubetkin E, Jia H, Franks P. Gender and the burden of disease attributable to obesity. Am J Public Health 2006;96(9):1662-8.

[80] White MA, O'Neil PM, Kolotkin RL, Byrne TK. Gender, race, and obesity-related quality of life at extreme levels of obesity. Obes Res 2004;12(6):949-55.

[81] Kolotkin RL, Crosby RD, Gress RE, Hunt SC, Engel SG, Adams TD. Health and health-related quality of life: differences between men and women who seek gastric bypass surgery. Surg Obes Relat Dis 2008;4(5):651-9.

[82] Sitton S, Blanchard S. Men's preferences in romantic partners: obesity vs addiction. Psychol Rep 1995;77(3 Pt 2):1185-6.

[83] Fallon EM, Tanofsky-Kraff M, Norman AC, McDuffie JR, Taylor ED, Cohen ML, et al. Health-related quality of life in overweight and nonoverweight black and white adolescents. J Pediatr 2005;147(4):443-50.

[84] Modi AC, Loux TJ, Bell SK, Harmon CM, Inge TH, Zeller MH. Weight-specific health-related quality of life in adolescents with extreme obesity. Obesity (Silver Spring) 2008;16(10):2266-71.

[85] Van den Berg P, Neumark-Sztainer D, Eisenberg ME, Haines J. Racial/ethnic differences in weight-related teasing in adolescents. Obesity (Silver Spring) 2008;16(Suppl 2):S3-10.

[86] Reynolds SL, McIlvane JM. The impact of obesity and arthritis on active life expectancy in older Americans. Obesity (Silver Spring) 2009;17(2):363-9.

[87] Zabelina DL, Erickson AL, Kolotkin RL, Crosby RD. The effect of age on weight-related quality of life in overweight and obese individuals. Obesity (Silver Spring) 2009;17(7):1410-3.

[88] Peluso L, Vanek VW. Efficacy of gastric bypass in the treatment of obesity-related comorbidities. Nutr Clin Pract 2007;22(1):22-8.

[89] Hager C. Quality of life after Roux-en-Y gastric bypass surgery. AORN J 2007;85(4):768-78.

[90] Bennett JC, Wang H, Schirmer BD, Northup CJ. Quality of life and resolution of co-morbidities in super-obese patients remaining morbidly obese after Roux-en-Y gastric bypass. Surg Obes Relat Dis 2007;3(3):387-91.

[91] Boan J, Kolotkin RL, Westman EC, McMahon RL, Grant JP. Binge eating, quality of life and physical activity improve after Roux-en-Y gastric bypass for morbid obesity. Obes Surg 2004;14(3):341-8.

[92] Kinzl JF, Traweger C, Trefalt E, Biebl W. Psychosocial consequences of weight loss following gastric banding for morbid obesity. Obes Surg 2003;13(1):105-10.

[93] Rea JD, Yarbrough DE, Leeth RR, Leath TD, Clements RH. Influence of complications and extent of weight loss on quality of life after laparoscopic Roux-en-Y gastric bypass. Surg Endosc 2007;21(7):1095-100.

[94] Fischer S, Chen E, Katterman S, Roerhig M, Bochierri-Ricciardi L, Munoz D, et al. Emotional eating in a morbidly obese bariatric surgery-seeking population. Obes Surg 2007;17(6):778-84.

[95] Herpertz S, Kielmann R, Wolf AM, Hebebrand J, Senf W. Do psychosocial variables predict weight loss or mental health after obesity surgery? A systematic review. Obes Res 2004;12(10):1554-69.

[96] van Hout GC, Hagendoren CA, Verschure SK, van Heck GL. Psychosocial predictors of success after vertical banded gastroplasty. Obes Surg 2009;19(6):701-7.

[97] Sanchez-Santos R, Del Barrio MJ, Gonzalez C, Madico C, Terrado I, Gordillo ML, et al. Long-term health-related quality of life following gastric bypass: influence of depression. Obes Surg 2006;16(5):580-5.

[98] van Hout GC, Verschure SK, van Heck GL. Psychosocial predictors of success following bariatric surgery. Obes Surg 2005;15(4):552-60.

[99] Green AE, Dymek-Valentine M, Pytluk S, Le Grange D, Alverdy J. Psychosocial outcome of gastric bypass surgery for patients with and without binge eating. Obes Surg 2004;14(7):975-85.

[100] Malone M, Alger-Mayer S. Binge status and quality of life after gastric bypass surgery: a one-year study. Obes Res 2004;12(3):473-81.

[101] Larsen JK, van Ramshorst B, Geenen R, Brand N, Stroebe W, van Doornen LJ. Binge eating and its relationship to outcome after laparoscopic adjustable gastric banding. Obes Surg 2004;14(8):1111-7.

[102] Kalarchian MA, Marcus MD, Wilson GT, Labouvie EW, Brolin RE, LaMarca LB. Binge eating among gastric bypass patients at long-term follow-up. Obes Surg 2002;12(2):270-5.

[103] de Zwaan M, Lancaster KL, Mitchell JE, Howell LM, Monson N, Roerig JL, et al. Health-related quality of life in morbidly obese patients: effect of gastric bypass surgery. Obes Surg 2002;12(6):773-80.

[104] Burgmer R, Grigutsch K, Zipfel S, Wolf AM, de Zwaan M, Husemann B, et al. The influence of eating behavior and eating pathology on weight loss after gastric restriction operations. Obes Surg 2005;15(5):684-91.

[105] Rohde P, Ichikawa L, Simon GE, Ludman EJ, Linde JA, Jeffery RW, et al. Associations of child sexual and physical abuse with obesity and depression in middle-aged women. Child Abuse Negl 2008;32(9):878-87.

[106] King TK, Clark MM, Pera V. History of sexual abuse and obesity treatment outcome. Addict Behav 1996;21(3):283-90.

[107] Larsen JK, Geenen R. Childhood sexual abuse is not associated with a poor outcome after gastric banding for severe obesity. Obes Surg 2005;15(4):534-7.

[108] Biorserud C, Olbers T, Fagevik Olsen M. Patients' experience of surplus skin after laparoscopic gastric bypass. Obes Surg 2009;21(3):273-7.

[109] Stuerz K, Piza H, Niermann K, Kinzl JF. Psychosocial impact of abdominoplasty. Obes Surg 2008;18(1):34-8.

[110] Potoczna N, Harfmann S, Steffen R, Briggs R, Bieri N, Horber FF. Bowel habits after bariatric surgery. Obes Surg 2008;18(10):1287-96.

[111] Mitchell JE, Lancaster KL, Burgard MA, Howell LM, Krahn DD, Crosby RD, et al. Long-term follow-up of patients' status after gastric bypass. Obes Surg 2001;11(4):464-8.

[112] Wang W, Yu PJ, Lee YC, Wei PL, Lee WJ. Laparoscopic vertical banded gastroplasty: 5-year results. Obes Surg 2005;15(9):1299-303.

[113] Poves I, Cabrera M, Maristany C, Coma A, Ballesta-Lopez C. Gastrointestinal quality of life after laparoscopic Roux-en-Y gastric bypass. Obes Surg 2006;16(1):19-23.

[114] Berarducci A. Bone loss. An emerging problem following obesity surgery. Orthop Nurs 2007;26(5):281-8.

[115] Bocchieri LE, Meana M, Fisher BL. Perceived psychosocial outcomes of gastric bypass surgery: a qualitative study. Obes Surg 2002;12(6):781-8.

[116] Ryan MA. My story: a personal perspective on bariatric surgery. Crit Care Nurs Q 2005;28(3):288-92.

[117] Garza SF. Bariatric weight loss surgery: patient education, preparation, and follow-up. Crit Care Nurs Q 2003;26(2):101-4.

[118] Walfish S. Self-assessed emotional factors contributing to increased weight gain in pre-surgical bariatric patients. Obes Surg 2004;14(10):1402-5.

SECTION 6: END OF LIFE

In: Food, Nutrition and Eating Behavior
Editors: Joav Merrick and Sigal Israeli

ISBN: 978-1-62948-233-0
© 2014 Nova Science Publishers, Inc.

Chapter 22

NUTRIENTS AND FLUIDS AT THE END OF LIFE

Lee A Bricker*, MD, Barry M Kinzbrunner, MD,
Kevin J Kavanaugh, MD
and Donald E Greydanus, MD, DrHC (ATHENS)

Department of Internal Medine, Department of Pediatric and Adolescent Medicine,
Western Michigan University School of Medicine, Kalamazoo, Michigan and Vitas
Innovative Hospice Care, Miami, Florida, US

ABSTRACT

Controversy over how and whether to provide nutrition and fluid support to patients at
the end of life has raged across medical, legal, ethical and religious disciplines for years,
largely unaided by agreed-upon scientifically established guidelines. Many terminally ill
patients are anorexic and may wish to be spared food and liquid beyond their own limited
preferences, raising questions, particularly on the part of family members, as to whether,
when, and how to initiate artificial feeding and administration of fluids. This chapter
outlines common techniques and consequences of such support. It reviews some unique
biochemical features of terminal illness, including the role of inflammatory cytokines in
anorexia and cachexia, and proposes tentative physiological mechanisms as to how those
processes in terminal phases of diseases, cancer-associated and others, may lead to
adverse effects when artificial nutrition and fluids are employed inappropriately. In
managing a patient nearing death, the ethical physician, acting within the constraints of
known physiology, should provide the patient, caregivers, and surrogate decision makers
with the best available information regarding the benefits and burdens of such artificial
support. The properly informed patient's decisions should be held as first priority when
possible.

---

* Correspondence: Professor Lee A Bricker, MD, Department of Medicine, Western Michigan University School of
Medicine, 1000 Oakland Drive, D48G, Kalamazoo, MI 49008-1284, United States. E-mail:
lee.bricker@med.wmich.edu.

INTRODUCTION

In recent years there has been much debate over whether, how and when to provide fluids and nutrition to terminally ill patients, i.e., patients with far-advanced illnesses of various types, no longer amenable to primary therapy directed at cure or remission. In general, treatment for those patients focuses on relief of symptoms and providing comfort (1). Administered fluids and nutrition fit with more difficulty into this paradigm and may spawn ethical dilemmas (2-5), since few scientific standards for estimating their requirements in these settings have been established. Physicians and other care givers, often abetted by family members (6-9), facing this paucity of guiding data, may experience a need to "help" and thus administer such substances, even after the decision may have been made to stop other therapies. This paper reflects the authors' experiences, and those of others, with patients in both hospice and hospital settings over the past several years.

In patients close to death, symptoms ordinarily associated with hunger and thirst may be overshadowed by other symptoms. Curtis et al. (10) examined this issue, and found that pain (89%), weight loss (58%), and dyspnea, early satiety and fatigue (40%) are more frequent and pressing than is hunger (generally uncommon in the terminal setting). "Thirst," also uncommon, rarely results from altered sodium levels or true deficit of volume or of free water (11), is usually mild, and may be manageable with sips of water or ice chips and meticulous mouth care. Volume repletion may help an occasional ambulatory patient with postural hypotension (12). Cognitive impairment (13) and delirium (14) are, by contrast, rather commonly encountered.

The general lack of urgency associated with use of artificial nutrition and volume/fluid repletion in terminally ill patients allows a more deliberate approach and a consideration of the related ethical and clinical issues. Utilizing artificial nutrition and fluid support in a patient nearing death requires careful evaluation of his/her probable true physiological needs and state of awareness and affect and individual wishes, mindful of the possibility of doing harm.

Definition of "terminal" status

Table 1 summarizes objective guidelines by which patients may be adjudged "terminal," i.e., "hospice-appropriate." Patients meeting these criteria do not regularly survive beyond six months (15), though some remain reasonably functional and able to nourish themselves over much of this time. The prognostic value of the criteria is more limited in patients with non-cancer diagnoses. The guidelines are based on well-accepted observations, but continue to evolve, influenced by changing fiscal and regulatory policies.

Many physicians believe that fluids and nutrition must always be supplied to a terminally ill patient, even when demise is imminent; and that failing to use them is equivalent to hastening death (16). A critical goal for the physician, rather, is to reach a reasoned decision as to whether artificial nutritional or fluid support might be harmful to such a patient.

Table 1. Criteria for determining terminal status

Cancer:	Continuing and irreversible decline after all appropriate forms of therapy (Some may be appropriate for investigational therapy)

Heart disease: New York Heart Association Class IV (Irreversible congestive
        heart failure)
    Symptomatic at rest
    Refractory to vasodilators, inotropics, and diuretics
    Intractable angina resistant to nitrates, beta-blockers and
    calcium channel blockers

Chronic pulmonary disease:
    Pulmonary disease both severe and progressive, with
        either hypoxemia ($PO_2 < 55$ mm Hg, on ABG* or
            pulse oximetry of <88%)
            or hypercapnia ($PCO_2 > 50$ mm Hg) on ABG*
    Evidence of cor pulmonale
    Weight loss > 10% in 6 months
    Resting tachycardia of > 100/min

Liver disease:
    One or more of these associates of advanced liver failure:
    Clinical:
        Diuretic-resistant ascites
        Hepatorenal syndrome
        Spontaneous bacterial peritonitis
        Lactulose-refractory hepatic encephalopathy
        Refractory variceal bleeding
    Laboratory:
        Prothrombin time over 5 seconds > control
        Hypoalbuminemia < 2.5 g/dL

AIDS: Patients have both:
        CD4+ (T-cell) $< 25/mm^3$
        Viral load > 100,000 copies/ml
    and one or more of:
        Refractory, or central nervous system, lymphoma
        Wasting, with > 33% loss of lean body mass
        Mycobacterium avium bacteremia
        Progressive multifocal leukoencephalopathy
        Refractory visceral Kaposi sarcoma
        Renal failure
        Refractory cryptosporidium or toxoplasmosis

General criteria for determining terminal status, i.e., hospice-appropriateness, in cancer and in selected
    non-cancer situations: an illustrative outline, not intended to be exhaustive. After Stuart (*136,137*);
    and Wright and Kinzbrunner (*138*).
*ABG = Arterial blood gases.

Table 2. Metabolic Alterations: "Simple" Starvation vs. Cancer Cachexia

	Starvation	Cancer Cachexia
METABOLIC RATE		
Resting energy exp.	Decreased	Normal / Increased
Respiratory quotient	Decreased	Normal / Increased
O_2 consumption, CO_2 prod.	Decreased	Unchanged
CARBOHYDRATE		
Insulin Resistance	Increased	Increased
Glucose turnover / utilization	Decreased	Increased (tumor effect)
Hepatic Gluconeogenesis	Increased	Increased (from tumor lactate)
Serum insulin	Decreased	Unchanged
Serum Lactate	Unchanged	Increased (tumor effect)
Cori Cycle Activity	Unchanged	Increased (tumor effect)
FAT		
Lipolysis	Increased	Increased
Lipoprotein Lipase Act.	Unchanged	Decreased (TNF-α-mediated?)
Serum Triglycerides	Decreased /	Increased /Unchanged
PROTEIN		
Protein Turnover	Decreased	Unchanged / Increased
Urinary nitrogen excr. rate	Decreased	Unchanged / Increased
Skeletal Muscle Catabolism	Decreased	Increased
Skeletal Muscle Anabolism	Decreased	Decreased
Nitrogen balance	Negative	Negative

Adapted from Gentilini et al. (20). This table contrasts metabolic sequelae of "simple" starvation with those seen in the cachexia of cancer. The latter is a hypermetabolic event, whereas in remediable starvation, the body attempts to adopt a mode of conservation.
(With Permission: Elsivier Science, Ltd)

Distinguishing terminal anorexia/cachexia from "simple" starvation

The patient with terminal cachexia associated with an incurable disease may look very similar to the patient with potentially remediable protein-calorie starvation (i.e., "concentration camp syndrome," or anorexia nervosa) with no underlying terminal illness. Despite their similar physical appearances, they are clinically distinguishable, with sharp differences in their physiology and management. Both states manifest negative nitrogen balance and weight loss (17). Table 2 illustrates principal differences between them, using cancer cachexia as the prototype model for the terminal cachexia syndrome. One key difference, for example, is that terminal cachexia is associated with increased resting energy expenditure and of rates of carbohydrate, fat, and protein metabolism, the extent dictated by tumor type (18, 19); while in starvation, energy expenditure and rates of metabolism of nutrients are generally conserved. Further, in starvation skeletal muscle is relatively spared whereas in the cachexia of terminal illness fat, muscle and bone all tend to be catabolized avidly (20). In "simple" starvation, nutrients can ultimately heal the defect. In terminally ill patients, by contrast, administered nutrients and fluids do little for the underlying illness and are likely to generate harmful results.

Table 3. Possible adverse fates of elemental nutrients administered to patients with terminal illnesses

Administered nutrient:	Desired fate of nutrient:	Possible adverse effects:
Glucose / Carbohydrate	ATP Generation	Hyperglycemia(D) Osmotic Diuresis (D, R) Metabolic acidosis (D, R) Resp acidosis (H,P) Hyponatremia (D) Hypertriglyceridemia (D) Cerebral Edema (D)
Amino acid / protein	New Protein Synthesis Increased Strength	Azotemia (D,R,H,L) Aminoaciduria (R,L) Ammonia Prod (R,L) Encephalopathy (P, L) Hyperchloremic Acidosis (L)
Fatty acid / fat	Energy	Fat deposition: liver, periphery (D,R,H,P,L) Pancreatitis (D,R,H,P,L) Fat overload syndrome (D,R,H,P,L) Hypertriglyceridemia (D)

Index end-stage diseases: D = diabetes; R = renal failure; H = heart disease; P = pulmonary disease; L = liver disease.

Possible consequences of administered nutrient components in non-cancer terminal illnesses in the setting(s) of the disease(s) indicated by the letters under "Index end-stage diseases." Events listed in the "possible adverse consequences" section may be also seen in some imminently terminal cancer patients.

In terminal cachexia, administered nutrients thus may not be effectively usable for production of energy or new protein. Amino acids may be disproportionately converted to urea, ammonia and other nitrogenous wastes, and carbohydrates to carbon dioxide and water, often with detrimental effects, including respiratory acidosis (21,22). Infused fat may deposit in, and impair function of, the liver. In the periphery, it may produce useless weight gain and may also produce acute pancreatitis or the uncommon fat overload syndrome. The latter may manifest in hypertriglyceridemia, coagulopathy, fever, or hepatosplenomegaly, with the administered fat accumulating in liver, kidneys, spleen, lungs, and brain.

Table 3 summarizes possible fates of nutrient components, contrasted with their desired goals, in anorexia / cachexia syndromes seen both in cancer and in non-cancer terminal diseases.

Table 4 lists some of the biochemical bases underlying the adverse effects produced by nutrients in these patients.

Table 4. Physiologic factors underlying possible adverse consequences of fluids and nutrients given in terminal non-cancer illnesses: selected examples

Disease State	Underlying Physiologic Defects	"Support" Measure	Possible Adverse Consequences
Cardiac or Pulmonary cachexia	Heart or lung failure ↑ Intravascular volume CO_2 retention	Glucose	Respiratory acidosis aggravated dyspnea Hypoxemia
Liver Failure	Hypoalbuminemia	Amino Acid, Protein	Ammonia/ urea production
	↓ intravascular volume ↓ intravascular oncotic pressure	Protein	Encephalopathy, pre-renal azotemia
	Fat overload syndrome	Lipid	Fat overload syndrome pancreatitis
	2° aldosteronism ↑ ECF* volume	Volume (saline)	Edema, ascites, restrictive pulm complications Hepatorenal syndrome
		Free Water	Hyponatremia, confusion
		Glucose	Osmotic diuresis (may palliate terminal hypoglycemia)
Diabetes Mellitus	Related to cardiac, renal, infectious, or other complications	Volume saline	Congestive failure in patients with cardiomyopathy ESRD†
		Glucose Fat	Hyperosmolar syndrome ↑ insulin resistance

Examples of adverse effects of fluid and nutrients in selected terminal non-cancer illnesses. The list expands concepts described in Table 3, and is not intended to be exhaustive. * ECF = Extracellular Fluid; † ESRD = End-stage renal disease. ↑ = increase; ↓ = decrease.

The physiological basis of the terminal anorexia / cachexia syndrome remains enigmatic, and current clinical application of principles extracted from it are tentative. Laviano et al. have proposed that in advanced cancer anorexigenic substances, including increased blood and cerebrospinal levels of tryptophan, stimulate the ventromedial hypothalamic serotoninergic system, augmenting hypothalamic serotonin synthesis and mediating anorexia (23). They have also implicated tumor-generated cytokines, including interleukin-1 (IL-1), as facilitators of tryptophan supply to the brain. Tryptophan, possibly by augmenting brain serotonin neurotransmission, inhibits closely linked neuropeptide Y (NPY), in the orexigenic process (24).

They showed that peripheral infusion of IL-1 increases brain concentrations of tryptophan and serotonin and induces anorexia in rats. Thyrotropin-releasing hormone (TRH) is similarly involved (25).

Cytokines, molecules with some hormone-like properties, are involved in mediating other disease-associated processes including apoptosis and inflammation. Tumor necrosis factor alpha (TNF-a) is probably a primary regulatory cytokine (26), and is involved, at least circumstantially, in the pathologic sequelae of many terminal illnesses. It is a likely factor in rendering ineffective attempts directed at metabolic remediation. This topic has been recently reviewed by Braun and Marks (27).

CLINICAL SYNDROMES

Cancer

Cachexia occurs in 50-80% of cancer patients (28) and more often in some cancers (e.g., lung and gastrointestinal lesions) than in others (29). In some cancers there are associated identifiable processes that may play a role in terminal wasting. Patients with gastrointestinal malignancies may develop an hepatic acute phase response (30) useful in monitoring for tumor recurrence or advance (31-33) and that may be associated with an increase in overall resting energy expenditure and reduced survival time. Interleukin-6 (IL-6), another inflammatory cytokine, may be important in producing acute phase (C-reactive) protein synthesis in hepatocytes in vitro (34), and thus possibly in cancer patients. Involved cytokines may circulate independently or be delivered to metabolically active target tissues by peripheral blood mononuclear cells (35), may activate other anorexigenic neuropeptides (such as corticotropin-releasing factor) acting through inhibition of appetite-stimulating NPY, and may share an anorexigenic signaling pathway with leptin (36). Laviano and Maguid (37) summarized the metabolic effects of four often-examined cytokines (Table 5). These products of the immune system act at multiple points to facilitate the anorexia associated with terminal illness (38, 39). Other cancer-related factors associated with cachexia appear able to mobilize fatty acids from adipose tissue and amino acid from muscle. One such factor is a class of proteoglycans that acts on skeletal muscle to promote release of amino acids (40-42) that are then brought to the liver and converted to glucose, or are metabolized by the tumor. Further, a "futile" anorexigenic energy-consuming Cori cycle between tumor-produced lactate and glucose resynthesis in the liver may occur (43).

Metabolic products of those processes tend to appear in the urine of patients with terminal cancer but not in that of persons with remediable starvation. Other metabolic hallmarks of deranged metabolism unique to cancer have been described. Tisdale has shown an association of cancer-related protein degradation with an increased activity of an ATP-ubiquitin-proteasome pathway, an effect blunted by eicosapentanoic acid, but not by other artificially supplied nutrients (Tables 3 and 4). This fatty acid may lessen the rate of weight and fat loss in patients with advanced pancreatic cancer (44,45) and AIDS (46). Tisdale has reviewed in detail current knowledge of the physiology of cancer cachexia (47).

Do nutrients given to terminal cancer patients stimulate tumor growth? No controlled studies have examined this, and suspicion to that effect remains without firm foundation. As Copeland has observed anecdotally, "Many thousands of cancer patients have been nutritionally replenished by both enteral and parenteral nutrition...without the scientific community noting tumor growth to be a clinical problem" (48). More recent work has continued unable to show convincingly that such stimulation occurs.

AIDS

End-stage AIDS is characterized by increased resting energy expenditure and negative nitrogen balance similar to that seen in other terminal illnesses, and is likewise not significantly remediable by nutritional repletion (49). Severe wasting may be less marked in AIDS than in other terminal illnesses until near the end of its course (50), then resulting from hypermetabolism as well as inability to consume or use calories. AIDS patients not yet terminal seem to decrease physical activity to protect themselves against wasting (51); but when wasting develops in AIDS, the final stage of the illness is likely close at hand (52).

End-stage pulmonary disease

Patients with terminal lung ailments often develop cachexia associated with a significant increase in the work of breathing (53). Tissue wasting is frequent among patients with chronic obstructive pulmonary disease (COPD). Its mechanism, not fully understood, involves cytokines, increased dietary thermogenesis, hypermetabolism, increased oxygen cost of ventilation, and chronic acidosis (54). With or without hypercapnia, patients with end-stage lung disease may reach a point where nutrients beyond a certain level produce an adverse effect on ventilatory status (55-57). These patients appear to do best when selecting their own diets (57).

Table 5. Cytokine-mediated effects on metabolism

Cytokine	Protein	Carbohydrate	Lipid
TNF-	Muscle proteolysis ↑ Liver protein synth* ↑ Skeletal wasting ↑	Glycogenolysis ↑ Gluconeogenesis ↑ Lactate production ↑	Lipogenesis ↓
IL-1	Liver protein synth* ↑ Skeletal wasting ↑	Gluconeogenesis ↑	Lipolysis ↑ LPL† synth* / act‡ ↓ Fatty Acid Synth ↑
IL-6	Liver protein synth* ↑		Lipolysis ↓ Fatty Acid Synth* ↑
INF-γ			Lipogenesis ↓ Lipolysis ↓ LPL synth* / act ‡ ↓

Cytokines related to the presence of many tumors and to many non-cancer terminal states exert effects that accelerate intermediate metabolism and promote tissue catabolism. These are not correctable by repletion of fuel substrate.

* synth = synthesis   ↑ = increased.
† LPL = lipoprotein lipase   ↓ = decreased.
‡ act = action/activity.
¶ INF-γ = Interferon gamma.
From: Laviano A and Meguid MM (*37*) reproduced with permission (Elsevier Science).

Cardiac cachexia

A multisystem, multifactorial syndrome is associated with advanced congestive heart failure. In this syndrome some patients experience generalized wasting with loss of fat, muscle and bone. As in other disease-specific terminal anorexia/ cachexia syndromes excess nutrient and fluid introduces substances that may be anabolically ineffective and potentially harmful. Once cachexia develops in a patient for whom transplant or support is unfeasible, remaining life span is usually short. Neuroendocrine and immunological abnormalities, including elevated TNF alpha in plasma (58, 59), have been found in these patients, though its precise role in the process remains unclear. Abnormal reflex control within cardiovascular and respiratory systems is also seen and portends a poor prognosis (50% at 18 months)(60). In this syndrome, as in cancer, AIDS, etc., overzealous administration of nutrients and fluids may introduce useless and often harmful outcomes.

Diabetes

Patients dying with diabetes present widely varied terminal pictures and usually succumb to one or more of the disease's complications, including end-stage cardiac and/or renal disease, sepsis, macrovascular disease, osteomyelitis and others. Forced fluid and nutrition in terminal patients with diabetes may aggravate problems associated with those of its complications.

Liver failure

End-stage liver disease may present in any of several ways; and patients not amenable to transplantation require terminal management. Advanced cirrhosis or a large tumor burden in the liver may cause significant hypoalbuminemia with diminished intravascular oncotic pressure, resulting in edema, and anasarca, complicated by abnormal renal sodium handling from secondary aldosteronism. Restriction of dietary protein and sodium may lessen the likelihood of hepatic encephalopathy and may reduce ascites (61-63). Restricting free water may lessen the extent of hyponatremia and cerebral edema. Response to the administration of fluids or nutrients beyond carefully selected basal amounts may be poor, though in some severely glycogen-depleted patients with end stage liver disease infusions of concentrated glucose may forestall hypoglycemia-associated coma.

End-stage renal disease

Death from renal failure is commonly delayed in the United States, owing to transplantation and dialysis. When advanced uremia dominates the terminal scenario it may be associated with hypoalbuminemia and an augmented inflammatory response, contributing to anorexia and wasting partly via cytokine-mediated mechanisms (64).

Inappropriately salt-restricted patients with terminal renal disease and critically-reduced nephron populations may crave salt in the service of re-expansion of plasma volume that has occurred in response to loss of urinary concentrating power and attendant sodium wasting (65). This salt craving, a seeming exception to the pattern of anorexia, may be seen among terminally ill renal patients and may have significant palliative value.

Volume repletion and hydration: Relevance to parenteral nutrition

Repletion of fluids, either intravenously or otherwise, with or without added elemental nutritional components, has major, practical implications in terms of body fluid spaces (Table 6) that should be considered when intravenous or enteral feeding is contemplated. Total parenteral nutrition (TPN) solutions are often composed of significant quantities of free-water-rich, hypo-osmolal materials that, on infusion, may lead not only to nutrient-associated complications (Tables 3 and 4), but also to increased volumes of gastrointestinal and urine output. This often produces maceration of the skin and the eventual need for bladder catheterization; and a risk of hyponatremia and cerebral edema with their attendant ill effects on sensorium.

Table 6. Possible adverse effects of artificially-administered volume and free water in terminally ill patients

Possible Effect	Administered Fluid	
	Isotonic saline ("volume")	Free water
↑ pulmonary / bronchial secretion ↑ dyspnea, cough,	+	
Congestive heart failure	+	
Pulmonary, peripheral, edema	+	
Ascites, effusion	+	
Cerebral edema, hyponatremia		+
↑ urine output; increased need for bladder catheter;		
maceration of perisacral skin	+	+
Headache	+	+
Increased GI output / diarrhea	+	+

This table focuses on separate predominant hazards of isotonic sodium-containing (i.e., "volume"), and of free water-containing, fluids (e.g., 5-20% glucose in water) administered to patients with terminal illnesses outside of carefully-identified clinical indications. Fluids such as 0.45 % (half-normal) saline and 5% glucose in 0.45% saline, which combine volume and free water, thereby combine the potential hazards of both types of fluid.

Table 6 summarizes possible consequences of inappropriate fluids given to patients who may be deficient in cardiovascular, pulmonary, hepatic, and/or renal reserve. It separately outlines potential ill effects of free water and of isotonic sodium-containing fluids. Either, given to a terminally ill patient may be hazardous.

A distinction between "volume repletion" and "rehydration" (66) (Table 6) thus carries practical clinical implications. Gentle volume repletion in terminally ill persons may be useful in managing troublesome orthostasis and in preserving cognitive function in patients on opioids (10). True dehydration (i.e., free water deficit with hypernatremia) is uncommon and is addressable, when necessary, with water drinking or ice chips (67), or by intravenous glucose in water.

Table 7. Results of prospective randomized controlled trials: Use of TPN* in cancer patients on chemotherapy (1978-1987)

Use of TPN* in cancer patients on chemotherapy (1978-1987)									
Study	Number of Patients		Infection Rate (%)		Tumor Response (%)		Survival (%)		Tumor Investigated
	TPN	Control	*TPN*	Control	*TPN*	Control	*TPN*	Control	
Issell et al. *(78)*	13	14	---	---	*31*	8	---	---	Lung/ squamous cell
Van Eys et al. *(91)*	10	10	**0.71** †	**0.01** †	---	---	---	---	Various / childhood
Popp et al. *(79, 80)*	20	21	---	---	---	---	69	66 (2 years)	Lymphoma
Nixon et al. *(86, 87)*	20	25	5	4	15	12	**79**	**308** (days)	Colon / rectal
Samuels et al. *(92)*	18	15	**17**	**4**	63	79	72	77 (2.5 yrs)	Testis
Jordan et al. *(81)*	19	24	**32**	**8**	**12**	**30**	**22**	**40** (wk)	Lung / aden
Hays et al. *(88)*	5	5	---	---	60	80	**80**	**100** *(post ctx)* ‡	Acute Leukemia
Shamberger et al. *(84, 85)*	14	18	42	33	14	50	**13**	**44** (4 yrs)	Sarcomas
Clamon et al. *(93)*	57	62	**35**	**5**	48	43	51	57 (1 year)	Lung/ small cell
Valdivieso et al. *(82, 83)*	30	35	27	18	43	66	11 mo	12 mo	Lung/ small cell

From: *(76)* Klein S and Koretz, RL: in Nutrition support in patients with cancer: what do the data really show? Nutrition in Clinical Practice 9: 91-100, 1994. **Bold underline**: apparent net harm; ***bold italics:*** apparent net benefit from TPN

Adapted with permission, American Society of Parenteral and Enteral Nutrition.

* TPN = total parenteral nutrition.

† Rate of sepsis per 100 days on protocol.

‡ ctx= chemotherapy.

It has been speculated that, should some dehydration occur in a dying patient, a natural analgesia rather than thirst may occur (68). Such an effect may be related to endogenous cerebral opioid production in patients, as suggested by opioid production in the brains of water-deprived experimental animals (69); alternatively, some analgesia may result from the ketogenesis that may accompany cessation of eating (70).

Parenteral nutrition in terminally ill patients

In the 1970's there was early optimism that TPN might prevent wasting and preserve muscle mass and strength in patients with terminal malignancies. This optimism was sparked by reports such as those of Copeland et al. (71), who examined the effects of TPN in 406 cancer patients over 3 years, in whom it appeared to facilitate anti-cancer therapy. Other reports showed TPN-associated improvement in delayed hypersensitivity, suitability for chemotherapy and radiotherapy, and improved well being and strength in cancer patients (72-75).

Other work from that era showed less favorable or consistent results (76-78)(see table 7). Data comparing effects of TPN with non-TPN-managed controls have often demonstrated the modality to be of limited value and sometimes harmful in cancer management (79-88), albeit of possible limited benefit in selected patients with obstructive bowel cancer (89) and for symptom reduction in patients with problematic dehydration (90). Increases in rates of infection associated with TPN are commonly observed (91-94). Though TPN appears not to directly stimulate tumor growth, it has been suggested that a nutrition regimen exceeding basal needs may complicate a patient's general anorexia-associated adaptive responses to the tumor, a viewpoint that has been supported by subsequent biochemical and clinical evidence (95).

Sakurai and Klein (21) enumerated disappointing results from attempting to improve clinical outcomes in cancer with artificial nutritional support and concluded that tumor-induced alterations in intermediate metabolism were responsible for the cachexia. Moreover, intravenous nutrition in terminal patients, a major financial expense (96), rarely improves either quality or length of life (97).

Enteral feeding

Enteral techniques require the use of nasogastric tubes, percutaneous gastrostomy, or percutaneous tube insertions directly into the duodenum or jejunum. Adverse events unique to enteral alimentation, aside from discomfort, include nasal and esophageal problems including aspiration, esophagitis, ulceration and fistula. Leakage with percutaneous techniques may produce peritonitis. Enteric-feeding-associated problems of nausea and vomiting, maldigestion, osmotic diarrhea, and fecal impaction, as well as the unwanted effects of absorption of the infused substances (tables 3 and 7), also must be considered. Furthermore, downstream implantation of a feeding tube does not preclude aspiration.

Tube feeding does not simulate the sensory aspects of eating and drinking. There is little evidence that it prolongs life in dying patients or can reverse terminal anorexia / cachexia. Aside from its supportive role in non-terminal patients temporarily unable to eat or drink, we believe that enteral techniques have limited applicability. Some advocate their use in upper gastrointestinal (non terminal) cancer patients (98), in whom intravenous support may also be of benefit. Others employ it in selected nursing home patients with dementia. However, once dementia becomes advanced, tube feeding does not prolong life or enhance apparent comfort, is no more effective than spoon-feeding, and is thus of little constructive value (99,100).

Ahronheim reached similar conclusions (101). More recent studies have been largely confirmatory of the idea that tube feeding in dementia, while common and widespread, is usually a result of a need to "do something helpful" whereas a sound scientific basis for it remains lacking (102). Scott and Austin (103) studied severely dysphagic patients with amyotrophic lateral sclerosis, finding no difference in survival times or in ages of death between the groups with and without feeding tubes. Their observations highlight the importance of continuing to try to use hand feeding even in patients with advanced neurological disorders. Sampson has discussed the benefits and problems associated with enteral tube feeding in these settings (104).

Subcutaneous infusion: hypodermoclysis

Many patients near the end of life do not have access to intravenous lines and have peripheral veins that make intravenous therapy impractical or impossible. Fluids and medications can nonetheless sometimes be given in effective variety and amounts via hypodermoclysis, i.e., the infusion of these materials directly into the subcutaneous space via a small Teflon canola or butterfly needle. Hyaluronidase is added to the infusate to lessen resistance to absorption in the interstitial space (105,106). This important and effective technique should be used with the same cautions and restraints that apply to other methods.

Ancillary methods

Anabolic agents used to stimulate appetites of patients with terminal anorexia have produced varied results (107-109). Currently several are available, with helpful effects seen in selected patients, usually for a limited time. Of these, megestrol acetate (Megace ®) is of particular interest. Used in patients with both cancer and AIDS, it may increase appetite and sense of well-being and may produce a delayed gain in non-edema weight that may persist as long as the medication is continued; and, in cancer, may effectively stimulate appetite and objective measures of nutrition (110). However, its anti-anorexigenic effects may dissipate within a few weeks. Side effects include deep-vein thrombosis, mild vaginal bleeding, and impotence (111). The drug may have significant corticosteroid-like effects, including Cushing syndrome and adrenocortical suppression over time that reveals itself when the drug is withdrawn (112).

Other corticosteroid analogs may transiently enhance mood, but usually are not associated with weight gain (113, 114). They may also promote edema and cushingoid stigmata. Human growth hormone may have symptomatic benefits; clinical observations suggest that it may stimulate some recovery of lean body mass relatively early in a wasting illness. However, it is costly and does not prolong life (115).

Ghrelin, a hormone produced in the stomach, is a natural ligand for the growth hormone secretagogue receptor and is the only known natural stimulator of appetite in man. It exhibits anti-cachectic activity, acting in part by blocking production of proinflammatory cytokines, and is under study for use in cancer as well as several other terminal states (116-118), though early results in cancer have been disappointing (119). It has shown interesting preliminary results in chronic obstructive disease (120) and congestive heart failure (121). Other agents, such as melanocortin antagonists eicosapentanoic acid, and antimyostatin agents, have been examined as possible means of managing cachexia in several chronic illnesses (122)

These, and other agents under investigation, may have palliative value in certain settings. None has been shown to impact favorably on the basic underlying disease process. Relatively simple ancillary measures can sometimes enhance a patient's desire to eat and are a vital part of management. These include sensitive dietary counseling, easing of other medical restrictions on eating such as sodium restriction (2), careful mouth care and management of thrush, and providing frequent small meals.

CLINICAL CONSIDERATIONS

Terminally ill patients ideally are shifted from aggressive management to comfort measures, directed in large part by the patient. When questions arise regarding methods of delivering fluids and nutrients to dying patients it should be kept in mind that there is no currently known way of estimating the optimal requirements of these substances, or, indeed, if such requirements exist.

Patients have a right to be provided with "information from physicians" within this framework, and full discussion of "benefits, risks, and costs of appropriate treatment alternatives" (123). Such discussion should include, where feasible, information relevant to the patient's condition, communicated in terms easily understood by the patient and his/her caregivers; and should include consideration about how various approaches are likely to affect survival as well as symptoms and social relationships. Additional benefits of such discussion may include reinforcement of relationships between the patient, the family, and the health care professionals involved that need to be sustained though the dying process.

If careful analysis of the situation suggests that the patient is more likely to be harmed than benefited from an intervention such as fluid administration or nasogastric feeding, either in terms of survival or symptom management, the physician should recommend against the intervention. The physician should review the natural history of a patient's specific disorder, as well as medical literature regarding known benefits and burdens of possible interventions. In such situations, the patient, family, and involved health care professionals, may need to explicitly acknowledge, and carefully set aside, assumptions they may have made about the role of food as a physical, social, and moral imperative.

If conflict develops over the potential value of using artificial support, acceding to the patient's wishes or those of the surrogate decision-maker may be the preferred route (123). For example, if a patient with a tracheo-esophageal fistula prefers to eat with his/her family in spite of being advised of the risk of aspiration, this preference might be honored. Likewise, a patient with locally advanced stomach cancer who chooses multiple uncomfortable procedures in the hope that artificial nutrition will prolong his life should be supported in attempting that course of treatment.

If it appears that the patient is more likely, in terms of survival and symptom management, to benefit from an intervention, the physician should recommend it. However, the fact that the patient has a terminal illness should not necessarily prevent the physician or others from considering a noninvasive treatment whose benefit is mainly to the patient's morale or psychological well-being. Careful consideration of the clinical situation and the patient's needs and wishes are required. Further, in this charged setting, depression may dominate and needs to be sought out and dealt with as expeditiously as possible.

Other problems may be encountered by adhering to a patient-directed approach. A common example is the sudden appearance on the scene of an indignant relative, making his/her view forcefully clear that the patient in question is "obviously starving to death" and demanding that the situation be corrected at once, usually by administering intravenous fluids. Reconciling the relative's demands with the physician's understanding of the practical limitations imposed by the events of the dying process may be resistant to negotiation.   Yet another problem may be the support team member who is adamant that any form of withdrawal/withholding of treatment, including patient-requested cessation of feeding or fluids, equals assisting suicide, or committing euthanasia (if the patient is comatose or delirious)(16). This stance may deny the right of an incurably ill patient who may be ready for death to be afforded the most comfortable exit possible.

Physicians and staff who are uncomfortable with patient-directed withdrawal of support or who equate it with assisting suicide should strongly consider transfer care to another physician. The patient's (or decision-maker's) election to withhold/withdraw fluids or feeding should not violate the physician's moral- or religious-based principles of conscience.

Quill and Byock (124) carefully confronted the question: when a terminally ill patient decides to stop eating and drinking in what the care team may perceive as an attempt to hasten death, is the physician supporting that decision assisting suicide? They described a patient dying from a brain tumor, who, witnessing his own deterioration, had adamantly made such a decision, with no input from his physicians. The authors, in describing the doubts and difficulties experienced by family and support team members in that and similar situations, set out guidelines for handling a patient's refusal or directed withdrawal/withholding of food and drink: the physician managing the basic illness must encourage open communication and consensus from close family members and from other physicians and staff, as well with hospice/palliative care specialists.

This is necessary for coordinating care and for minimizing the chance of doing harm by not acceding to the dying patient's wishes to be spared unwanted eating and drinking. Many believe that the two terms, withdrawing and withholding, are not distinguishable in terminal situations and connote no ethical difference (125, 126). Physicians have often observed, rather, that allowing dying patients to exercise their own preferences seems to maximize comfort and ease the process of dying (127). The literature is replete with anecdotal examples of patients who fared better when allowed to dictate their own intakes than when feeding and hydration were forced on them.

Eddy (128) described the peaceful death of his 85 year-old mother, whose entreaties not to be fed beyond her own limited desires were observed with gratifying effect. In a period of a year, McCann et al. (129) examined 32 terminally ill patients on a "comfort care unit" in which food and liquids were offered but never forced; and when given in quantities beyond what patients had asked for, played no evident role in enhancing comfort. In every case, ice chips and sips of liquid relieved the reported symptoms.

We would suggest that physicians should recognize patients' described levels of hunger and thirst with the same objectivity routinely afforded to their pain levels, considering that it is irrelevant whether the dying patient's directions to withhold food and drink are verbalized as part of a desire for a more peaceful demise, or perhaps result from a less formally expressed consequence of disease-induced, possibly cytokine/neuropeptide-generated anorexia. In whatever manner the dying patient may make known a wish to curtail eating and drinking, that wish may reflect an underlying biochemical process. Though pathophysiological evidence in support of this remains tentative, we believe it supports the notion that the physician acceding to a dying patient's wish to be spared unwanted food and fluid is acting in an ethical manner (130).

In their essay on potential legal barriers to end-of-life care, Meisel et al. (131) discussed several "myths," including that of the illegality of non-provision of artificial fluids and nutrition to terminally ill patients. In their follow up section, "Grains of Truth," they noted that "states with high legal standards about withholding and/or withdrawing feeding tubes or *other life-sustaining therapy* (italics ours) may effectively preclude these options from being legally available to patients who have not explicitly refused [them]," and that many nursing homes, fearing legal sanction, may not permit such withholding.

Nursing home policies are thus often problematic with regard to standards involving patients with dementia. They are often subjects of controversy based on the geographic location in which they operate (132,133), the ethnicity of patients in question (134) and other factors unrelated to a patient's actual clinical status. Though use of feeding tubes in demented, dysphagic patients in nursing homes may prolong life slightly (135), such "life-sustaining therapy" in these patients is in practicality no such thing. Their use in those who have "not explicitly refused" them, however, is subject to the same restraints that apply to those who have. "High legal standards" mandating their use in dying patients need to be reconsidered.

Physicians who "forge ahead" with aggressive measures on "ethical" grounds, howsoever well-intentioned, may be acting in a manner contrary to contemporary medical ethics and that fails to grasp the feasible limitations of Medicine. A proper balance of benefits and burdens and of ranges of choices by patients (or their decision makers) is required for clarifying the complexities of ethical problems at the end of life. This balance should be grounded as solidly as possible on known physiology. Valiant attempts to carry the battle out to the patient's last breath may run a significant risk of hastening it.

CONCLUSION

Many, if not most, terminal illnesses, whether cancer-related or not, are associated with a late anorexia not commonly accompanied by subjective senses of hunger or thirst, and not therefore requiring symptomatic relief. Patients themselves, where possible, should provide input as to how severe their symptoms are. Their wishes for nutrients and fluids should be paramount among the relevant guides to their use, since their administration is not likely to improve either the clinical course of an end-of-life scenario or its accompanying cachexia. Rather, these expensive substances, if not used with thoughtful deliberation in a setting in which precise guidelines for their use have not been established, have real capacity to do damage and to erode both the quality and the duration of what life may remain.

This paper highlights some known pathophysiologic mechanisms that appear associated irremediably with the process of dying and that are able to interfere with the terminal patient's ability to benefit from such intercessions. This mandates that such intercessions be carefully considered on a patient-by-patient basis, with attention to detail and to the avoidance of complications. The implications of that pathophysiology, although imperfectly understood, would seem to be a relevant component of an ethical approach to the clinical management of a patient near the end of life.

ACKNOWLEDGMENTS

The authors are indebted to Daniel M Lane, MD, PhD, and Richard Alan Shapiro, MD, for their reviews and comments on earlier drafts of the manuscript.

REFERENCES

[1]   Caring connections: National Hospice and Palliative Care Organization. Accessed 2011 Aug 20. URL: http://.www.caringinfo.org.

[2]   Kinzbrunner BM. Ethical dilemmas in hospice and palliative care. Support Care Cancer 1995;3:28-36.

[3]   Dunphy K, Finlay I, Rathbone G. Hicks F. Rehydration in palliative and terminal care: if not--why not? Palliat Med 1995;9:165-6.

[4]   Macdonald N. International Association for Hospice and Palliative Care. Accessed 2011 Aug 20. URL: http://www.hospicecare.com/Ethics/MacDoc.htm

[5]   Sihra L, Kinzbrunner BM. Artificial nutrition and hydration. In: Kinzbrunner BM, Policzer JM, eds. End-of-life care: A practical guide, 2nd ed. New York: McGraw-Hill Med, 2011.

[6]   Alpert HR, Emanuel L. Comparing utilization of life-sustaining treatments with patient and public preferences. J Gen Intern Med 1998;13:175-81.

[7]   Craig GM. On withholding artificial hydration and nutrition from terminally ill sedated patients: The debate continues. J Med Ethics 1996; 22:147-53.

[8]   Viola RA, Wells GA, Peterson J. The effects of fluid status and fluid therapy on the dying: A systematic review. J Palliat Care 1997;15:77-84.

[9]   Morita T, Tsunoda J, Inoue S, Chihara S. Perceptions and decision-making on rehydration of terminally ill cancer patients and family members. Am J Hosp Palliat Care 1999;16:509-16.

[10]   Curtis, EB, Krech R, and Walsh TD. Common symptoms in patients with advanced cancer. J Palliat Care 1991;7:25-9.

[11]   Vullo-Navich K, Smith S, Andrews M, et al. Comfort and incidence of abnormal serum sodium, BUN, creatinine and osmolality in dehydration of terminal illness. Am J Hosp Palliat Care 1998;15:77-84.

[12]   Billings JA. Comfort measures for the terminally ill: is dehydration painful? J Am Geriatr Soc 1985;33:808-10.

[13]   Bruera E, Miller L, McCallion J, Macmillan K, Krefting L, Hanson J. Cognitive failure in patients with terminal cancer: a prospective study. J Pain Sympt Manage 1992;7:192-5.

[14]   Lawlor PG, Fainsinger RL, Bruera ED. Delirium at the end of life: Critical issues in clinical practice and research. JAMA 2000; 284:2427-9.

[15]   Christakis NA and Escarce JJ. Survival of Medicare patients after enrollment in hospice programs. N Engl J Med 1996;335:172-8.

[16] Solomon MZ, O'Donnell L, Jennings B, Guilfoy V, Wolf SM, Nolan K, et al. Decisions near the end of life: Professional views on life-sustaining treatments. Am J Public Health 1993;83:14-23.

[17] Torun B, Chew F. Protein-energy malnutrition. In: Shils ME, Olson JA, Shike M, eds. Modern nutrition in health and disease. Baltimore, Williams Wilkins, 1994: 222-32.

[18] Fredrix EW, Soeters PB, Wouters EF, Deerenberg IM, von Meyenfeldt MF, Saris WH. Effect of different tumor types on resting energy expenditure. Cancer Res 1991;51:6138-41.

[19] Falconer JS, Fearon KC, Ross JA, Elton R, Wigmore SJ, Garden OJ, Carter DC. Acute-phase protein response and survival duration of patients with pancreatic cancer. Cancer 1995;75:2077-82.

[20] Gentilini O, Fahey TJ 3rd, Daly JM. Nutrition and the cancer patient. In: Winchester DP, Jones RS, Murphy GP, eds. Cancer surgery for the general surgeon. Philadelphia, PA: Lippincott-Raven, 1998:568-89.

[21] Sakurai Y, Klein S. Metabolic alterations in patients with cancer: nutritional implications. Surg Today 1998;28:247-57.

[22] Lindholm M. Critically ill patients and fat emulsions. Minerva Anesthesiol 1998;58: 875-9.

[23] Laviano A, Meguid MM, Yang Z-J, Gleason JR, Cangiano C, Fanelli FR. Cracking the riddle of cancer anorexia. Nutrition 1996;12:706-10.

[24] Laviano A, Cangiano C, Fanelli FR. Pathogenesis of cancer anorexia: personal perspective. Nutrition 1997;13:557-60.

[25] Karydis I, Tolis G. Orexis, anorexia, and thyrotripin-releasing hormone. Thyroid 1998;8:947-50.

[26] Luster MI, Simeonova PP, Gallucci R, Matheson J. Tumor necrosis factor alpha and toxicology. Crit Rev Toxicol 1999;29:491-511.

[27] Braun TP, Marks DL. Pathophysiology and treatment of inflammatory anorexia in chronic disease. J Cachex Sarcopenia Muscle 2010;1: 135-45.

[28] Nixon DW, Heymsfield SB, Cohen AE, et al. Protein-calorie undernutrition in hospitalized cancer patients. Am J Med 1989;68: 683-90.

[29] DeWys WD, Begg C, Lavin PT, et al. Prognostic effect of weight loss prior to chemotherapy in cancer patients. Am J Med 1980;69:491-7.

[30] Cooper EH, Stone J. Acute phase reactant proteins in cancer. In: Klein G, Weinhouse S, eds. Advances in cancer research. Academic Press, New York, 1979:11-44.

[31] Ward MA, Cooper EH, Turner R, Anderson JA, Neville AM. Acute phase reactant   protein profiles: an aid to monitoring large bowel cancer by CEA and serum enzymes. Br J Cancer 1977;35:170-8.

[32] Falconer JS, Fearon KCH, Plester CE, Ross JA, Carter DC. Cytokines, the acute phase response, and resting energy expenditure in cachectic patients with pancreatic cancer. Ann Surg 1994;219:325-32.

[33] Falconer JS, Fearon KCH, Ross JA, Elton RE, Wigmore SJ, Garden OJ, et al. Acute-phase protein response and survival duration of patients with pancreatic cancer. Cancer 1995;75:2077-82.
    Castell JV, Gomez-Lechon MJ, David M, Fabra R, Trullenque R, Heinrich PC. Acute-phase response of human hepatocytes: regulation of acute phase protein synthesis by   interleukin-6.   Hepatology 1990;12: 1179-86.

[34] O'Riordain MG, Falconer JS, Maingay J, Fearon KCH, Ross JA. Peripheral blood cells from weight-losing cancer patients control the hepatic acute phase response by a primarily interleukin-6 dependent mechanism. Int J Oncol 1999;15:823-7.

[35] Inui A. Cancer anorexia-cachexia syndrome: are neuropeptides the key? Cancer Res 1999;59:4493-4501.

[36] Laviano A, Meguid MM. Nutritional issues in cancer management. Nutrition 1996;12:358-71.

[37] Laviano A, Renvyle T, Yang, Z-J. From laboratory to bedside: new strategies in the treatment of malnutrition in cancer patients. Nutrition 1996;12:112-22.

[38] Langstein HN, Norton JA. Mechanisms of cancer cachexia. Hematol Oncol Clin North Am 1991;5:103-23.

[39] Nabel GJ, Grunfeld C. Calories lost -- another mediator of cancer cachexia? Nature Med 1996;2: 397-8.

[40] Todorov PT, McDevitt TM, Cariuk P, Coles B, Tisdale MJ. Induction of muscle protein degradation and weight loss by a tumor product. Cancer Res 1996;56:1256-61.

[41]   Figueroa J, Vijayagopal P, Debata C, Prasad A, Prasad C. Azaftig, a urinary proteoglycan from a cachectic cancer patient, causes profound weight loss in mice. Life Sci 1999;64:1339-47.

[42]   Edén E, Edström S, Bennegård K, Scherstén T, Lundholm K. Glucose flux in relation to energy expenditure in malnourished patients with and without cancer during periods of fasting and feeding. Cancer Res 1984; 44:1718-24.

[43]   Tisdale MJ. Wasting in cancer. J Nutr 1999;129(suppl 1):234S-5.

[44]   Barber MD. Ross JA, Voss AC, Tisdale MJ, Fearon KCH. The effect of an oral   nutritional supplement enriched with fish oil on weight-loss in patients with pancreatic cancer. Br J Cancer 1999;81:80-6.

[45]   Corcoran C, Grinspoon S. Drug therapy: Treatments for wasting in patients with the acquired immunodeficiency syndrome. N Engl J Med 1999;340:1740-50.

[46]   Tisdale MJ. Mechanisms of cancer cachexia. Physiol Rev 2009;89: 381-410.

[47]   Copeland EM. Historical perspective on nutritional support of cancer patients. Cancer 1998;48:67-8.

[48]   Grunfeld C, Feingold KR. Metabolic disturbances and wasting in the acquired immunodeficiency syndrome. N Engl J Med 1992;327:329-37.

[49]   Hommes MJ, Romijn JA, Endert A, Sauerwein HP. Resting energy expenditure and sub-strate oxidation in human immunodeficiency virus (HIV)-infected asymptomatic men: HIV affects host metabolism in the early asymptomatic stage. Am J Clin Nutr 1991;54:   311-5.

[50]   Macallan DC, Noble C, Baldwin C, Jebb SA, Prentice AM, Coward WA, et al. Energy expenditure and wasting in human immunodeficiency virus infection. N Engl J Med 1995;333:83-8.

[51]   Macallan DC, Noble C, Baldwin C, Foskett M, McManus T, Griffin GE. Prospective analysis of patterns of weight change in stage IV human immunodeficiency virus infection. Am J Clin Nutr 1999;58:417-24.

[52]   Donahoe M, Rogers RM, Wilson DO, Pennock BE. Oxygen consumption of the respiratory muscles in normal and in malnourished patients with chronic obstructive pulmonary disease. Am Rev Respir Dis 1989;140: 385-91.

[53]   Farber MO, Mannix ET. Tissue wasting in patients with chronic obstructive pulmonary disease. Neurol Clin 2000;1:245-62.

[54]   Brown SE, Nagendran RC, McHugh JW, Stansbury DW, Fischer CE, Light RW. Effects of a large carbohydrate load on walking performance in chronic air-flow obstruction. Am Rev Resp Dis 1985;132:960-2.

[55]   Phillipson EA, Duffin J, Cooper JD. Critical dependence of respiratory rhythmicity on metabolic CO_2 load. J Appl Physiol 1981;50:45-54.

[56]   Minai OA, Maurer JR, Kesten S. Comorbidities in end-stage lung disease. J Heart Lung Transplant 1999;18:891-903.

[57]   Anker SD, Coats AJS. Cardiac cachexia: a syndrome with impaired survival and immune and neuroendocrine activation. Chest 1999;115: 836-47.

[58]   Bolger AP, Anker SD. Tumor necrosis factor in chronic heart failure: a peripheral view on pathogenesis, clinical manifestations and therapeutic implications. Drugs 2000;60:1245-57.

[59]   Ponikowski P, Piepoli M, Chua TP, Banasiak W, Anker SD, Coats SJ. The impact of cachexia on cardiorespiratory reflex control in chronic heart failure. Eur Heart J 1999;20:1667-75.

[60]   Epstein M. Renal sodium handling in liver disease. In: Epstein M, ed. The kidney in liver disease, 4th ed. Philadelphia, PA: Hanley Belfus, 1996: 1-31.

[61]   Gentilini P. Hepatorenal syndrome and ascites - an introduction. Liver 1999;19(suppl 1):5-14.

[62]   Bataller R, Arroyo V, Gines P. Management of ascites in cirrhosis. J Gastroenterol Hepatol 1997;12:723-33.

[63]   Don BR, Kaysen GA. Assessment of inflammation and nutrition in patients with end-stage renal disease. J Nephrol 2000;13:249-59.

[64]   Bricker NS, Klahr S, Lubowitz H, Rieselbach, RE. Renal function in chronic renal disease. Medicine 1965;44:263-88.

[65]   Mange K, Matsuura D, Cizman B, Soto H, Ziyadeh FN, Goldfarb S, et al. Language guiding therapy: the case of dehydration versus volume depletion. Ann Intern Med 1997;127:848-53.

[66]   McGee S, Abernethy, WB, III, Simel DL. Is this patient hypovolemic? JAMA 1999;281:1022-9.

[67] Oliver D. Terminal dehydration. Lancet 1984;11(8403): 631-3.

[68] Printz LA. Terminal dehydration: a compassionate treatment. Arch Int Med 1992;152:697-700.

[69] Majeed N, Lawson W, Przeulocka B. Brain and peripheral opioid peptides after changes in ingestive behavior. Neuroendocrinol 1986;42: 267-72.

[70] Copeland EM 3rd, Daly JM, Dudrick SJ. Nutrition as an adjunct to cancer treatment in the adult. Cancer Res 1977;37:2451-6.

[71] Copeland EM, MacFayden BV, Jr., Dudrick SJ. Effect of intravenous hyperalimentation on established delayed hypersensitivity in the cancer patient. Ann Surg 1976;170:60-4.

[72] Souchon EA, Copeland EM, Watson P, Dudrick SJ. Intravenous hyperalimentation as an adjunct to cancer chemotherapy with 5-fluorouracil. J Surg Res 1975;18:451-4.

[73] Dudrick SJ, MacFayden BV, Jr., Souchon EA, Englert DM, Copeland EM. Parenteral nutrition techniques in cancer patients. Cancer Res 1977; 37:2440-50.

[74] Copeland EM 3rd, Souba WW. Nutritional considerations in treatment of the cancer patient.Nutr Clin Pract 1988;3:173-4.

[75] Klein S, Koretz RL. Nutrition in patients with cancer: what do the data really show? Nutr Clin Pract 1994;9:91-100.

[76] McGeer AJ, Detsky AS, O'Rourke K. Parenteral nutrition in patients receiving cancer chemotherapy: position paper. Ann Intern Med 1989; 110:734-6.

[77] Issell BF, Valdivieso MD, Zaren HA, Dudrick SJ, Freireich EJ, Copeland EW, et al. Protection against chemotherapy toxicity by IV hyperalimentation. Cancer Treat Rep 1978;62:1139-43.

[78] Popp MB, Fisher RI, Wesley R, Aamodt R, Brennan MF. A prospective randomized study of adjuvant parenteral nutrition in the treatment of advanced, diffuse lymphoma: influence on survival. Surgery 1981;90: 195-203.

[79] Popp MB, Fisher RI, Simon RM. A prospective randomized study of adjuvant parenteral nutrition in the treatment of diffuse lymphoma. Effect on drug tolerance. Cancer Treat Rep 1981;65 (suppl 5):129-35.

[80] Jordan WM, Valdivieso M, Frankmann C, Gillespie M, Issell BF, Bodey GP, et al. Treatment of advanced adenocarcinoma of the lung with ftorafur, doxorubicin, cyclophosphamide, and cisplatin (FACP) and intensive IV hyperalimentation. Cancer Treat Rep 1981;65:197-205.

[81] Valdivieso M, Frankmann C, Murphy WK, Benjamin RS, Barkley HT Jr, McMurtrey MJ, et al. Long-term effects of intravenous hyperalimentation administered during intensive chemotherapy for small cell bronchogenic carcinoma. Cancer 1987;59:362-9.

[82] Valdivieso M, Bodey GP, Benjamin RS, Barkley HT, Freeman MB, Ertel M, et al. Role of intravenous hyperalimentation as an adjunct to intensive chemotherapy for small cell bronchogenic carcinoma. Cancer Treat Rep 1981;65(suppl 5):145-50.

[83] Shamberger RC, Brennan MF, Goodgame JT Jr, Lowry SF, Maher MM, Wesley RA, et al. A prospective, randomized study of adjuvant parenteral nutrition in the treatment of sarcoma: results of metabolic and survival studies. Surgery 1984;96:1-12.

[84] Shamberger RC, Pizzo PA, Goodgame JT Jr, Lowry SF, Maher MM, Wesley RA, et al. The effect of total parenteral nutrition on chemotherapy-induced myelo-suppression. Am J Med 1983;74:40-8.

[85] Nixon DW, Moffitt S, Lawson DH, Ansley J, Lynn MJ, Kutner MH, et al. Total parenteral nutrition as an adjunct to chemotherapy of metastatic colorectal cancer. Cancer Treat Rep 1981;l65(suppl 5):121-8.

[86] Nixon DW, Lawson DH, Kutner MH, Moffitt SD, Ansley J, Heymsfield SB, et al. Effect of total parenteral nutrition on survival in advanced colon cancer. Cancer Detect Prev 1989;4:421-7.

[87] Hays DM, Merritt RJ, White L, Ashley J, Siegel SE. Effect of total parenteral nutrition on marrow recovery during induction therapy for acute nonlymphocytic leukemia in childhood. Med Pediatr Oncol 1983; 11:134-40.

[88] Chermesh I, Mashiach T, Amit A, Haim N, Papier I, Efergan R, Lachter J, Eliakim R. Home parenteral nutrition (HTPN) for incurable patients with cancer with gastrointestinal obstruction: do the benefits outweigh the risks? Med Oncol 2010;28:83-8.

[89] Bruera E, Sala R, Rico MA, Moyano J, Centeno C, Willey J, Palmer JL. Effects of parenteral hydration in terminally ill cancer patients: a preliminary study. J Clin Oncol 2005;23:2366-71.

[90]   Van Eys J, Copeland EM, Cangir A, Taylor G, Teitell-Cohen B, Carter P, et al. A clinical trial of hyperalimentation in children with metastatic malignancies. Med Pediatr Oncol 1980;8:63-73.

[91]   Samuels ML, Selig DE, Ogden S, Grant C, Brown B. IV hyperalimentation and chemotherapy for stage III testicular cancer: a randomized study. Cancer Treat Rep 1989;65:615-27.

[92]   Clamon GH, Feld R, Evans WK, Weiner RS, Moran EM, Blum RH, et al. Effect of adjuvant central IV hyperalimentation on the survival and response to treatment of patients with small lung cancer: a randomized trial. Cancer Treat Rep 1985;69:167-77.

[93]   DeWys WD and Kubota TT. Enteral and parenteral nutrition in the care of the cancer patient. JAMA 1981;246:1725-7.

[94]   Palesty JA, Dudrick SJ. Cachexia, malnutrition, the refeeding syndrome, and lessons from Goldilocks. Surg Clin North Am 2011;91:653-73.

[95]   Tchekmedyian NS. Pharmacoeconomics of nutritional support in cancer. Semin   Oncol   1998;25: 62-9.

[96]   Torelli GF, Campos AC, Meguid MM. Use of TPN in terminally ill cancer patients. Nutrition 1999;15:665-7.

[97]   Daly JM, Weintraub FN, Shou J, Rosato EF, Lucia M. Enteral nutrition during multi-modality therapy in upper gastrointestinal cancer patients. Ann Surg 1995;221:327-38.

[98]   Gillick MR. Rethinking the role of tube feeding in patients with advanced dementia. N Engl J Med 2000;342:206-10.

[99]   Finucane TE, Christmas C, Travis K. Tube feeding in patients with advanced dementia: A review of the evidence. JAMA 1999;282: 1365-70.

[100]   Ahronheim JC. Nutrition and hydration in the terminal patient. Clin Geriatric Med 1996;12:379-91.

[101]   Finucane TE, Christmas C, Leff BA. Tube feeding in dementia: how incentives undermine health care quality and patient safety. J Am Med Dir Assoc 2007;8:205-8.

[102]   Scott AG, Austin HE. Nasogastric feeding in the management of severe dysphagia in motor neurone disease. Palliat Med 1994;8:45-7.

[103]   Sampson EL. Palliative care for people with dementia. Br Med Bull 2010;96:159-74.

[104]   Bruera E, Legris MA, Kuehn N, Miller MJ. Hypodermoclysis for the administration of fluids and narcotic analgesics in patients with advanced cancer. J Pain Symptom Manage 1990;5:218-20.

[105]   Bruera E, de Stoutz ND, Fainsinger RL, et al. Comparison of two different concentrations of hyaluronidase in patients receiving one-hour infusions of hypodermoclysis. J Pain Symptom Manage 1995;10:505-9.

[106]   Grauer PA. Appetite stimulants in terminal care: treatment of anorexia. Hospice J 1993;9:73-8.

[107]   Tchekmedyian NS, Heber D. Cancer and AIDS cachexia: mechanisms and approaches to therapy. Oncology 1993;7:55-9.

[108]   Beal JE, Olson R, Laubenstein L, Morales JO, Bellman P, Yangco B, et al. Dronanibol as a treatment for anorexia associated with weight loss in patients with AIDS. J Pain Symptom Manage 1995;10:89-97.

[109]   Navari RM, Brenner MC. Treatment of cancer-related anorexia with olanzapine and megestrol acetate: A randomized trial. Support Care Cancer 2010;18:951-6.

[110]   Loprinzi CL, Bernath AM, Schaid DJ, Malliard JA, Athmann LM, Michalak JC, et al. Phase III evaluation of four doses of megestrol acetate as therapy for patients with cancer anorexia and/or cachexia. J Clin Oncol 1993;11:762-7.

[111]   Leinung M, Koller EA, Fossler MJ. Corticosteroid effects of megestrol acetate. Endocrinologist 1998;8:153-9.

[112]   Moertel CG, Schutt AJ, Reitemeier RJ, Hahn RG. Corticosteroid therapy of preterminal gastrointestinal cancer. Cancer 1974;33:1607-9.

[113]   Bruera E, Roca E, Cedaro L, Carraro S, Chacon R. Action of oral methylprednisolone in terminal cancer patients: A prospective randomized double-blind study. Cancer Treat Rep 1985;69:751-4.

[114]   Tchekmedyian NS. Costs and benefits of nutrition support in cancer. Oncology 1995;9(suppl):79-84.

[115]   Akamizu T, Kangawa K. Ghrelin for cachexia. J Cachex Sarcopenia Muscle 2010;1:169–76.

[116]   Akamizu T., Kangawa K. Therapeutic applications of ghrelin to cachexia utilizing its appetite-stimulating effect. Peptides 2011;17:34-40.

[117] Gullett NP, Hebbar G, Ziegler TR. Update on clinical trials of growth factors and anabolic steroids in cachexia and wasting. Am J Clin Nutr 2010;91:1143S-7.

[118] Strasser F, Lutz TA, Maeder MT, Thuerlimann B, Bueche D, Tschöp M, et al. Safety, tolerability and pharmacokinetics of intravenous ghrelin for cancer-related anorexia/cachexia: A randomised, placebo-controlled, double-blind, double-crossover study. Br J Cancer 2008;98:300-8.

[119] Nagaya N, Itoh T, Murakami S, Oya H, Uematsu M, Miyatake K, et al. Treatment of cachexia with ghrelin in patients with COPD. Chest 2005; 128:1187-93.

[120] Nagaya N, Moriya J, Yasumura Y, Uematsu M, Ono F, Shimizu W, et al. Effects of ghrelin administration on left ventricular function, exercise capacity, and muscle wasting in patients with chronic heart failure. Circulation 2004;110:3674-9.

[121] Elamin E. Dietary and pharmacological management of severe catabolic conditions. Am J Med Sci 2011;342(6):513-8.

[122] American Medical Association. Code of Medical Ethics. Medical futility in end-of-life care. JAMA 1999;281:937-41.

[123] Quill TE, Byock IR. Responding to intractable terminal suffering: the role of terminal sedation and voluntary refusal of food and fluids. Ann Intern Med 2000;132:408-14.

[124] Snyder JW, Swartz SJ. Deciding to terminate treatment: a practical guide for physicians. Crit Care 1993;8:177-85.

[125] Callahan D. Persuing a peaceful death. Hastings Center Rep 1993;23: 33-8.

[126] Byock IR. Patient refusal of nutrition and hydration: walking the ever-finer lin Am J Hosp Palliat Care 1995;12:9-13.

[127] Eddy D. A conversation with my mother. JAMA 1994;272:179-81.

[128] McCann RM, Hall WJ, Groth-Juncker A. Comfort care for terminally ill patients: The appropopriate use of nutrition and hydration. JAMA 1994; 271:1263-6.

[129] Wanzer SH, Federman DD, Adelstein SJ, Cassel CK, Cassem EH, Cranford RE, et al. The physician's responsibility toward hopelessly ill patients. N Engl J Med 1989;320:844-9.

[130] Meisel A, Snyder JD, Quill T. Seven legal barriers to end-of-life care: myths, realities, and grains of truth. JAMA 2000;284:2495-2501.

[131] Aronheim JC, Mulvihill M, Sieger C, Park P, Fried BE. State practice variations in the use of tube feeding for nursing home patients with severe cognitive impairment. J Am Geriatr Soc 2001;49:148-52.

[132] Mitchell SL, Berkowitz RE, Lawson FM, Lipsitz LA. A cross-national survey of tube-feeding decisions in cognitively impaired older persons. J Am Geriatr Soc 2000;48:391-7.

[133] Gessert CE, Curry NM, Robinson A. Ethnicity and end-of-life care: the use of feeding tubes. Ethn Dis 2001;11:97-106.

[134] Rudberg MA, Egleston BL, Grant MD, Brody JA. Effectiveness of feeding tubes in nursing home residents with swallowing disorders. J Parenter Enteral Nutr 2000;24:97-102.

[135] Stuart B. The NHO medical guidelines for non-cancer disease and local medical review policy: hospice access for patients with diseases other than cancer. Hospice 1999;50:139-54.

[136] Stuart B, Connor S, Kinzbrunner BM, et al. Medical guidelines for determining medical prognosis in selected non-cancer diseases, 2nd ed. Arlington, DC: National Hospice Organization, 1996:222-32.

[137] Wright JB, Kinzbrunner BM. Predicting prognosis: How to decide when end-of-life care is needed. In: Kinzbrunner BM, Policzer JM, eds. End-of-life care: A practical guide, 2nd ed. New York: McGraw-Hill Med, 2011:111-23.

SECTION 7: ACKNOWLEDGMENTS

In: Food, Nutrition and Eating Behavior   ISBN: 978-1-62948-233-0
Editors: Joav Merrick and Sigal Israeli   © 2014 Nova Science Publishers, Inc.

Chapter 23

ABOUT THE EDITORS

Joav Merrick, MD, MMedSci, DMSc, is professor of pediatrics, child health and human development affiliated with Kentucky Children's Hospital, University of Kentucky, Lexington, Kentucky, United States and the Division of Pediatrics, Hadassah Hebrew University Medical Center, Mt Scopus Campus, Jerusalem, Israel, the medical director of the Health Services, Division for Intellectual and Developmental Disabilities, Ministry of Social Affairs and Social Services, Jerusalem, the founder and director of the National Institute of Child Health and Human Development in Israel. Numerous publications in the field of pediatrics, child health and human development, rehabilitation, intellectual disability, disability, health, welfare, abuse, advocacy, quality of life and prevention. Received the Peter Sabroe Child Award for outstanding work on behalf of Danish Children in 1985 and the International LEGO-Prize ("The Children's Nobel Prize") for an extraordinary contribution towards improvement in child welfare and well-being in 1987. E-mail: jmerrick@zahav.net.il

Sigal Israeli, RD, BScNutr, is a clinical nutritionist, the chief nutritionist, Ministry of Social Affairs and Social Services, Jerusalem and affiliated with the National Institute of Child Health and Human Development in Israel. She received her formal education at the Robert H. Smith Faculty of Agriculture, Food and Environment of the Hebrew University of Jerusalem in Rehovot, Israel.

She is a member of the Israeli Dietitian organization (ATID). She has worked as a clinical nutritionist at the Tel-Aviv Sourasky Medical Center, Tel-Aviv Municipality Adolescent Clinic, and Clalit Health Services before becoming the chief nutritionist of the Ministry. Lecturer in various areas connected to nutrition: proper nutrition, nutrition and feeding of individuals with special health care needs and disability. E-mail: sigalis@molsa.gov.il

In: Food, Nutrition and Eating Behavior   ISBN: 978-1-62948-233-0
Editors: Joav Merrick and Sigal Israeli   © 2014 Nova Science Publishers, Inc.

Chapter 24

ABOUT THE NATIONAL INSTITUTE OF CHILD HEALTH AND HUMAN DEVELOPMENT IN ISRAEL

The National Institute of Child Health and Human Development (NICHD) in Israel was established in 1998 as a virtual institute under the auspicies of the Medical Director, Ministry of Social Affairs and Social Services in order to function as the research arm for the Office of the Medical Director. In 1998 the National Council for Child Health and Pediatrics, Ministry of Health and in 1999 the Director General and Deputy Director General of the Ministry of Health endorsed the establishment of the NICHD.

MISSION

The mission of a National Institute for Child Health and Human Development in Israel is to provide an academic focal point for the scholarly interdisciplinary study of child life, health, public health, welfare, disability, rehabilitation, intellectual disability and related aspects of human development. This mission includes research, teaching, clinical work, information and public service activities in the field of child health and human development.

SERVICE AND ACADEMIC ACTIVITIES

Over the years many activities became focused in the south of Israel due to collaboration with various professionals at the Faculty of Health Sciences (FOHS) at the Ben Gurion University of the Negev (BGU). Since 2000 an affiliation with the Zusman Child Development Center at the Pediatric Division of Soroka University Medical Center has resulted in collaboration around the establishment of the Down Syndrome Clinic at that center. In 2002 a full course on "Disability" was established at the Recanati School for Allied Professions in the Community, FOHS, BGU and in 2005 collaboration was started with the Primary Care Unit of the faculty and disability became part of the master of public health course on "Children and society". In the academic year 2005-2006 a one semester course on "Aging with disability" was started as part of the master of science program in gerontology in our collaboration with the Center for Multidisciplinary Research in Aging. In 2010 collaborations with the Division of Pediatrics, Hadassah Hebrew University Medical Center, Jerusalem, Israel around the National Down Syndrome Center and teaching students and residents about intellectual and developmental disabilities as part of their training at this campus.

RESEARCH ACTIVITIES

The affiliated staff have over the years published work from projects and research activities in this national and international collaboration. In the year 2000 the International Journal of Adolescent Medicine and Health and in 2005 the International Journal on Disability and Human Development of De Gruyter Publishing House (Berlin and New York) were affiliated with the National Institute of Child Health and Human Development. From 2008 also the International Journal of Child Health and Human Development (Nova Science, New York), the International Journal of Child and Adolescent Health (Nova Science) and the Journal of Pain Management (Nova Science) affiliated and from 2009 the International Public Health Journal (Nova Science) and Journal of Alternative Medicine Research (Nova Science). All peer-reviewed international journals.

NATIONAL COLLABORATIONS

Nationally the NICHD works in collaboration with the Faculty of Health Sciences, Ben Gurion University of the Negev; Department of Physical Therapy, Sackler School of Medicine, Tel Aviv University; Autism Center, Assaf HaRofeh Medical Center; National Rett and PKU Centers at Chaim Sheba Medical Center, Tel HaShomer; Department of Physiotherapy, Haifa University; Department of Education, Bar Ilan University, Ramat Gan, Faculty of Social Sciences and Health Sciences; College of Judea and Samaria in Ariel and in 2011 affiliation with Center for Pediatric Chronic Diseases and National Center for Down Syndrome, Department of Pediatrics, Hadassah Hebrew University Medical Center, Mount Scopus Campus, Jerusalem.

INTERNATIONAL COLLABORATIONS

Internationally with the Department of Disability and Human Development, College of Applied Health Sciences, University of Illinois at Chicago; Strong Center for Developmental Disabilities, Golisano Children's Hospital at Strong, University of Rochester School of Medicine and Dentistry, New York; Centre on Intellectual Disabilities, University of Albany, New York; Centre for Chronic Disease Prevention and Control, Health Canada, Ottawa; Chandler Medical Center and Children's Hospital, Kentucky Children's Hospital, Section of Adolescent Medicine, University of Kentucky, Lexington; Chronic Disease Prevention and Control Research Center, Baylor College of Medicine, Houston, Texas; Division of Neuroscience, Department of Psychiatry, Columbia University, New York; Institute for the Study of Disadvantage and Disability, Atlanta; Center for Autism and Related Disorders, Department   Psychiatry,   Children's Hospital Boston, Boston; Department of Paediatrics,

Child Health and Adolescent Medicine, Children's Hospital at Westmead, Westmead, Australia; International Centre for the Study of Occupational and Mental Health, Düsseldorf, Germany; Centre for Advanced Studies in Nursing, Department of General Practice and Primary Care, University of Aberdeen, Aberdeen, United Kingdom; Quality of Life Research Center, Copenhagen, Denmark; Nordic School of Public Health, Gottenburg, Sweden, Scandinavian Institute of Quality of Working Life, Oslo, Norway; The Department of Applied Social Sciences (APSS) of The Hong Kong Polytechnic University Hong Kong.

TARGETS

Our focus is on research, international collaborations, clinical work, teaching and policy in health, disability and human development and to establish the NICHD as a permanent institute at one of the residential care centers for persons with intellectual disability in Israel in order to conduct model research and together with the four university schools of public health/medicine in Israel establish a national master and doctoral program in disability and human development at the institute to secure the next generation of professionals working in this often non-prestigious/low-status field of work.

Contact

Joav Merrick, MD, MMedSci, DMSc
Professor of Pediatrics, Child Health and Human Development
Medical Director, Health Services, Division for Intellectual and Developmental Disabilities,
    Ministry of Social Affairs and Social Services, POB 1260, IL-91012 Jerusalem, Israel.
E-mail: jmerrick@zahav.net.il

In: Food, Nutrition and Eating Behavior
Editors: Joav Merrick and Sigal Israeli

ISBN: 978-1-62948-233-0
© 2014 Nova Science Publishers, Inc.

Chapter 25

ABOUT THE BOOK SERIES "HEALTH AND HUMAN DEVELOPMENT"

Health and human development is a book series with publications from a multidisciplinary group of researchers, practitioners and clinicians for an international professional forum interested in the broad spectrum of health and human development. Books already published:

- Merrick J, Omar HA, eds. Adolescent behavior research. International perspectives. New York: Nova Science, 2007.
- Kratky KW. Complementary medicine systems: Comparison and integration. New York: Nova Science, 2008.
- Schofield P, Merrick J, eds. Pain in children and youth. New York: Nova Science, 2009.
- Greydanus DE, Patel DR, Pratt HD, Calles Jr JL, eds. Behavioral pediatrics, 3 ed. New York: Nova Science, 2009.
- Ventegodt S, Merrick J, eds. Meaningful work: Research in quality of working life. New York: Nova Science, 2009.
- Omar HA, Greydanus DE, Patel DR, Merrick J, eds. Obesity and adolescence. A public health concern. New York: Nova Science, 2009.
- Lieberman A, Merrick J, eds. Poverty and children. A public health concern. New York: Nova Science, 2009.
- Goodbread J. Living on the edge. The mythical, spiritual and philosophical roots of social marginality. New York: Nova Science, 2009.
- Bennett DL, Towns S, Elliot E, Merrick J, eds. Challenges in adolescent health: An Australian perspective. New York: Nova Science, 2009.
- Schofield P, Merrick J, eds. Children and pain. New York: Nova Science, 2009.
- Sher L, Kandel I, Merrick J, eds. Alcohol-related cognitive disorders: Research and clinical perspectives. New York: Nova Science, 2009.
- Anyanwu EC. Advances in environmental health effects of toxigenic mold and mycotoxins. New York: Nova Science, 2009.
- Bell E, Merrick J, eds. Rural child health. International aspects. New York: Nova Science, 2009.

- Dubowitz H, Merrick J, eds. International aspects of child abuse and neglect. New York: Nova Science, 2010.
- Shahtahmasebi S, Berridge D. Conceptualizing behavior: A practical guide to data analysis. New York: Nova Science, 2010.
- Wernik U. Chance action and therapy. The playful way of changing. New York: Nova Science, 2010.
- Omar HA, Greydanus DE, Patel DR, Merrick J, eds. Adolescence and chronic illness. A public health concern. New York: Nova Science, 2010.
- Patel DR, Greydanus DE, Omar HA, Merrick J, eds. Adolescence and sports. New York: Nova Science, 2010.
- Shek DTL, Ma HK, Merrick J, eds. Positive youth development: Evaluation and future directions in a Chinese context. New York: Nova Science, 2010.
- Shek DTL, Ma HK, Merrick J, eds. Positive youth development: Implementation of a youth program in a Chinese context. New York: Nova Science, 2010.
- Omar HA, Greydanus DE, Tsitsika AK, Patel DR, Merrick J, eds.　Pediatric and adolescent sexuality and gynecology: Principles for the primary care clinician. New York: Nova Science, 2010.
- Chow E, Merrick J, eds. Advanced cancer. Pain and quality of life. New York: Nova Science, 2010.
- Latzer Y, Merrick, J, Stein D, eds. Understanding eating disorders. Integrating culture, psychology and biology. New York: Nova Science, 2010.
- Sahgal A, Chow E, Merrick J, eds. Bone and brain metastases: Advances in research and treatment. New York: Nova Science, 2010.
- Postolache TT, Merrick J, eds. Environment, mood disorders and suicide. New York: Nova Science, 2010.
- Maharajh HD, Merrick J, eds. Social and cultural psychiatry experience from the Caribbean Region. New York: Nova Science, 2010.
- Mirsky J. Narratives and meanings of migration. New York: Nova Science, 2010.
- Harvey PW. Self-management and the health care consumer. New York: Nova Science, 2011.
- Ventegodt S, Merrick J. Sexology from a holistic point of view. New York: Nova Science, 2011.
- Ventegodt S, Merrick J. Principles of holistic psychiatry: A textbook on holistic medicine for mental disorders. New York: Nova Science, 2011.
- Greydanus DE, Calles Jr JL, Patel DR, Nazeer A, Merrick J, eds. Clinical aspects of psychopharmacology in childhood and adolescence. New York: Nova Science, 2011.
- Bell E, Seidel BM, Merrick J, eds. Climate change and rural child health. New York: Nova Science, 2011.
- Bell E, Zimitat C, Merrick J, eds. Rural medical education: Practical strategies. New York: Nova Science, 2011.
- Latzer Y, Tzischinsky. The dance of sleeping and eating among adolescents: Normal and pathological perspectives. New York: Nova Science, 2011.
- Deshmukh VD. The astonishing brain and holistic consciousness: Neuroscience and Vedanta perspectives. New York: Nova Science, 2011.

- Bell E, Westert GP, Merrick J, eds. Translational research for primary healthcare. New York: Nova Science, 2011.
- Shek DTL, Sun RCF, Merrick J, eds. Drug abuse in Hong Kong: Development and evaluation of a prevention program. New York: Nova Science, 2011.
- Ventegodt S, Hermansen TD, Merrick J. Human Development: Biology from a holistic point of view. New York: Nova Science, 2011.
- Ventegodt S, Merrick J. Our search for meaning in life. New York: Nova Science, 2011.
- Caron RM, Merrick J, eds. Building community capacity: Minority and immigrant populations. New York: Nova Science, 2012.
- Klein H, Merrick J, eds. Human immunodeficiency virus (HIV) research: Social science aspects. New York: Nova Science, 2012.
- Lutzker JR, Merrick J, eds. Applied public health: Examining multifaceted Social or ecological problems and child maltreatment. New York: Nova Science, 2012.
- Chemtob D, Merrick J, eds. AIDS and tuberculosis: Public health aspects. New York: Nova Science, 2012.
- Ventegodt S, Merrick J. Textbook on evidence-based holistic mind-body medicine: Basic principles of healing in traditional Hippocratic medicine. New York: Nova Science, 2012.
- Ventegodt S, Merrick J. Textbook on evidence-based holistic mind-body medicine: Holistic practice of traditional Hippocratic medicine. New York: Nova Science, 2012.
- Ventegodt S, Merrick J. Textbook on evidence-based holistic mind-body medicine: Healing the mind in traditional Hippocratic medicine. New York: Nova Science, 2012.
- Ventegodt S, Merrick J. Textbook on evidence-based holistic mind-body medicine: Sexology and traditional Hippocratic medicine. New York: Nova Science, 2012.
- Ventegodt S, Merrick J. Textbook on evidence-based holistic mind-body medicine: Research, philosophy, economy and politics of traditional Hippocratic medicine. New York: Nova Science, 2012.
- Caron RM, Merrick J, eds. Building community capacity: Skills and principles. New York: Nova Science, 2012.
- Lemal M, Merrick J, eds. Health risk communication. New York: Nova Science, 2012.
- Ventegodt S, Merrick J. Textbook on evidence-based holistic mind-body medicine: Basic philosophy and ethics of traditional Hippocratic medicine. New York: Nova Science, 2013.
- Caron RM, Merrick J, eds. Building community capacity: Case examples from around the world. New York: Nova Science, 2013.
- Steele RE. Managed care in a public setting. New York: Nova Science, 2013.
- Srabstein JC, Merrick J, eds. Bullying: A public health concern. New York: Nova Science, 2013.
- Pulenzas N, Lechner B, Thavarajah N, Chow E, Merrick J, eds. Advanced cancer: Managing symptoms and quality of life. New York: Nova Science, 2013.

- Stein D, Latzer Y, eds. Treatment and recovery of eating disorders. New York: Nova Science, 2013.
- Sun J, Buys N, Merrick J. Health promotion: Community singing as a vehicle to promote health. New York: Nova Science, 2013.

Contact

Professor Joav Merrick, MD, MMedSci, DMSc
Medical Director, Health Services
Division for Intellectual and Developmental Disabailities
Ministry of Social Affairs and Social Services
POBox 1260, IL-91012 Jerusalem, Israel
E-mail: jmerrick@zahav.net.il

SECTION 8: INDEX

INDEX

B

C

G

H

I

J

O

P

S

U

V

X

Y

W

Z